Characterization of Bacteria-Dental Materials Interactions

Characterization of Bacteria-Dental Materials Interactions

Editor: Reynaldo Brito

AMERICAN
MEDICAL PUBLISHERS
www.americanmedicalpublishers.com

AMERICAN
MEDICAL PUBLISHERS
www.americanmedicalpublishers.com

Cataloging-in-Publication Data

Characterization of bacteria-dental materials interactions / edited by Reynaldo Brito.
p. cm.
Includes bibliographical references and index.
ISBN 978-1-63927-627-1
1. Teeth--Diseases--Microbiology. 2. Mouth--Microbiology. 3. Bacteria. 4. Dental hygiene.
5. Teeth--Care and hygiene. 6. Mouth--Care and hygiene. I. Brito, Reynaldo.
RK305 .C43 2023
617.522--dc23

American Medical Publishers,
41 Flatbush Avenue,
1st Floor, New York,
NY 11217, USA

ISBN 978-1-63927-627-1 (Hardback)

Contents

Preface

The world is advancing at a fast pace like never before. Therefore, the need is to keep up with the latest developments. This book was an idea that came to fruition when the specialists in the area realized the need to coordinate together and document essential themes in the subject. That's when I was requested to be the editor. Editing this book has been an honour as it brings together diverse authors researching on different streams of the field. The book collates essential materials contributed by veterans in the area which can be utilized by students and researchers alike.

Bacteria are a complex group of living microorganisms. They can be broadly classified on the basis of shape into different types such as cocci (spherical bacteria), bacilli (rod-shaped bacteria), and spirilla (spiral bacteria). The bacterial adhesion to a surface is a multi-step process through which single bacterial cells initially attach to the biomaterial followed by creation of biofilm, which is the primary cause of bacteria-related infections. Resin, composites, titanium alloys, and zirconia are some of the major dental biomaterials. An understanding of the interactions of the bacteria with the biomaterials is necessary for the growth of surgical intervention strategies. These strategies might be helpful in decreasing BCBIs and coatings which have the ability to prevent bacterial adhesion to biomaterials. This book unravels the recent studies on the interactions between bacteria and dental materials. It covers in detail some existent and innovative concepts revolving around the characterization of these interactions. This book will serve as a reference to a broad spectrum of readers.

Each chapter is a sole-standing publication that reflects each author´s interpretation. Thus, the book displays a multi-facetted picture of our current understanding of application, resources and aspects of the field. I would like to thank the contributors of this book and my family for their endless support.

Editor

1

Pilot Study Using a Chitosan-Hydroxyapatite Implant for Guided Alveolar Bone Growth in Patients with Chronic Periodontitis

Fabiola Vaca-Cornejo [1], Héctor Macías Reyes [2], Sergio H. Dueñas Jiménez [1], Ricardo A. Llamas Velázquez [3] and Judith M. Dueñas Jiménez [1,*]

1 Department of Physiology, University Center of Health Sciences ,University of Guadalajara, Guadalajara, Jalisco 44100, Mexico; sidlc@hotmail.com (F.V.-C.); sduenas@cucs.udg.mx (S.H.D.J.)
2 Department of Clinical Surgery, Fray Antonio Alcalde Hospital, University of Guadalajara, Guadalajara, Jalisco 44100, Mexico; hectormaciasr@gmail.com
3 Sophia Laboratories, Guadalajara 45010, Jalisco, México; drricardollamas@gmail.com
* Correspondence: mduenas@cucs.udg.mx

Academic Editor: Christine Knabe-Ducheyne

Abstract: Periodontitis is an infectious and inflammatory disease associated with significant loss of alveolar crest and soft tissue attached to the teeth. Chitosan and hydroxyapatite are biomaterials used for bone tissue repair because of their biodegradability and biocompatibility in nature. The present study evaluated the effects of chitosan (CH) in combination with hydroxyapatite (HAP) to promote alveolar bone growth. A chitosan implant mixed with hydroxyapatite was implanted into the affected area of 9 patients suffering chronic periodontitis. Patients were evaluated through X-ray images and a millimetric slide over a one year period. The application of CH/HAP produced an average alveolar bone growth of 5.77 mm ($\pm$1.87 mm). At the onset of the study, the dental pocket exhibited a depth level (DPDL) of 8.66 mm and decreased to 3.55 mm one year after the implant. Tooth mobility grade was 2.44 mm at the onset and 0.8 mm at the end of the study with a significant difference of $p < 0.001$. Moreover, the bone density in the affected areas was similar to the density of the bone adjacent to it. This result was confirmed with the software implant viewer from Anne Solutions Company. In conclusion, the CH/HAP implant promoted alveolar bone growth in periodontitis patients.

Keywords: chitosan; hydroxyapatite; periodontitis; guided bone regeneration

1. Introduction

Chronic periodontitis is caused by aerobic and anaerobic microorganisms. Clinical manifestations depend on the host´s response to the bacterial invasion. Chronic periodontitis also produces bone loss as well as damage to the soft tissue attached to it, which is accompanied by an inflammatory tissue reaction and extracellular matrix breakdown. At the present time, the most common periodontitis treatment is Emdogain, a protein derived from developing pork enamel. This protein promotes alveolar bone growth and the periodontal mucous membrane restitution [1]. The combined treatment of Emdogain with the bovine lyophilized bone protein has a better outcome compared to individual treatments [2]. However, this combined treatment is expensive for most people living in low-income countries. An alternative inexpensive treatment is guided bone regeneration. It consists in the insertion of a membrane separation between the soft tissue and the bone defect in order to allow bone regeneration and thus, avoid mucous invagination [3].

A 3D scaffold embedded in a synthetic extracellular matrix (ECM) environment could be a good biomaterial to produce tissue regeneration. Furthermore, it should be biodegradable, easy to apply and effective for bone repair [4]. Chitosan is a partially N-deacetylated biomaterial, a derivative of chitin (2-acetamido-2-deoxy-β-D-glucose through a β (1–4) linkage). Macrophages, convert chitosan into chitooligomers. In vivo, these oligomers stimulate fibroblasts to produce collagen and ECM [5]. The combination of collagen and hydroxyapatite $Ca_{10}(PO4)_6(OH)_2$ works as a guide for converting chitosan into an osteoinductor [6]. In rats, powder chitosan has been used as a material to fill a tibia bone defect, where bone repair was faster in the chitosan group compared with the control group after four weeks of treatment. This biomaterial was also used to promote human bone repair [7]. Hydroxyapatite has also been used as a substitute in bone grafting [8] and it is designed to work as a temporary template for migration, proliferation, and differentiation of osteoblasts. Calcium deficient hydroxyapatite (CDHA) and silicon substituted hydroxyapatite (SiHA) macroporous scaffolds favor the adequate interaction with osteoblast-like cells and pre-osteoblast-like cells producing a higher bone cell proliferation and differentiation [9].

The effects of the combination of HAP and chitosan to promote alveolar bone regeneration in local chronic periodontitis patients are unknown. Therefore, the present study evaluates chitosan in combination with hydroxyapatite in guided bone regeneration of periodontitis patients.

2. Results

At the onset of the clinical study, nine patients with chronic periodontitis exhibited a dental pocket depth level (DPDL) of 8.66 ± 0.52 mm. A year after the implant with CH/HAP, DPDL changed to 3.55 ± 0.47 mm. Data were analyzed by Student's t-test. This change has a statistically significant difference of $p < 0.001$ (Figure 1).

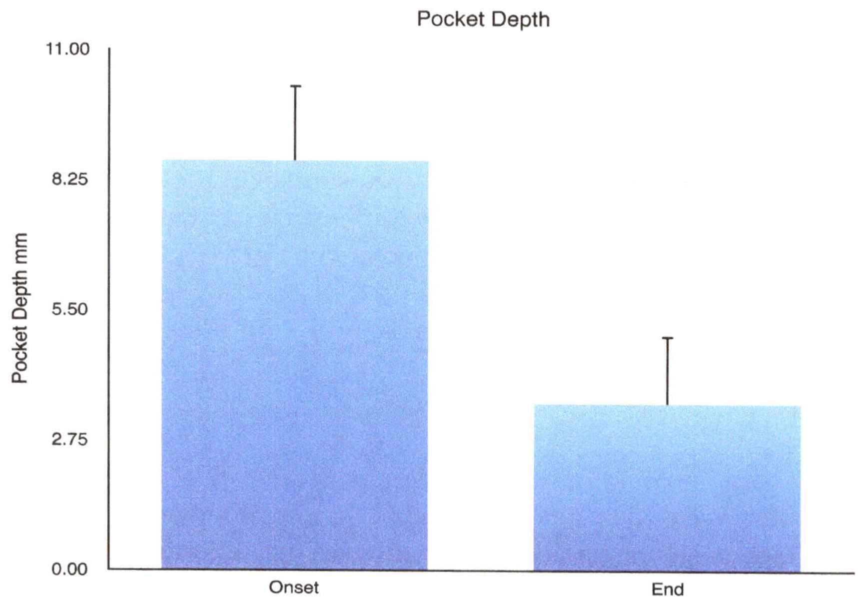

Figure 1. Pocket depth (mm) in patients with chronic periodontitis. Data are expressed as mean ± standard deviation (X ± SD). Left bar shows the pocket depth (mm) in periodontitis patients measured at the onset of the study, and the right bar exhibits the pocket at the end of the study. Data were analyzed by Student's t-test. This change has a statistically significant difference of $p < 0.001$ (Figure 1).

At the onset of the study, tooth mobility grade was of 2.44 ± 0.17 mm, and one year after CH/HAP treatment the dental mobility grade was reduced to 0.88 ± 0.20 mm. This reduction has a statistically significant difference of $p < 0.001$ (Student's t-test) (Figure 2).

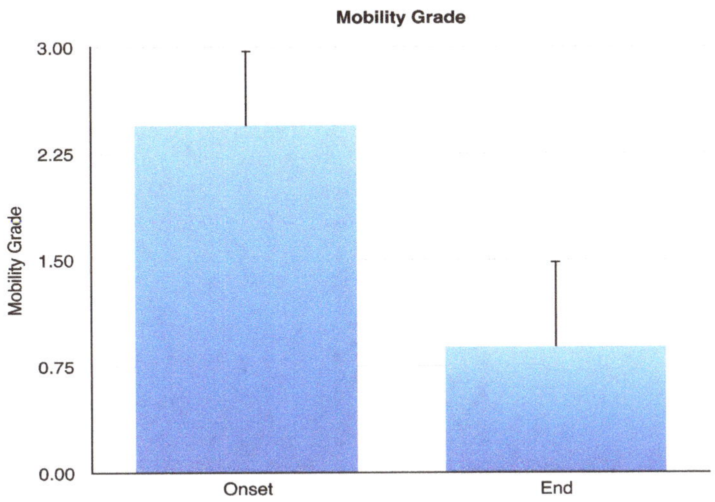

Figure 2. Tooth mobility grade (mm) in periodontitis patients. Data is shown as mean ± SD and the results were compared at the onset and at the end of the study. Mobility grade in pp at the onset of study was of 2.44 mm ± 0.1757 and at the end of the end of the evaluation it decreased to 0.8889 ± 0.2003 mm (gray bar) with a statistically significant difference of $p < 0.001$ evaluated by Student's t-test. SD: Standard Deviation.

The alveolar bone growth was measured at 1, 3, 6, 9 and 12 months after treatment. This data is exhibited in (Figure 3). The values shown in the table for each patient observed must be added together to obtain the final growth; in patient number five, there was an increase of 10 mm at the end of the study.

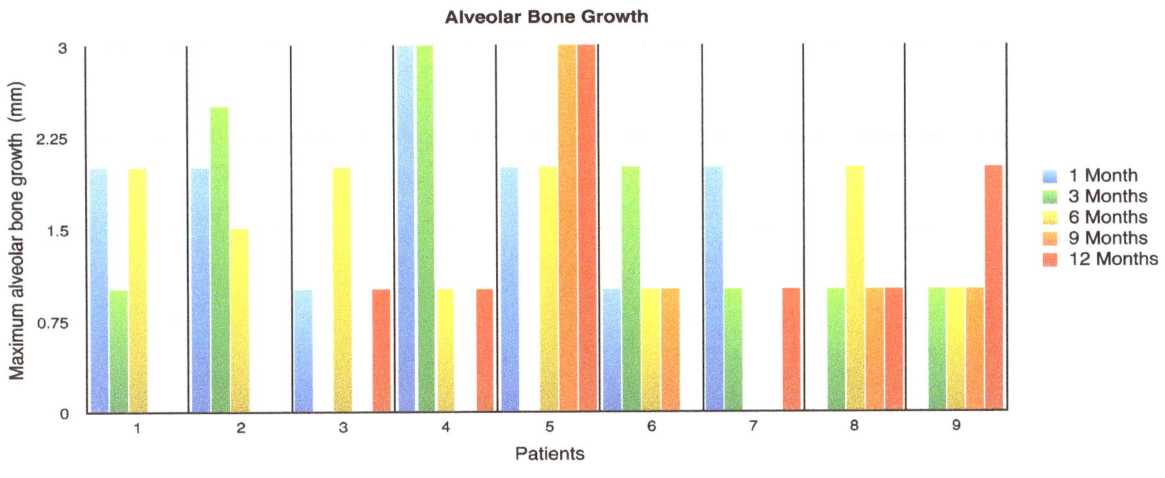

Figure 3. Maximum alveolar bone growth (mm) in periodontitis patients treated with the CH/HAP implant. Periodontitis patients treated with the CH/HAP implant were evaluated after the first month of treatment and subsequently every three months post-implant (pi), for a period of twelve months. Note that in patient 5, the highest level of alveolar bone growth (10 mm) occurred at twelve months pi (green bar) and some patients (1, 2, 3, 4 and 7) presented different alveolar bone growth after a period of six months pi. CH: Chitosan; HAP: Hydroxyapatite.

In seven patients, the maximum alveolar bone growth was reached between the third and sixth month, post implant (pi). In two patients, alveolar bone grew beyond the sixth month, in one of the patients, it reached a maximal growth at the twelfth month. At the onset of the study, patients had a depth oral defect of 12.44 ± 3.12 mm without supporting bone. After a year of treatment, the depth defect was reduced to 5.77 ± 1.98. In other words, the bone grew about 6–7 mm. The oral defect reduction had a significant difference of $p < 0.001$ (Figure 4).

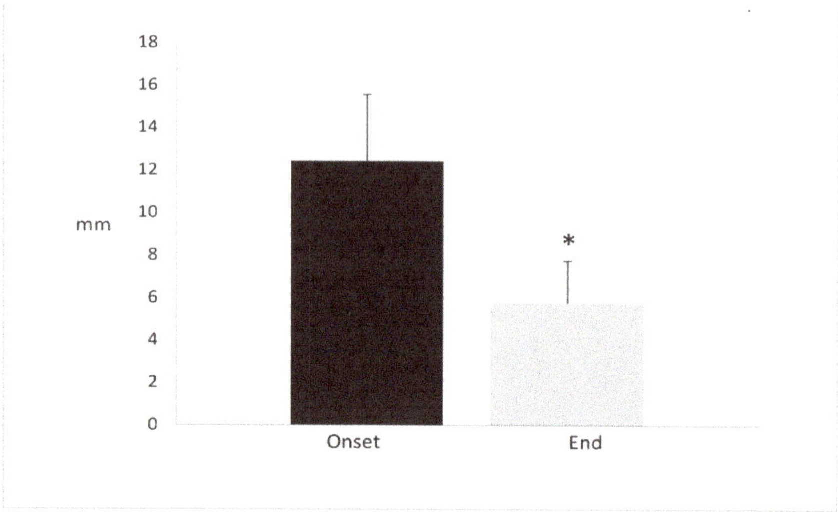

Figure 4. Alveolar bone size (mm) in local chronic periodontitis patients. The left bar represents the alveolar bone lost at the onset of the clinical study and the right bar represents the alveolar bone growth recovery at the end of the study. Data are expressed as the mean ± SD. The bone size defect at the onset of the study was larger than at the end of study with a statistically significant difference of * $p < 0.001$ (Student's *t*-test).

These results confirm that chitosan and hydroxyapatite treatment in chronic periodontitis patients promotes alveolar regeneration. Figure 5c,d shows the X-rays taken from one patient at the onset of the study and after one year of treatment with CH/HAP. Figure 5a exhibits the bone defect and Figure 5d shows the alveolar bone regeneration as indicated by an arrow. Figure 5b illustrates the recuperation of the gingival mucosa after treatment as compared with gingival mucosa before treatment Figure 5a.

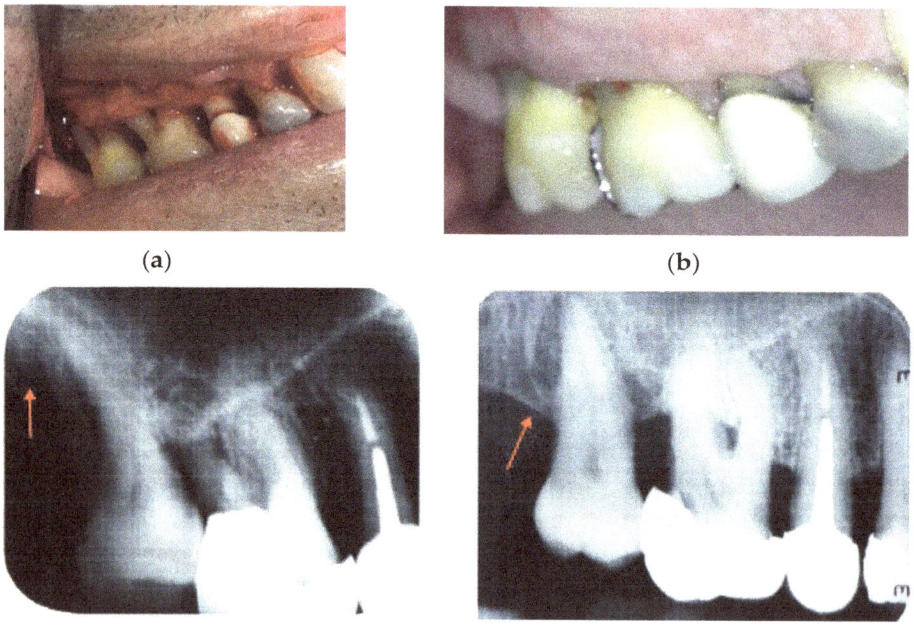

(a) (b) (c) (d)

Figure 5. X-rays of one patient with local chronic periodontitis, at the onset of the CH/HAP implant and at the end of the treatment (12 months). The arrows show the alveolar bone growth (**c**) compared to the oral defect before the implant of the biomaterial (**d**). In (**a**) a considerable loss of mucous tissue is observed in the oral defect. In (**b**) a repair of mucous tissue on the implanted oral defect is observed. CH: Chitosan; HAP: Hydroxyapatite.

The biomaterial of CH/HAP was analyzed three months after the implant in periodontitis patients. The biopsy of the biomaterial exhibited a high activity of fibroblasts with a large content of collagen in the presence of osteoblasts and it did not have an inflammatory infiltrate (Figure 6).

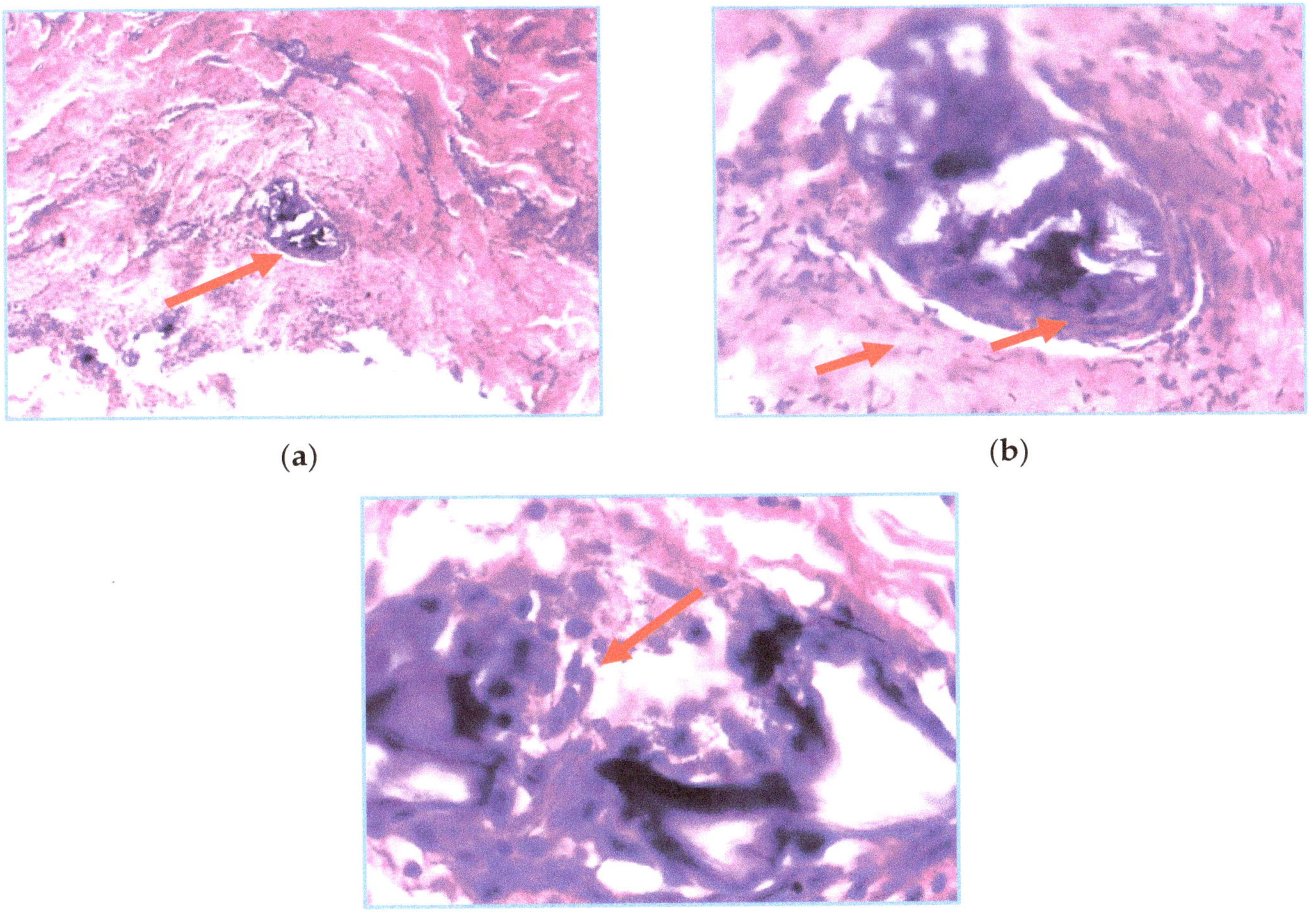

(a) (b) (c)

Figure 6. Histologic analysis of the biomaterial of CH/HAP taken three months after the implant in periodontitis patients. The biomaterial was stained with hematoxylin-eosin. In (**a**), the biomaterial is indicated by the arrow; the microphotography was taken with a 10× objective; in (**b**), the microphotography was taken at 40× amplification, where the collagen can be observed surrounding the biomaterial (pink color). The fibroblasts are stained in purple and are fusiform in shape, osteoblasts are purple rounded cells and they are infiltrated into biomaterial, these histological characteristics are indicated by the arrows; in (**c**), the biomaterial is stained in dark purple and the osteoblasts can be appreciated by the arrow. CH: Chitosan; HAP: Hydroxyapatite.

Figure 7 illustrates bone density and includes the image of dental organ 37 from a periodontitis patient; the organ treated with CH/HAP exhibits an adequate density and growth compared to dental organ 36.

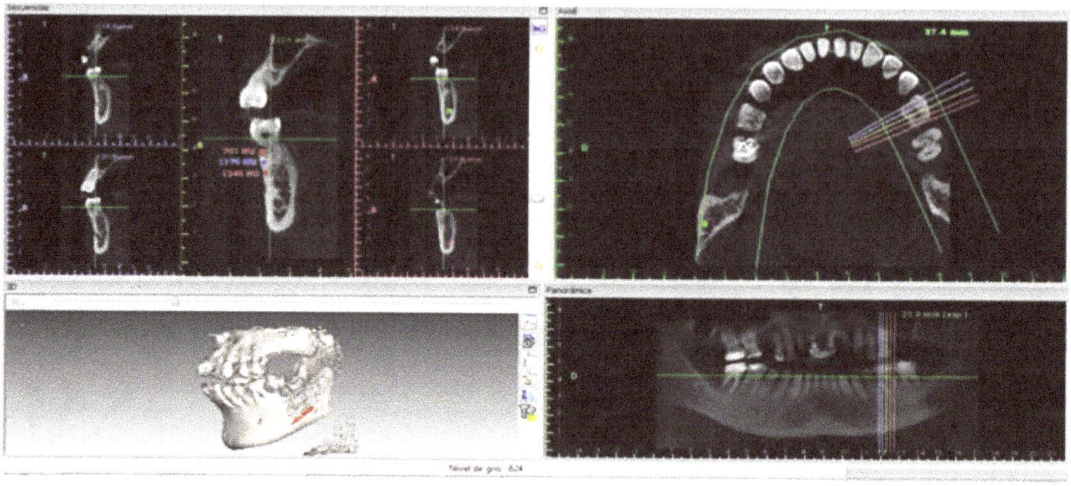

Figure 7. Image in 3D of one patient after the treatment was complimented. Bone density in tooth 37 in a treated patient is illustrated in the top left panel, five cuts were made every 2 mm, following the shape of the dental arch in order to evaluate the amount of bone by the vestibular side. Three measures were taken, one at the crest level, another in the middle zone and the third one at the apical level. The density is given in Hounsfield units. In the upper right panel a mandibular axial cut is illustrated. The 5 lines are shown as a reference to indicate the zone where the cuts were made. In the lower left panel, a 3D reconstruction of the oral cavity is shown. The lower right panel illustrates a panoramic lateral mandibular reconstruction of 20 mm wide.

Table 1 shows the bone density in Hounsfield units in treated patients, Patient 1 had a higher density in the lateral superior right tooth treated than the central superior tooth, in the three measured zones: apical, middle and crest. In contrast, patient 2 treated with CH/HAP exhibited a lower density in the second right molar compared to the untreated first right molar. This result can be explained because the maxillary angle has a minor bone density. Patient 3 presented a higher bone density in the inferior first treated right molar than the untreated second right molar.

Table 1. The bone density in Hounsfield (UH) units in patients treated with a CH/HAP implant. The bone density in UH units of dental organs (do) 12, 17 and 36 compared to do 11, 16 and 37 respectively, is shown. The bone density was measured in three zones: apical, middle and crest. Note that patients 1 and 3 had a higher density in the oral bone defect compared with the untreated nearest tooth. Patient 2 had a low density in the treated oral defect compared to the nearest untreated tooth. All data were obtained at one year of treatment. CH: Chitosan; HAP: Hydroxyapatite.

Patients	Tooth	Hounsfield (UH) Apical	UH Middle	Crest
Patient 1	Tooth #12 (Treated)	1201	1080	587
	Tooth #11	1044	647	451
Patient 2	Tooth #16	914	814	409
	Tooth #17 (Treated)	729	632	285
Patient 3	Tooth #36 (Treated)	893	1334	944
	Tooth #37	801	944	747

3. Discussion

In this pioneer clinical pilot study, we used an innovative procedure for the treatment of periodontitis by implanting CH/HAP. At the onset of the present study, the group of periodontitis patients had a significant oral defect with an important loss of alveolar bone of 12.44 mm; one-year post-implant the treated patients had an important alveolar bone growth of 5.77 ± 1.87 mm. This beneficial outcome for teeth preservation improved patient quality of life.

The biomaterial exhibited the presence of osteoblasts, fibroblasts and connective tissue without inflammatory infiltrate. The presence of osteoblasts seems to promote the alveolar bone growth filling the oral defect.

The inorganic phase of the biomaterial integrated to the alveolar bone must be chemically and structurally similar to the mineral phase that forms the bone. In a previous study [10], the bioactivity of HAP and the presence of N-acetyl glucosamine in the chitosan analog of glycosaminoglycans (GAG), promoted bone growth [10]. When chitosan is mixed with hydroxyapatite it is difficult to achieve uniform distribution in the polymeric matrix. This situation sometimes limits its applicability, particularly with tissue inflammation, producing a voluminous fibrotic capsule and inducing a biomaterial rejection [11]. In this study, there was no such rejection, this could be attributed to an absence of an inflammatory infiltrate.

In diabetic rats with an oral defect, the oral inflammation was regulated using a combination of 2% Chitosan, type 1 collagen, and antibody anti-tumor necrosis factor α (anti-TNFα). In this implant, TNFα and the factor nuclear kappa B (NFkB) levels decreased. Furthermore, these implants produced an increase in osteogenesis which was associated with proteins that promoted the alveolar bone restoration [12]. In our results, Chitosan (3%) in combination with Hydroxyapatite (3%) promoted the alveolar bone growth. This combination of biomaterials could be inducing a decrease in the inflammation by the decrease in TNFα or NFkB. Additional studies should be made to corroborate this premise.

Huang et al. (2011) using an implant of chitosan/hydroxyapatite/collagen (CH/HAC) combined with allogeneic mesenchymal stem cells (MSC) in a rabbit's femur bone defect, found larger areas of new bone and collagen fibrous tissues. The new bone was observed after twelve weeks post implant. The size and structure of alveolar bone in teeth is different to a large bone, therefore our scaffold is good enough to repair the lost alveolar bone [13].

Chitosan has an important microbicide activity [14–17]. Chitosan exhibits a potent oral plaque reduction action as well as an antibacterial activity against several oral pathogens such as Actinobacilus actinomycetemcomitans, Streptococcus mutans, and Porphyromonas gingivalis, all of which are implicated in plaque formation in periodontitis [18–20]. This antibacterial chitosan effect could also contribute to the repair of the oral defect.

Hoemann (2005), found that chitosan hydrogels guide macrophages to the wounds, thus contributing to repair the wounds in vivo. Macrophages are also responsible for chitosan degradation in vivo through the release of cytokines as tumor necrosis factor α (TNFα) and interleukin-1β (IL-1 β), which attract fibroblast into the wound to initiate a reconstruction process. In the present study, chitosan was absorbed approximately in three months, with moderate alveolar bone growth. However, no macrophages were observed in the biomaterial analysis [21,22]. Chatelet (2001), showed that fibroblasts do not proliferate on chitosan films, independently of chitosan deacetylation grade, because of a great cellular adhesion to the biomaterial, thus inhibiting their proliferation [23]. In the present clinical study, the CH/HAP biomaterial was implanted in a paste. This biomaterial form may contribute to fibroblast proliferation and collagen formation and thus, induce the alveolar bone growth.

The biomaterial of CH/HAP is cheaper than Emdogain, which supports its use in clinical odontology in low-income countries. Furthermore, the bone density was similar to that found in normal neighboring teeth, except for patient 2; this observation could be due to the position of the dental organ. In this case, the molar was in the maxillary angle, which has a spongier bone.

The bone density in the oral defect treated with CH/HAP was larger in younger male patients than that in adult women patients. Perhaps this result is the consequence of calcium levels and is related to patient gender. This premise deserves to be confirmed.

4. Materials and Methods

Nine patients with chronic periodontitis were studied, six men and three women, with ages ranging from 20 to 70 years old. All patients were treated in accordance with the 2013 Declaration of Helsinki. All patients agreed to participate in the study and signed the informed consent form.

4.1. Inclusion Criteria

Patients who exhibited localized chronic periodontitis with a pocket depth of 7–14 mm, accompanied by two wall intra-bone defects, without the presence of systemic diseases and who were non-smokers.

4.2. Exclusion Criteria

Patients with any periodontal treatment (one year before the study), pregnant women, and subjects with other chronic diseases, such as diabetes or cancer.

4.3. Elimination Criteria

Uncooperative study subjects and those individuals with any adverse reaction to the biomaterials.

4.4. Chitosan and Hydroxyapatite Implant

All patients presented localized chronic two-wall periodontitis with a vertical bone loss of seven millimeters or more. An implant of 3% chitosan and 3% hydroxyapatite was applied to each patient. Chitosan was obtained from Sigma-Aldrich with catalog number 448877. This molecule is 75–85% deacetylated, its viscosity is of 200–800 centipoise (cps), and it has a medium molecular weight. Hydroxyapatite (HAP) was obtained from Sigma with catalog number 289396. 3% deacetylated chitosan was dissolved in 10 ml of 2% acetic acid and then was mixed with 3% hydroxyapatite (HAP) under sterile conditions. That suspension was placed in a Petri cage. The material was dried for 24 h using sterile air into a laminar flow hood for 24 h. Later, 3 ml of saline physiologic solution (0.9%) was added to the CH/HAP to obtain a paste, the suspension had a final concentration of 0.0143 M. This paste was made immediately before making the implant for patients. The humidified CH/HAP paste was applied to the oral bone defect by filling the injured area completely. The membrane had the following size: 15.44 $\pm$ 4.79 mm large $\times$ 15.88 mm $\pm$ 2.50 high, with an average total surface of 245.18 mm^2 and 1 mm^2 of thickness; this size could change depending on the oral defect. The biomaterial elasticity, which was measured by a water column system, was of 82.3 $\pm$ 2.5 Kg and had a pressure of 58.3 $\pm$ 6.23 Pascals. Surgery was performed as follows: A full thickness flap was performed and elevated, followed by scaling and root planning in preparation; afterwards, the biomaterial was applied to the injured zone. The flap was closed and stitched up. Stitches were removed after 14 days.

Three months after the biomaterial implantation, a small sample was removed to study the distribution of fibroblasts, collagen, and osteoblasts and it was stained with hematoxylin-eosin. Ten sagittal cuts were obtained from the implanted biomaterial. The biomaterial was cut into 10 μm sections and these were mounted on slides. Hematoxylin solution was used for 5 min per slide and then alcoholic Eosin solution (0.5% eosin in 90% ethanol) was added for a period of 30 s. Then, slides were washed with deionized water for 5 min. Subsequently, an ethanol dehydration protocol was applied and the slides were covered with Entellan resin.

To measure the bone growth, a millimetric slide was used in the periapical radiography behind the tooth. Then, an X-ray was taken from each patient in the oral defect. The X-ray image was measured from the crown to the root of the tooth. To evaluate the level of teeth insertion, mucosa clinical photographs were taken of each patient. Periodontal probes with William´s markings at 1, 2, 3, 5, 7, 8, 9 and 10 mm were used to measure the pocket deep by introducing this instrument between the mucosa and the tooth.

To evaluate the tooth mobility grade, we employed a dental mirror and a dental tweezer generating a weak pressure in a horizontal direction. Then, we used the classification of dental mobility from 0 to 3 of American Academy of Periodontology.

To analyze the bone density of the oral defect from periodontitis patients treated with CH/HAP, a Computerized Tomography was taken and analyzed with the software Implant Viewer from Anne Solutions Company using the lateral tooth density as a control.

4.5. Statistics

All data are expressed as Mean ± SE. The U-Mann Whitney test was used to compare data among patients. To compare the data of alveolar bone growth among patients a paired Student's *t*-test was used.

5. Conclusions

The CH/HAP implant is a therapeutic strategy for chronic periodontitis patients that allows guided bone regeneration at a low cost, expanding the opportunity of their use for people in countries with a low socioeconomic grade.

The CH/HAP implant reduced the pocket depth of the supporting tissue. It also reduced the grading of tooth mobility and promoted alveolar bone growth.

The patients conserved the dental organ, favoring a better quality of life.

It is important to highlight that there was no inflammation surrounding the implant.

Author Contributions: Fabiola Vaca Cornejo did the actual work and collected the data and design experiments. Sergio H. Dueñas Jiménez contributed to the statistical analysis and writing. Ricardo A. Llamas Velázquez contributed to the graphical designs. Héctor Macías Reyes reviewed the experiments. Judith M. Dueñas Jiménez participated in the experimental design and wrote the paper.

References

1. Majzoub, Z.; Bobbo, M.; Atiyeh, F.; Cordioli, G. Two patterns of histologic healing in an intrabony defect following treatment with enamel matrix derivative: A human case report. *Int. J. Periodontics Restor. Dent.* **2005**, *25*, 283–294.
2. Sculean, A.; Windisch, P.; Keglevich, T.; Chiantella, G.C.; Gera, I.; Donos, N. Clinical and Histologic Evaluation of Human Intrabony Defects Treated with an Enamel Matrix Protein Derivative Combined with a Bovine-Derived Xenograft. *Int. J. Periodontics Restor. Dent.* **2003**, *23*, 47.
3. Bernabéu Martínez, E.; López-Oliva Muñoz, F.; Larena Pellejero, A.; Tur Gil, A.; de la Piedra Gordo, M.C.; Montero Escobar, M. Estudio de la composición ósea para su apropiada regeneración con materiales implantados. *Patología del Aparato Locomotor* **2006**, *4*, 202–207.
4. Jun, S.H.; Lee, E.J.; Jang, T.S.; Kim, H.E.; Jang, J.H.; Koh, Y.H. Bone morphogenic protein-2 (BMP-2) loaded hybrid coating on porous hydroxyapatite scaffolds for bone tissue engineering. *J. Mater. Sci. Mater. Med.* **2013**, *24*, 773–782. [CrossRef] [PubMed]
5. Ueno, H.; Nakamura, F.; Murakami, M.; Okumura, M.; Kadosawa, T.; Fujinaga, T. Evaluation effects of chitosan for the extracellular matrix production by fibroblasts and the growth factors production by macrophages. *Biomaterials* **2001**, *22*, 2125–2130. [CrossRef]
6. Yamaguchi, I.; Iizuka, S.; Osaka, A.; Monma, H.; Tanaka, J. The effect of citric acid addition on chitosan/hydroxyapatite composites. *Coll. Surf. A* **2003**, *214*, 111–118. [CrossRef]
7. Ezoddini-Ardakani, F.; Navabazam, A.; Fatehi, F.; Danesh-Ardekani, M.; Khadem, S.; Rouhi, G. Histologic evaluation of chitosan as an accelerator of bone regeneration in microdrilled rat tibias. *Dent. Res. J.* **2012**, *9*, 694–699.

8. Meseguer-Olmo, L.; Muñoz-Ruiz, J.; Bernabeu-Esclapez, A.; Clavel-Sainz Nolla, M.; Arcos-Pérez, D.; Vallet-Regí, M.; López-Prats, F.; Lax-Pérez, A.; Meseguer-Ortiz de Villajos, C.L. Cinética de crecimiento in vitro de osteoblastos humanos sobre cerámica porosa de hidroxiapatita. *ROT Revista de Ortopedia y Traumatología* **2006**, *50*, 224–232. [CrossRef]
9. de la Concepción Matesanz, M.; Feito, M.J.; Ramírez-Santillán, C.; Lozano, R.M.; Sánchez-Salcedo, S.; Arcos, D.; Vallet-Regí, M.; Portolés, M.T. Signaling pathways of immobilized FGF-2 on silicon-substituted hydroxyapatite. *Macromol. Biosci.* **2012**, *12*, 446–453. [CrossRef] [PubMed]
10. Wu, J.Q.; Liu, Y.; Yang, T.F.; Mu, Y.H.; Guo, T.; Li, Y.B. Porous polyvinyl alcohol hydrogel composite prepared and studied initially for biocompatibility. *J. Sichuan Univ. Med. Sci. Ed.* **2007**, *38*, 705–708.
11. Davidenko, N.; García, R.; Peniche, C.; Solís, Y. Chitosan/hydroxyapatite-based composites. *Biotecnología Aplicad* **2010**, *27*, 202–210.
12. Wang, Q.; Li, H.; Xiao, Y.; Li, S.; Li, B.; Zhao, X.; Ye, L.; Guo, B.; Chen, X.; Ding, Y.; Bao, C. Locally controlled delivery of TNFa antibody from a novel glucose-sensitive scaffold enhances alveolar bone healing in diabetic conditions. *COREL J. Control. Release* **2015**, *206*, 232–242. [CrossRef] [PubMed]
13. Huang, Z.; Chen, Y.; Feng, Q.-L.; Zhao, W.; Yu, B.; Tian, J.; Li, S.-J.; Lin, B.-M. In vivo bone regeneration with injectable chitosan/hydroxyapatite/collagen composites and mesenchymal stem cells. *Front. Mater. Sci.* **2011**, *5*, 301–310. [CrossRef]
14. Martinez, L.R.; Mihu, M.R.; Han, G.; Frases, S.; Cordero, R.J.; Casadevall, A.; Friedman, A.J.; Friedman, J.M.; Nosanchuk, J.D. The use of chitosan to damage Cryptococcus neoformans biofilms. *Biomaterials* **2010**, *31*, 669–679. [CrossRef] [PubMed]
15. Muzzarelli, R.; Tarsi, R.; Filippini, O.; Giovanetti, E.; Biagini, G.; Varaldo, P.E. Antimicrobial properties of N-carboxybutyl chitosan. *Antimicrob. Agents Chemother.* **1990**, *34*, 2019–2023. [CrossRef] [PubMed]
16. Rhoades, J.; Roller, S. FOOD MICROBIOLOGY—Antimicrobial Actions of Degraded and Native Chitosan against Spoilage Organisms in Laboratory Media and Foods. *Appl. Environ. Microbiol.* **2000**, *66*, 80. [CrossRef] [PubMed]
17. Jeon, Y.-J.; Park, P.-J.; Kim, S.-K. Antimicrobial effect of chitooligosaccharides produced by bioreactor. *Carbohydr. Polym.* **2001**, *44*, 71–76. [CrossRef]
18. No, H.K.; Park, N.Y.; Lee, S.H.; Meyers, S.P. Antibacterial activity of chitosans and chitosan oligomers with different molecular weights. *Int. J. Food Microbiol.* **2002**, *74*, 65–72. [CrossRef]
19. Choi, B.K.; Kim, K.Y.; Yoo, Y.J.; Oh, S.J.; Choi, J.H.; Kim, C.Y. In vitro antimicrobial activity of a chitooligosaccharide mixture against Actinobacillus actinomycetemcomitans and Streptococcus mutans. *Int. J. Antimicrob. Agents* **2001**, *18*, 553–557. [CrossRef]
20. Ikinci, G.; Senel, S.; Akincibay, H.; Kas, S.; Ercis, S.; Wilson, C.G.; Hincal, A.A. Effect of chitosan on a periodontal pathogen Porphyromonas gingivalis. *Int. J. Pharm.* **2002**, *235*, 121. [CrossRef]
21. Hoemann, C.D.; Sun, J.; Légaré, A.; McKee, M.D.; Buschmann, M.D. Tissue engineering of cartilage using an injectable and adhesive chitosan-based cell-delivery vehicle. *Osteoarthr. Cartil.* **2005**, *13*, 318–329. [CrossRef] [PubMed]
22. Chellat, F.; Tabrizian, M.; Dumitriu, S.; Chornet, E.; Magny, P.; Rivard, C.H.; Yahia, L. In vitro and in vivo biocompatibility of chitosan-xanthan polyionic complex. *J. Biomed. Mater. Res.* **2000**, *51*, 107–116. [CrossRef]
23. Chatelet, C.; Damour, O.; Domard, A. Influence of the degree of acetylation on some biological properties of chitosan films. *Biomaterials* **2001**, *22*, 261–268. [CrossRef]

2

Dental Composite Formulation Design with Bioactivity on Protein Adsorption Combined with Crack-Healing Capability

Chen Chen [1,2,†], Junling Wu [2,3,†], Michael D. Weir [2], Lin Wang [2,4], Xuedong Zhou [1], Hockin H. K. Xu [2,5,6] and Mary Anne S. Melo [2,*]

1 State Key Laboratory of Oral Diseases, West China Hospital of Stomatology, Sichuan University, Chengdu 610041, China; Cchen@umaryland.edu (C.C.); zhouxd@scu.edu.cn (X.Z.)
2 Department of Prosthodontics, Endodontics and Operative Dentistry, University of Maryland School of Dentistry, Baltimore, MD 21201, USA; JWu@umaryland.edu (J.W.); MWeir@umaryland.edu (M.D.W.); LWang@umaryland.edu (L.W.); Hxu@umaryland.edu (H.H.K.X.)
3 Shandong Provincial Key Laboratory of Oral Biomedicine, Jinan 250012, China
4 VIP Integrated Department, Stomatological Hospital of Jilin University, Changchun 130011, China
5 Center for Stem Cell Biology & Regenerative Medicine, University of Maryland School of Medicine, Baltimore, MD 21201, USA
6 Department of Mechanical Engineering, University of Maryland, Baltimore County, MD 21250, USA
* Correspondence: mmelo@umaryland.edu
† These authors contributed equally to this work.

Abstract: Fracture and secondary caries are the primary reasons for the failure of dental restorations. To face this omnipresent problem, we report the formulation design and synthesis of a protein-resistant dental composite composed of 2-methacryloyloxyethyl phosphorylcholine (MPC) that also can self-repair damage and recover the load-bearing capability via microencapsulated triethylene glycol dimethacrylate (TEGDMA) and *N,N*-dihydroxy ethyl-*p*-toluidine (DHEPT). The bioactivity of the resulting MPC-microencapsulated TEGDMA-DHEPT was evaluated on protein adsorption through early bacterial attachment. Its mechanical properties were also investigated, including self-healing assessment. Microcapsules of poly (urea-formaldehyde) (PUF) were synthesized by incorporating a TEGDMA-DHEPT healing liquid. A set of composites that contained 7.5% of MPC, 10% of microcapsules, and without MPC/microcapsules were also prepared as controls. The two distinct characteristics of strong protein repellency and load-bearing recovery were achieved by the combined strategies. The novel dual composite with a combination of protein-repellent MPC and PUF microcapsules for restoring microcracks is a promising strategy for dental restorations to address the two main challenges of fracture and secondary caries. The new dual composite formulation design has the potential to improve the longevity of dental restorations significantly.

Keywords: self-healing; microcapsules; mechanical property; protein repellent; dental composite

---

1. Introduction

In a range of materials available for the restoration of the tooth cavity, composites are the predominantly selected choice as they offer advantages in their aesthetics and less invasive preparation techniques [1,2]. Prospective randomized controlled trials (RCTs) and systematic reviews have highlighted that even though the overall survival rates were satisfactory, there are high annual failure rates associated with composites [3,4]. The replacement of a failed composite restoration leads to an increase in cavity size and destruction of the remaining tooth structure [5,6]. Replacement costs represent an enormous annual expense in the United States, considering that the annual cost for tooth cavity restorations in the United States was $46 billion in 2005 [7].

The predominant reasons for composite restoration failures are secondary caries and restoration fractures, which represent more than 90% of recorded failures [8]. Short-term survival rates report secondary caries often occurred after three years or later, which contribute to the high annual failure rates related to this material [9]. Besides the lack of suitable mechanical properties reflected by fracture, the incidence rate for biological complications represented by secondary caries, with or without fracture of the restoration, has been reported to be close to twice as high as technical complications [9]. New rational materials design based on prior knowledge have been developed for finding advanced designs to address these ongoing problems of dental composites [10].

One step on this path addresses the inhibition of nonspecific adsorption of proteins at the surface of dental restorative materials [11]. Since protein adsorption is believed to be the first step in the salivary pellicle formation, which also leads to bacterial attachment and biofilm formation, the inhibition of this process is a potential target for antibacterial approaches. Among the many strategies for imparting high resistance to protein adsorption so far investigated, the polymer 2-Methacryloylothelxyethyl-phosphorylcholine (MPC), in particular, has been one of the most promising approaches [12,13]. Since proteins are hydrophobic, MPC shows a high resistance toward protein adsorption due to the low polymer–water interfacial energy and high hydrophilicity [14,15]. This feature plays a critical role in reducing protein adsorption and preventing the formation of any conditioning layer that might otherwise enable the bacteria to gain anchorage to the surface [15,16]. The excellent biocompatibility of MPC-containing polymers has also been confirmed [17]. To date, recently resin-based direct restorative materials modified with MPC have shown lower protein adsorption, which has been associated with oral bacterial reduction [18–23].

Given the major requirements of clinical services and materials after fracture, an autonomous crack-healing ability has recently captured a lot of attention due to the recovery strength of biomaterials after being forced to break [24]. This approach employs a liquid healing agent encapsulated in a polymeric shell to form microcapsules, which are then incorporated into a matrix material [25]. When cracking occurs, the propagating crack will rupture the microcapsules, release the healing liquid that has its polymerization trigger when in contact with capsules, and lead to the healing of the composite [26,27]. More recently, novel self-healing poly (urea-formaldehyde) (PUF) microcapsules containing polymerizable TEGDMA and *N*,*N*-dihydroxy ethyl-*p*-toluidine (DHEPT) were synthesized and incorporated into dental resin good self-healing efficacy [28,29].

A combination of adequately selected strategies can bring synergistic effect that can help to overcome the two most predominant reasons for failures in composite restorations. The design and development of a protein-repellent dental composite with autonomous crack-healing ability would have a significant impact on the longevity of the composite, which would be reflected in their service lives. However, while these two approaches are successful individually, they have never been evaluated together. In the present study, we report for the first time the design formulation of a dual-loaded dental composite that combines and provides both high protein repellency and self-healing simultaneously in their core and surface.

2. Materials and Methods

2.1. Chemicals and Reagents

Bisphenol A glycidyl dimethacrylate (Bis-GMA) and triethylene glycol dimethacrylate (TEGDMA) were obtained from Esstech (Essington, PA, USA) and used as received. *N*,*N*-dihydroxy ethyl-*p*-toluidine (DHEPT), ethylene-maleic anhydride (EMA), ammonium chloride, resorcinol, formaldehyde, bovine serum albumin (BSA), camphorquinone (CQ), ethyl 4-(diamethylamino) benzoate (4E), 2-Methacryloylothelxyethyl-phosphorylcholine (MPC), 3 methacryloxypropyltrimethoxysilane, and N-propylamine purchased from Sigma-Aldrich (Saint Louis, MO, USA) were used without further purification. Barium boroaluminosilicate glass particles were obtained from Caulk/ Dentsply (Milford, DE, USA).

2.2. *Synthesis of Self-Healing Microcapsules*

Microcapsules (MCS) were prepared using an in-situ polymerization of formaldehyde via the urea method, as described previously [28]. First, DHEPT was added to the TEGDMA monomer at 1 wt %. A mixture of 50 mL of distilled water and 13 mL of a 2.5% aqueous solution of EMA copolymer was prepared in a 250 mL-Erlenmeyer flask. The flask was suspended in a water bath on a hot plate. Second, the shell-forming material urea (1.25 g), ammonium chloride (0.125 g), and resorcinol (0.125 g) were added into the solution under 300 rpm agitation by a magnetic stir bar (Ø = 7.8 mm, length = 50 mm, Fisher Scientific). Resorcinol was added in the reaction of shell formation to enhance the rigidity of the shell [30]. The pH was adjusted to 3.5 by the drop-wise addition of 1 M NaOH. Then, the agitation rate was increased to 400 rpm, and 30 mL of the TEGDMA-DHEPT liquid was added into the flask [31]. After 10 min of agitation, a stabilized emulsion of fine TEGDMA-DHEPT droplets were formed. Then, 3.15 g of a 37% aqueous solution of formaldehyde was added. The stirring was continued with heating to 55 °C for 4 h [28]. In this process, ammonium chloride catalyzed the reaction of urea with formaldehyde to form PUF at the oil–water interface to develop the shell [29]. The resulting microcapsules were rinsed with water and acetone, vacuum filtered, and air dried for 24 h. The microcapsules' structure was confirmed by optical microscope 4× (TE2000-S, Nikon, Japan) and SEM (Quanta 200, FEI, Hillsboro, OR, USA), as shown in Figure 1.

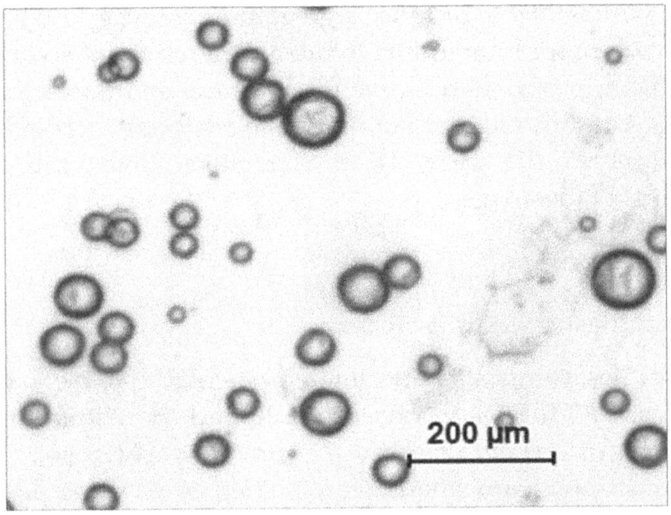

Figure 1. Transmitting optical image of resulting poly (urea-formaldehyde) (PUF) microcapsules loaded with polymerizable TEGDMA and *N,N*-dihydroxy ethyl-*p*-toluidine (DHEPT) (an average diameter of 73 ± 31 μm).

2.3. *Concepting MPC and Self-Healing Microcapsules into Composite*

A parental composite formulation was made by mixing the following components: Bis-GMA and TEGDMA at a mass ratio of 1:1, 0.2% camphorquinone, 0.8% ethyl 4-*N,N*-dimethylamino benzo, and barium boroaluminosilicate glass (mean particle size of 1.4 mm) silanized with 4% 3-methacryloxypropyltrimethoxy silane and 2% n-propylamine. MPC, a methacrylate with a phospholipid polar group in the side chain, was used as the protein-repellent agent. MPC was synthesized according to a reported method [15].

The MPC powder was mixed with photo-activated BisGMA-TEGDMA resin at mass fractions of 7.5%. Then, the composite was then mixed with microcapsules at microcapsule mass fractions of 10%.

The chosen mass fractions were selected considering previous investigations of the relationship between the MPC and microcapsules mass fraction and the mechanical properties of the composite [21,28].

2.4. Protein Repellence Essay

For the protein adsorption and live/dead essays, each composite paste was placed into disc molds (Ø = 9 mm; 2 mm in thickness). They were light-cured, stored in distilled water at 98.6 °F for 24 h, and sterilized by ethylene oxide, following a previous study [20].

The amount of protein adsorbed on the composite discs was determined by the micro bicinchoninic acid method [32]. Six disks were evaluated for each group. Each disk was immersed in phosphate buffered saline (PBS) for 2 h before immersing in 4.5 g/L bovine serum albumin (BSA) solutions at 37 °C for 2 h. The disks then were rinsed with fresh PBS by stirring method (300 rpm for 5 min). The adsorbed protein was detached in sodium dodecyl sulfate (SDS) 1 wt % in PBS by sonication for 20 min. A protein analysis kit (Micro BCA protein assay kit, Fisher Scientific, Pittsburgh, PA, USA) was used to determine the BSA concentration in the SDS solution. The amount of protein adsorbed on the resin disk surface was calculated from the concentration of protein [22].

2.5. Live/Dead Staining of Biofilms

Fluorescence microscopy via live/dead assay was used to directly visualize the early bacterial attachment (4 h after inoculum) over the studied materials. A dental plaque microcosm biofilm model using human saliva was used to promote the biofilm grown over the composites, according to a previous report [33]. The biofilms on the disks were gently washed three times with phosphate-buffered saline (PBS), and then stained using a live/dead bacterial viability kit (Molecular Probes, Eugene, OR, USA). Live bacteria were stained with Syto 9 to produce a green fluorescence, and bacteria with compromised membranes were stained with propidium iodide to produce a red fluorescence [19]. The corresponding images were acquired using appropriate selective filters in the epifluorescence microscope (TE2000-S, Nikon, Melville, NY, USA). The area of green staining (live bacteria) was computed with NIS-Elements imaging software (Nikon, Melville, NY, USA). The area fraction of live bacteria was calculated based on green staining area/total area of the image.

2.6. Assessment of Mechanical Properties

2.6.1. Flexural Strength and Elastic Modulus Testing

Following previous studies, composites specimens were placed in metal molds, photo-cured (Triad 2000, Dentsply, York, PA, USA) for 1 min on each side and then smoothed, which produced bar specimens with dimensions of 2 mm× 2 mm× 25 mm (n = 6) [29,34]. Twenty-four hours after manufacturing and water storage, specimens were subjected to three-point flexural testing using a computer-controlled Universal Testing Machine—UTM (5500R, MTS, Cary, NC, USA). All tests were performed using a span of 10 mm and a crosshead speed of 1 mm/min. Flexural strength (FS) was measured as $FS = 3PmaxL/(2bh^2)$, where P max is the load-at-failure, L is a span, b is specimen width, and h is thickness. Elastic modulus (E) was measured as E = (P/d)(L3/[4bh3]), where load P divided by displacement d is the slope in the linear elastic region of the load-displacement curve [34,35].

2.6.2. Fracture Toughness and Self-Healing Assessment

Fracture toughness (K_{IC}) was measured using a single edge V-notched beam (SEVNB) method [24]. The SEVNB composite bars specimens for fracture toughness measurement were prepared following a previous protocol [28,29]. After notching the bending bars with a razor blade and 3 µm-diamond suspensions (average notch: depth 700–800 µm; tip radius = 20 µm), the fracture toughness was determined by the same three-point bending test. The photo-cured composites containing the MPC and microcapsules as well the related controls were tested. This yielded the original virgin K_{IC} of the specimens ($K_{IC\text{-virgin}}$).

Before testing the self-healing assessment, the two halves of the specimen were attached to the metal mold and placed in a humidor at 37 °C for 24 h. After the fracture, the healing process was trigged [30]. In this period, the disrupted microcapsules released the healing agent TEGDMA-DHEPT, which reacts with the BPO in the resin matrix. The mix of these two components would cause the polymerization of the released liquid to heal and bond the two cracked planes into one cohesive specimen. The sample was fractured again using the same method, and the new fracture toughness ($K_{IC\ healed}$) was calculated [31]. The self-healing efficiency ($\acute{\eta}$) was assessed as the percentage of fracture toughness after the healing in comparison with the virgin ($\acute{\eta} = K_{IC\text{-healed}}\ K_{IC\text{-virgin}} \times 100$).

2.7. Statistical Analysis

Statistical evaluations were performed with SigmaStat 3.5 (Systat, San Jose, CA, USA). The normality distribution of the data and equality of variances were checked using the Kolmogorov–Smirnov test and Levene's test, respectively. As the data were normally distributed, analysis of variance (ANOVA) and the Tukey test were applied at a significance level of $p < 0.05$.

3. Results

The amounts of protein adsorption on composite disc surfaces are plotted in Figure 2 ($n = 6$). Adding MPC to composites significantly decreased the protein adsorption ($p < 0.05$). The resin composite with 7.5% MPC had the lowest amount of protein adsorption, which was nearly 5% that of the control and the composite without MPC ($p < 0.05$).

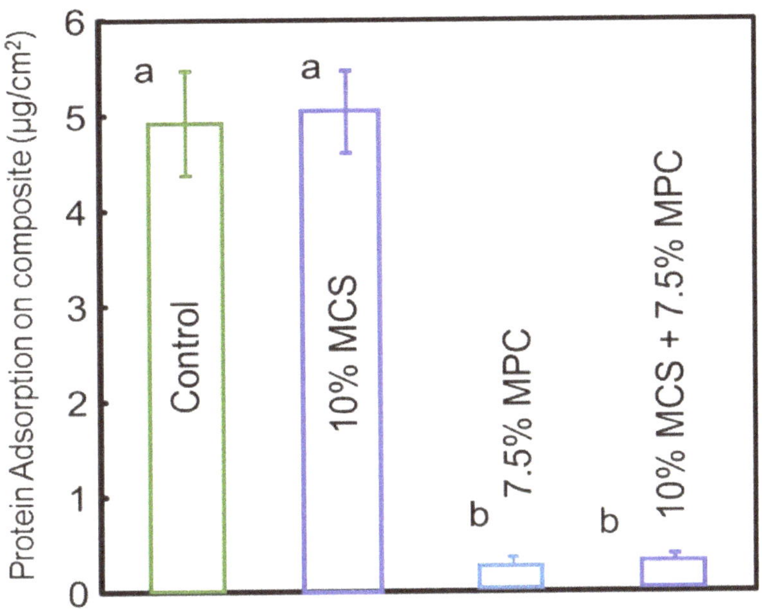

Figure 2. Protein adsorption onto composite surfaces. The composite with 7.5% 2-methacryloyloxyethyl phosphorylcholine (MPC) had the lowest amount of protein adsorption, which was approximately 1/16 those of the composite control and the composite with 10% microcapsules (MCS) ($p < 0.05$). Different letters indicate values that are significantly different from each other ($p < 0.05$).

Figure 3 shows the early bacterial attachment onto composite surfaces by representative live/dead staining images after 4 h of the inoculum. Live bacteria were stained green, and dead bacteria were stained red. The composite discs had primarily live bacteria, with few dead bacteria. Both the control composite and the composite with 10% MCS but without MPC had noticeably more bacteria coverage than the composites containing MPC. The quantification of the area fraction of the composite surface covered by live bacteria is plotted in Figure 3E, and corroborates with the outcome found in the qualitative evaluation of images where composites with 7.5% MPC had great bacterial adhesion reduction.

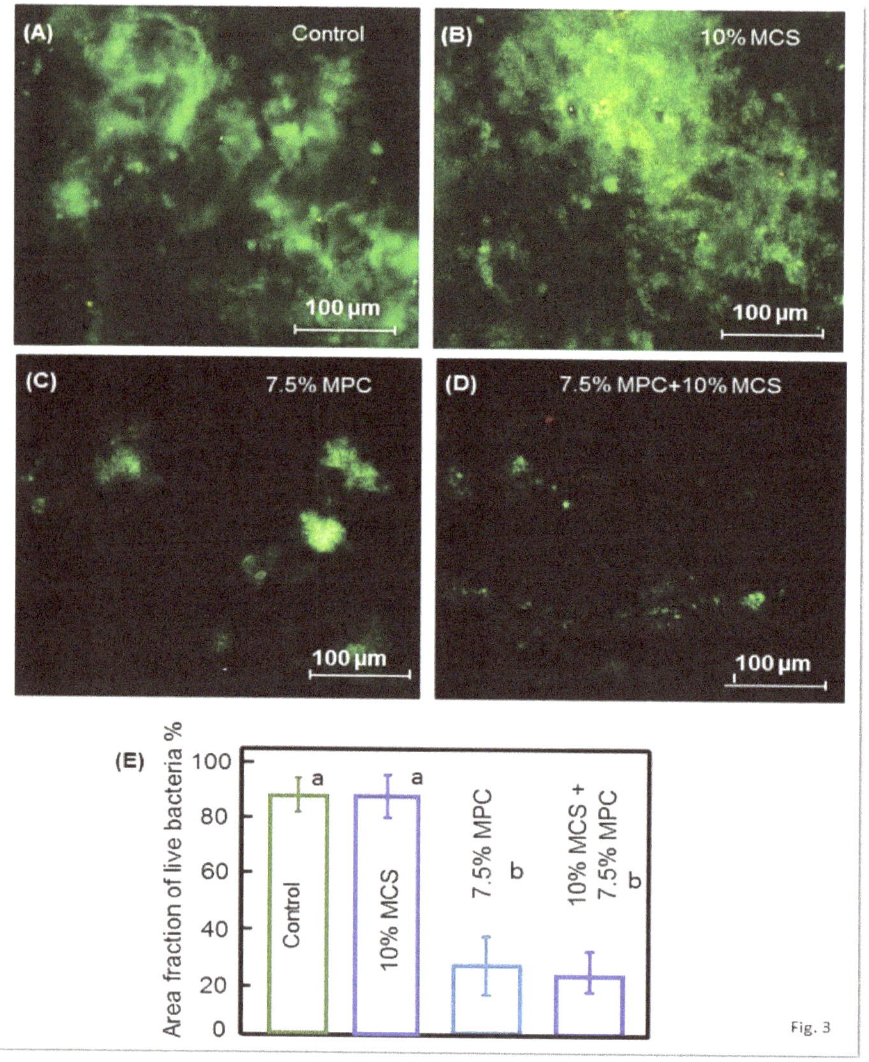

Figure 3. Representative live/dead staining images on the early attachment of oral biofilms of the disks (**A**–**D**). Live bacteria showed green, while dead bacteria showed red, and (**E**) shows the area fraction of the green staining of live bacteria coverage on composite surfaces (mean ± SD; $n = 6$). The composite control had much more bacterial attachment. All groups were covered with live bacteria and few dead bacteria; the images (**C**,**D**) show that the composite with incorporated MPC had noticeably fewer bacteria on the cover zone than the images of composites without MPC (**A**,**B**). Different letters in (**E**) indicate values that are significantly different from each other ($p < 0.05$).

The flexural strength and elastic modulus of composites with combined and isolated tested components were evaluated after one day of water storage, and are plotted in Figure 4 (mean ± SD; $n = 6$). The flexural strength and elastic modulus of a composite containing 10% microcapsules and 7.5% MPC were not significantly different from controls ($p > 0.5$).

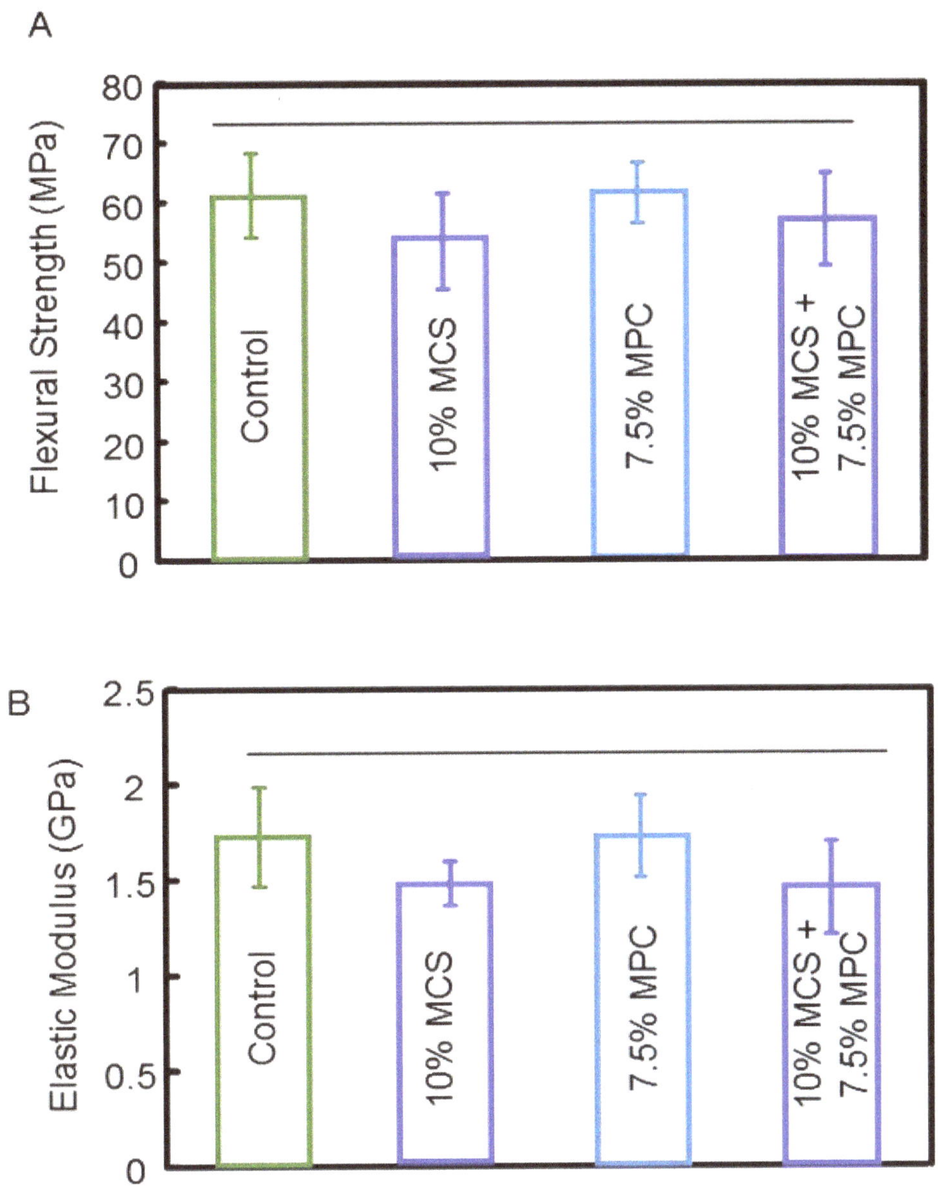

Figure 4. Mechanical properties of resin-containing microcapsules of various concentrations: (**A**) flexural strength, and (**B**) elastic modulus (mean ± SD; $n = 6$). The addition of up to 10% of microcapsules and/or 7.5% MPC resulted in no significant decrease in strength or the elastic modulus of the composite. Horizontal line indicates statistically similar values ($p > 0.5$).

The critical stress-intensity value, or plane-strain fracture toughness, denoted K_{IC} were expressed in MPa-$m^{1/2}$.The results for all tested composites after one day of water storage are shown in Figure 5. The virgin-healed K_{IC} and the percentage of damage recovery of the composites are expressed for each material. The virgin K_{IC} of the composite to which the microcapsules were added was about 36% higher than that at 0% microcapsules ($p < 0.05$; one-way ANOVA). The healed K_{IC} were similar for the composites containing 10% microcapsules with and without the addition of MPC. The MPC incorporation did not compromise the healed K_{IC} ($p < 0.05$). The self-healing efficiency of 57–71% in damage recovery was obtained in both composites where the microcapsules were present.

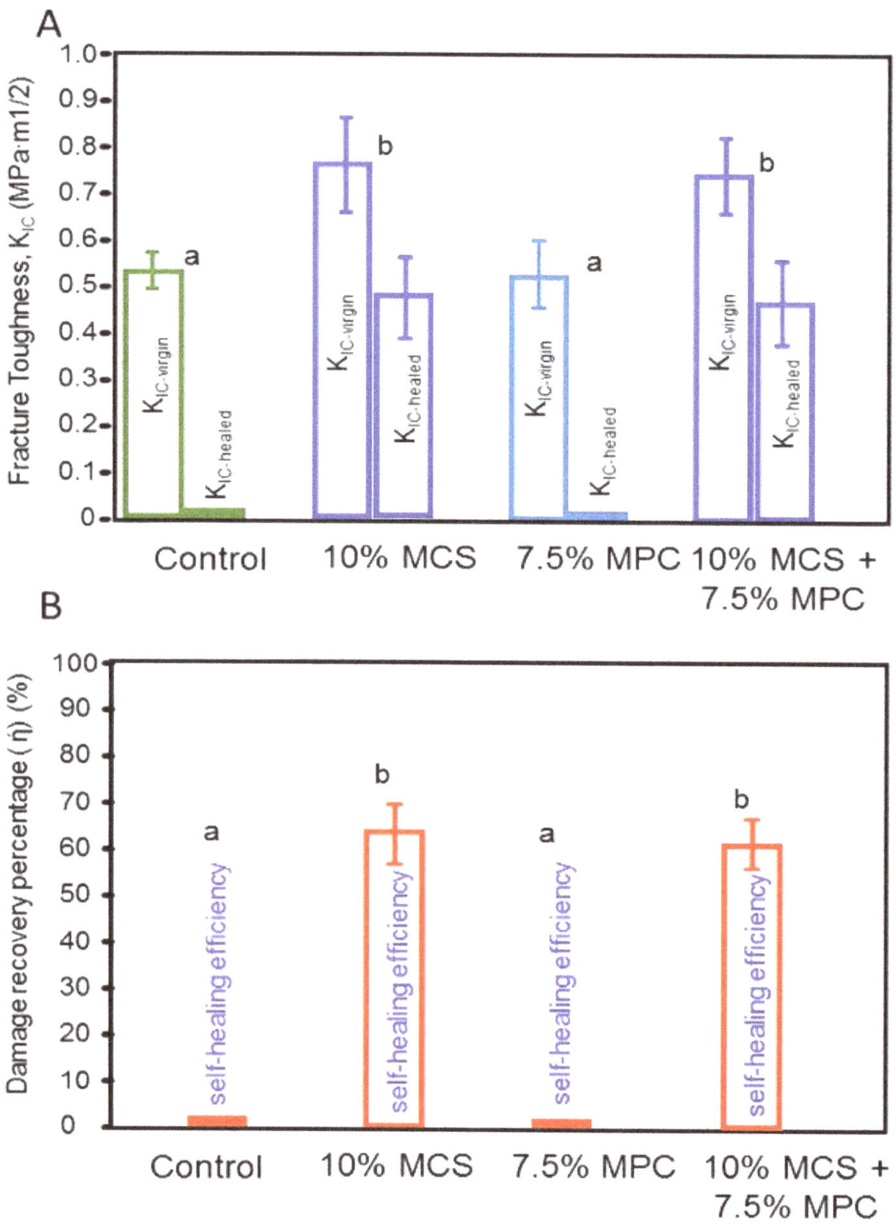

Figure 5. Fracture toughness and self-healing of a composite containing microcapsules and MPC. (**A**) Initial and post-healing fracture toughness (K_{IC}), and (**B**) the damage recovery for K_{IC} according to the formulation designed for each tested composite. In each plot, values with dissimilar letters are significantly different from each other ($p < 0.05$).

4. Discussion

Significant advancements in mechanical strength and surface roughness have been achieved in dental composites. Nevertheless, microcracking induced by fatigue and biofilm accumulation are long-standing problems in dental resin composites, and current strategies are non-responsive. In this study, we present an innovative strategy that involves the combination of a protein-repellant approach and the simultaneous targeting healing of the microcracks that eventually lead to the failure of restorations. More specifically, we aimed to design a composite that can fight the recurrence of dental caries around the composite, as well as help elicit mechanisms for the self-correction of many initial micro-cracks without a dentist's operative intervention. The facets of this approach complement each other for optimal efficacy and increased clinical life service.

The self-healing approach has been investigated in previous reports, which indicate that healing efficiency is relative to the matrix used, and can vary tremendously due to different matrix-healed network interactions [24,30,31]. By concept, the self-healing polymeric materials have the built-in capability to substantially recover their load-transferring ability after damage. Such recovery can occur autonomously or be activated after an application of a particular stimulus (e.g., heat, radiation)[36,37]. Research into producing self-healing dental composites has been based on the release of a healing liquid after cracking produced via fatigue[38]. In the present study, microcapsules with a healing liquid of TEGDMA plus 1% DHEPT surrounded by a PUF shell were used via an in situ polymerization technique in an oil-in-water emulsion [28]. This method allowed the production of microcapsules with an average diameter of 70 ± 24 μm [29], which respond to a massive rupture of the PUF shell when stress is required to propagate a pre-existing flaw. We proposed that this effect was efficient due to sufficient microcapsule stability inside the resin matrix promoted by the roughness of the external surface of microcapsule wall and a suitable thickness of the wall, which also protects the encapsulated healing agent from premature polymerization [29]. Approximately 65% of the original strength was recovered after repair with TEGDMA-DHEPT as a healing liquid. Efficient self-healing has been also demonstrated in previous studies using the applied method of fabrication of microcapsules [29,31]. The microencapsulated healing is quite stable and durable, which broadens the process window for fabricating self-healing composites and prevents the deterioration of the healing capability of the composites during storage [32]. The successful demonstration of this healing system will open pathways for healing in dental composites.

The incorporation of additives with different purposes into a resin matrix would inevitably affect its intrinsic properties. The fraction of each element is critical for the current system to achieve the highest healing efficiency. One major goal of this study was to combine the best performance of those two elements (healing system and protein repellent) without detrimental effects on their highlighted properties. High healing efficiency can be acquired at 10% capsules content so that the fundamental mechanical properties of the matrix are insignificantly affected. Previous studies showed a positive correlation between microcapsule content incorporation and the fracture toughness of the polymer matrix [26,27]. In a previous study, a nearly 40% increase in the original virgin KIC was achieved when the microcapsule mass fraction was increased from 0 to 10%, and slightly reduced when increased to 15% [29]. This finding was also consistent with a previous study showing that the incorporation of up to 6% of microcapsules into a host material did not affect the original flexural strength [30]. Mechanistically, we show that the addition of 10% microcapsules into the composite did not decrease its properties, and can be used as an optimal concentration that reaches up to 70% of healing efficiency. Also, because the healing agent possesses high flow ability and reactivity and belongs to the same family as the matrix polymer, crack healing is automatically conducted at or below room temperature, which offers satisfactory repair effectiveness.

Our results highlight composites for dental restorations that satisfy the characteristics of autonomous recovery after damage and ultra-low protein adsorption, and also, that low bacterial adhesion thereon was successfully achieved. The incorporation of 2-Methacryloylothelxyethyl-phosphorylcholine (MPC) into dental composites displays antibiofilm potential properties regulated by reduced protein adsorption, since the attachment of oral bacteria to a material's surface is moderated by adsorbed proteins [23]. A recent report has first demonstrated the contribution of MPC as an excellent agent for reducing bacterial adhesion [19]. The present study also confirmed that MPC-containing composite could repel proteins, which indicated that the composite could potentially also reduce biofilm attachment.

The polymer MPC has been shown to be highly hydrophilic and capture the surrounding water that is credited to detach proteins efficiently, thereby repelling protein adsorption [36,37]. Based on this mechanism, it would have the higher mass fraction of MPC in the resin composite to reach the protein-repellent potency. The current study showed for the first time that while the composite containing MPC was indeed strongly protein-repellent, its potency was not compromised via a dual method (MPC & MCS). The addition of MPC at a mass fraction of 7.5% did not adversely affect the mechanical strength of the newly designed material.

The set of tests performed here significantly revealed reduced oral biofilm attachment and a triggered a self-healing response, which prove that our approach was feasible and efficient in vitro, and suggest that this combined strategy may indeed help overcome recurrent caries and material fracture in dental composites.

5. Conclusions

This preliminary study demonstrates the feasibility of preparing a self-healing dental composite formulation by embedding the TEGDMA-DHEPT healing agent into microcapsules combined with an antibiofilm surface. High healing efficiency can be acquired at optimal capsules content so that the basic mechanical properties of the matrix are insignificantly affected. In this research, the design and development of a protein-repellent dental composite formulation with autonomous crack-healing ability was successfully performed. The dual strategies for overcoming the most commons problem of composites can provide a new platform for anticaries dental materials.

Acknowledgments: This study was supported by NIH R01 DE17974 (HX), a bridge fund from the Department of Endodontics, Prosthodontics and Operative Dentistry (HX), and a seed grant from the University of Maryland Baltimore (HX).

Author Contributions: Hockin H. K. Xu and Mary Anne S. Melo conceived and designed the experiments; Chen Chen, Junling Wu and Lin Wang performed the experiments; Michael D. Weir and Mary Anne S. Melo analyzed the data; Mary Anne S. Melo wrote the paper; Xuedong Zhou discussed the paper.

References

1. Ferracane, J.L. Resin composite—State of the art. *Dent. Mater.* **2011**, *27*, 29–38. [CrossRef] [PubMed]
2. Ali, Z.; Eliyas, S.; Vere, J.W. Choosing the Right Dental Material and Making Sense of the Options: Evidence and Clinical Recommendations. *Eur. J. Prosthodont. Restor. Dent.* **2015**, *23*, 150–162.
3. Krämer, N.; Reinelt, C.; Frankenberger, R. Ten-year Clinical Performance of Posterior Resin Composite Restorations. *J. Adhes. Dent.* **2015**, *17*, 433–441. [PubMed]
4. Ástvaldsdóttir, Á.; Dagerhamn, J.; van Dijken, J.W.; Naimi-Akbar, A.; Sandborgh-Englund, G.; Tranæus, S.; Nilsson, M. Longevity of posterior resin composite restorations in adults—A systematic review. *J. Dent.* **2015**, *43*, 934–954. [CrossRef] [PubMed]
5. Forss, H.; Widstrom, E. Reasons for restorative therapy and the longevity of restorations in adults. *Acta Odontol. Scand.* **2004**, *62*, 82–86. [CrossRef] [PubMed]
6. Brantley, C.F.; Bader, J.D.; Shugars, D.A.; Nesbit, S.P. Does the cycle of restoration lead to larger restorations? *J. Am. Dent. Assoc.* **1995**, *126*, 1407–1413. [CrossRef] [PubMed]
7. Beazoglou, T.; Eklund, S.; Heffley, D.; Meiers, J.; Brown, L.J.; Bailit, H. Economic impact of regulating the use of amalgam restorations. *Public Health Rep.* **2007**, *122*, 657–663. [CrossRef] [PubMed]
8. Demarco, F.F.; Corrêa, M.B.; Cenci, M.S.; Moraes, R.R.; Opdam, N.J. Longevity of posterior composite restorations: Not only a matter of materials. *Dent. Mater.* **2012**, *28*, 87–101. [CrossRef] [PubMed]
9. Chauhan, R. Good short-term survival rates for posterior resin composite restorations. *Evid. Based Dent.* **2015**, *16*, 114–115. [CrossRef] [PubMed]
10. Potyrailo, R.; Rajan, K.; Stoewe, K.; Takeuchi, I.; Chisholm, B.; Lam, H. Combinatorial and high-throughput screening of materials libraries: A review of state of the art. *ACS Comb. Sci.* **2011**, *13*, 579–633. [CrossRef] [PubMed]
11. Cross, M.C.; Toomey, R.G.; Gallant, N.D. Protein-surface interactions on stimuli-responsive polymeric biomaterials. *Biomed. Mater.* **2016**, *11*, 022002. [CrossRef] [PubMed]
12. Sibarani, J.; Takai, M.; Ishihara, K. Surface modification on microfluidic devices with 2-methacryloyloxyethyl phosphorylcholine polymers for reducing unfavorable protein adsorption. *Colloids Surf. B Biointerfaces* **2007**, *54*, 88–93. [CrossRef] [PubMed]

13. Lewis, A.L.; Tolhurst, L.A.; Stratford, P.W. Analysis of a phosphorylcholine-based polymer coating on a coronary stent pre- and post-implantation. *Biomaterials* **2002**, *23*, 1697–1706. [CrossRef]
14. Huang, X.D.; Yao, K.; Zhang, H.; Huang, X.J.; Xu, Z.K. Surface modification of silicone intraocular lens by 2-methacryloyloxyethyl phosphoryl-choline binding to reduce Staphylococcus epidermis adherence. *Clin. Exp. Ophthalmol.* **2007**, *35*, 462–467. [CrossRef] [PubMed]
15. Ishihara, K. Bioinspired phospholipid polymer biomaterials for making high-performance artificial organs. *Sci. Technol. Adv. Mater.* **2000**, *1*, 131–138. [CrossRef]
16. Moro, T.; Takatori, Y.; Ishihara, K.; Konno, T.; Takigawa, Y.; Matsushita, T.; Ung-Il, C.; Nakamura, K.; Kawaguchi, H. Surface grafting of artificial joints with a biocompatible polymer for preventing periprosthetic osteolysis. *Nat. Mater.* **2004**, *3*, 829–836. [CrossRef] [PubMed]
17. Willis, S.L.; Court, J.L.; Redman, R.P.; Wang, J.H.; Leppard, S.W.; Obyrne, V.J.; Small, S.A.; Lewis, A.L.; Jones, S.A.; Stratford, P.W. A novel phosphorylcholine-coated contact lens for extended wear use. *Biomaterials* **2001**, *22*, 3261–3272. [CrossRef]
18. Zhang, N.; Chen, C.; Weir, M.D.; Bai, Y.; Xu, H.H. Antibacterial and protein-repellent orthodontic cement to combat biofilms and white spot lesions. *J. Dent.* **2015**, *43*, 1529–1538. [CrossRef] [PubMed]
19. Zhang, N.; Ma, J.; Melo, M.A.; Weir, M.D.; Bai, Y.; Xu, H.H. Protein-repellent and antibacterial dental composite to inhibit biofilms and caries. *J. Dent.* **2015**, *43*, 225–234. [CrossRef] [PubMed]
20. Zhang, N.; Melo, M.A.; Bai, Y.; Xu, H.H. A novel protein-repellent dental adhesive containing 2-methacryloyloxyethyl phosphorylcholine. *J. Dent.* **2014**, *42*, 1284–1291. [CrossRef] [PubMed]
21. Zhang, N.; Zhang, K.; Melo, M.A.; Chen, C.; Fouad, A.F.; Bai, Y.; Xu, H.H. Novel protein-repellent and biofilm-repellent orthodontic cement containing 2-methacryloyloxyethyl phosphorylcholine. *J. Biomed. Mater. Res. B Appl. Biomater.* **2016**, *104*, 949–959. [CrossRef] [PubMed]
22. Zhang, N.; Weir, M.D.; Romberg, E.; Bai, Y.; Xu, H.H. Development of novel dental adhesive with double benefits of protein-repellent and antibacterial capabilities. *Dent. Mater.* **2015**, *31*, 845–854. [CrossRef] [PubMed]
23. Zhang, N.; Chen, C.; Melo, M.A.; Bai, Y.X.; Cheng, L.; Xu, H.H. A novel protein-repellent dental composite containing 2-methacryloyloxyethyl phosphorylcholine. *Int. J. Oral Sci.* **2015**, *7*, 103–109. [CrossRef] [PubMed]
24. Huyang, G.; Debertin, A.E.; Sun, J. Design and development of self-healing dental composites. *Mater. Des.* **2016**, *94*, 295–302. [CrossRef] [PubMed]
25. Jones, A.S.; Rule, J.D.; Moore, J.S.; Sottos, N.R.; White, S.R. Life extension of self-healing polymers with rapidly growing fatigue cracks. *J. R. Soc. Interface* **2007**, *4*, 395–403. [CrossRef] [PubMed]
26. Jones, A.S.; Rule, J.D.; Moore, J.S.; White, S.R.; Sottos, N.R. Catalyst morphology and dissolution kinetics of self-healing polymers. *Chem. Mater.* **2006**, *18*, 1312–1317. [CrossRef]
27. Dry, C. Procedures developed for self-repair of polymer matrix composite materials. *Compos. Struct.* **1996**, *35*, 263–269. [CrossRef]
28. Wu, J.; Weir, M.D.; Melo, M.S.; Zhang, Q.; Zhou, C.; Xu, H.H. Novel self-healing dental resin with microcapsules of polymerizable trimethylene glycol dimethacrylate and *N,N*-dihydroxy ethyl-*p*-toluidine. *Dent. Mater.* **2016**, *32*, 294–304. [CrossRef] [PubMed]
29. Wu, J.; Weir, M.D.; Melo, M.S.; Xu, H.H. Development of novel self-healing and antibacterial dental composite containing calcium phosphate nanoparticles. *J. Dent.* **2015**, *43*, 317–326. [CrossRef] [PubMed]
30. Brown, E.N.; Kessler, M.R.; Sottos, N.R.; White, S.R. In situ poly (urea-formaldehyde) microencapsulation of dicyclopentadiene. *J. Microencapsul.* **2003**, *20*, 719–730. [CrossRef] [PubMed]
31. Hillewaerea, X.K.D.; Preza, F.E.D. Fifteen chemistries for autonomous external self-healing polymers and composites. *Prog. Polym. Sci.* **2015**, *49–50*, 121–153. [CrossRef]
32. Wu, J.; Weir, M.D.; Melo, M.A.; Strassler, H.E.; Xu, H.H. Effects of water-aging on self-healing dental composite containing microcapsules. *J. Dent.* **2016**, *47*, 86–93. [CrossRef] [PubMed]
33. Melo, M.A.; Cheng, L.; Weir, M.D.; Hsia, R.C.; Rodrigues, L.K.; Xu, H.H. A novel dental adhesive containing antibacterial agents and calcium phosphate nanoparticles. *J. Biomed. Mater. Res. B Appl. Biomater.* **2013**, *101*, 620–629. [CrossRef] [PubMed]
34. Xu, H.H.; Moreau, J.L.; Sun, L.; Chow, L.C. Novel CaF(2) nanocomposite with high strength and fluoride ion release. *J. Dent. Res.* **2010**, *89*, 739–745. [CrossRef] [PubMed]

35. O'Donnell, J.N.; Schumacher, G.E.; Antonucci, J.M.; Skrtic, D. Adhesion of amorphous calcium phosphate composites bonded to dentin: A study in failure modality. *J. Biomed. Mater. Res. B Appl. Biomater.* **2009**, *90*, 238–249. [CrossRef] [PubMed]
36. Tateishi, T.; Kyomoto, M.; Kakinoki, S.; Yamaoka, T.; Ishihara, K. Reduced platelets and bacteria adhesion on poly (ether ether ketone) by photoinduced and self-initiated graft polymerization of 2-methacryloyloxyethyl phosphorylcholine. *J. Biomed. Mater. Res. A* **2014**, *102*, 1342–1349. [CrossRef] [PubMed]
37. Goda, T.; Konno, T.; Takai, M.; Ishihara, K. Photoinduced phospholipid polymer grafting on Parylene film: Advanced lubrication and anti-biofouling properties. *Colloids Surf. B Biointerfaces* **2007**, *54*, 67–73. [CrossRef] [PubMed]
38. Wu, D.Y.; Meurer, S.; Solomon, D. Self-healing polymeric materials: A review of recent developments. *Prog. Polym. Sci.* **2008**, *33*, 479–522. [CrossRef]

3

Novel Chlorhexidine-Loaded Polymeric Nanoparticles for Root Canal Treatment

Gina Quiram [1], Francisco Montagner [2], Kelli L. Palmer [3], Mihaela C. Stefan [1,4], Katherine E. Washington [4] and Danieli C. Rodrigues [1,*]

[1] Department of Bioengineering, University of Texas at Dallas, 800 W Campbell, Richardson, TX 75080, USA; Gina.Quiram@utdallas.edu (G.Q.); mihaela@utdallas.edu (M.C.S.)
[2] Department of Conservative Dentistry, Dental School, Federal University of Rio Grande do Sul, Rua Ramiro Barcelos 2492, 90460-001 Porto Alegre, Brazil; francisco.montagner@ufrgs.br
[3] Department of Biological Sciences University of Texas at Dallas, 800 W Campbell, Richardson, TX 75080, USA; Kelli.Palmer@utdallas.edu
[4] Department of Chemistry, University of Texas at Dallas, 800 W Campbell, Richardson, TX 75080, USA; katherine.washington@utdallas.edu
* Correspondence: danieli@utdallas.edu

Abstract: Persistence of microorganisms in dentinal tubules after root canal chemo-mechanical preparation has been well documented. The complex anatomy of the root canal and dentinal buffering ability make delivery of antimicrobial agents difficult. This work explores the use of a novel trilayered nanoparticle (TNP) drug delivery system that encapsulates chlorhexidine digluconate, which is aimed at improving the disinfection of the root canal system. Chlorhexidine digluconate was encapsulated inside polymeric self-assembled TNPs. These were self-assembled through water-in-oil emulsion from poly(ethylene glycol)-*b*-poly(lactic acid) (PEG-*b*-PLA), a di-block copolymer, with one hydrophilic segment and another hydrophobic. The resulting TNPs were physicochemically characterized and their antimicrobial effectiveness was evaluated against *Enterococcus faecalis* using a broth inhibition method. The hydrophilic interior of the TNPs successfully entrapped chlorhexidine digluconate. The resulting TNPs had particle size ranging from 140–295 nm, with adequate encapsulation efficiency, and maintained inhibition of bacteria over 21 days. The delivery of antibacterial irrigants throughout the dentinal matrix by employing the TNP system described in this work may be an effective alternative to improve root canal disinfection.

Keywords: chlorhexidine; dentin permeability; dentin tubules; drug encapsulation; polymeric nanoparticles; poly(ethylene glycol)-*b*-poly(lactic acid)

---

1. Introduction

The translation of controlled drug delivery technologies in dentistry, especially in Endodontics, has been somewhat limited. The applications of nanoparticles as vehicles for drug delivery during root canal treatment procedures have been particularly concentrated in the blending of nanocomposites, such as zinc oxide, into endodontic sealers or root filling assemblies [1]. Recently, Shrestha and Kishen (2016) revised the current application of nanoparticles in Endodontics and reported that they were tested as solutions for irrigation, medication and as additive within sealers/restorative materials [2]. Nevertheless, further studies on drug release from loaded nanoparticles have not been tested as part of the presently intracanal medicament systems that are used to promote the reduction of residual microorganisms. An extensive variety of drugs can be conveyed through a number of avenues using degradable nanoparticles [3,4]. These nanocarriers can be utilized to carry and distribute hydrophilic and hydrophobic drugs, and other biological macromolecules [5–10]. Nanoparticles can thus be tailored to transport different drugs that are important in root canal treatment, such as chlorhexidine (CHX).

Chlorhexidine (CHX) is widely used in dentistry due to its broad-spectrum and potent antimicrobial action [11]. It is a strong antiseptic bisguanide with a di-cationic structure (positively charged) at pH levels above 3.5 that has bactericidal and bacteriostatic effects [12,13]. Furthermore, CHX demonstrates substantivity properties, which permits it to reside attached to different tissues and provide a long-lasting antibacterial activity of 8 to 12 h [14]. CHX has been used previously in two different forms, hydrogel or liquid, to create formulations that are designed to accompany chemo-mechanical preparation, as a mean of reducing the bacterial load within the complex root canal system. CHX has been proved highly effective as an intracanal treatment alone or combined with calcium hydroxide. Gomes et al. (2003), in an in vitro study, observed that chlorhexidine gel completely inhibited the growth of *Enterococcus faecalis* after 1, 2, 7, and 15 days [15]. Furthermore, Rosenthal et al. (2004) showed that bovine root dentine can retain CHX and can release it in concentrations that can inhibit *E. faecalis* for up to 12 weeks [16]. Siqueira et al. (2007) demonstrated that chemomechanical preparation with 0.12% CHX solution significantly reduced the number of intracanal bacteria in teeth from patients with primary intraradicular infections and chronic apical periodontitis [17]. However, it failed to render the canal free of cultivable bacteria in 50% of the cases. The application of a 7-day intracanal dressing with $Ca(OH)_2$/CHX paste increased significantly the number of cases yielding negative cultures.

To improve bacterial reduction in infected root canal systems and to generate an environment that is optimal for periapical healing, it is required to prolong the time release of CHX beyond the current delivery systems currently available. Nanoencapsulation could offer a better medicament release control while further lengthening the delivery period of the bactericidal in dentinal tissues [18]. Thus, the aim of this study is to develop an innovative approach to extend the antimicrobial action of CHX by encapsulating the drug in poly(ethylene glycol)-*b*-poly(lactic acid) (PEG-*b*-PLA) nanoparticles. Poly(lactide) (PLA) and its derivatives are the most widely used polymers for the self-assembly of synthetic nanoparticles [19]. These polymers are known for both their biocompatibility, resorbability through natural physiological pathways, and their ability to transport a diverse range of drugs that can be lipophilic, hydrophilic, or amphiphilic [20]. Nanoparticle size distribution and encapsulation efficiency are significantly correlated to the molecular weight of the polymer and the ratio used of drug-to-polymer during self-assembly [21].

Thus, deploying nanoparticles that are specifically designed to encapsulate the drug, is expected to allow for the delivery of the bactericidal for a prolonged period of time and in a continuous manner, which will directly target the dentinal matrix. Prior work by Haseeb et al. demonstrated that poly(ethylene glycol)-*block*-poly(lactic acid) (PEG-*b*-PLA) bilayer nanoparticles (BNPs) for CHX encapsulation can be effectively self-assembled to enhance drug bioavailability and target drug distribution to the complex dentinal matrix [22]. The previous study demonstrated that self-assembly of these nanoparticles achieved sustained inhibition of bacteria, which could potentially be promoted for use in the treatment of root canal systems. The BNPs presented a hydrophilic corona with a hydrophobic interior space that encapsulated CHX. However, the synthesis of this kind of nanoparticle was experimentally difficult to reproduce due to the low solubility of CHX in water (800 mg/L) and in most solvents [22,23].

This study aimed to improve the physiochemical properties of poly(ethylene glycol)-*b*-poly(lactic acid) (PEG-*b*-PLA) nanoparticles through self-assembly of a trilayer nanoparticles (TNPs) system that were loaded with chlorhexidine digluconate (CHX-digluconate), a stable salt form of chlorhexidine (CHX). It was hypothesized that TNPs would provide prolonged drug release of up to 21 days, improving the antimicrobial effect of intracanal bactericidals. The TNPs encapsulated hydrophilic drugs that produced nanoparticles with a relatively packed structure in the range of 140–295 nm. In this study, TNPs encapsulated with CHX-digluconate were chemically and physically characterized and their antimicrobial efficiency estimated.

2. Results

2.1. Molecular Weight and Ratio of Polymeric Chains Estimation

Synthesized PEG-*b*-PLA block copolymer was analyzed by ^{1}H NMR. The PEG-*b*-PLA block copolymer number-average molecular weight was 4690 Daltons and the structure configuration of the block copolymer was 43 mol % PEG and 57 mol % PLA (Figure 1). The peaks at 3.64 ppm and 3.38 ppm corresponded to methylene units and CH_3O– in the PEG block, respectively. Signals at 1.47 ppm and 5.16 ppm are attributed to the hydrogen atoms in CH_3– and CH– groups from PLA segments, respectively [24].

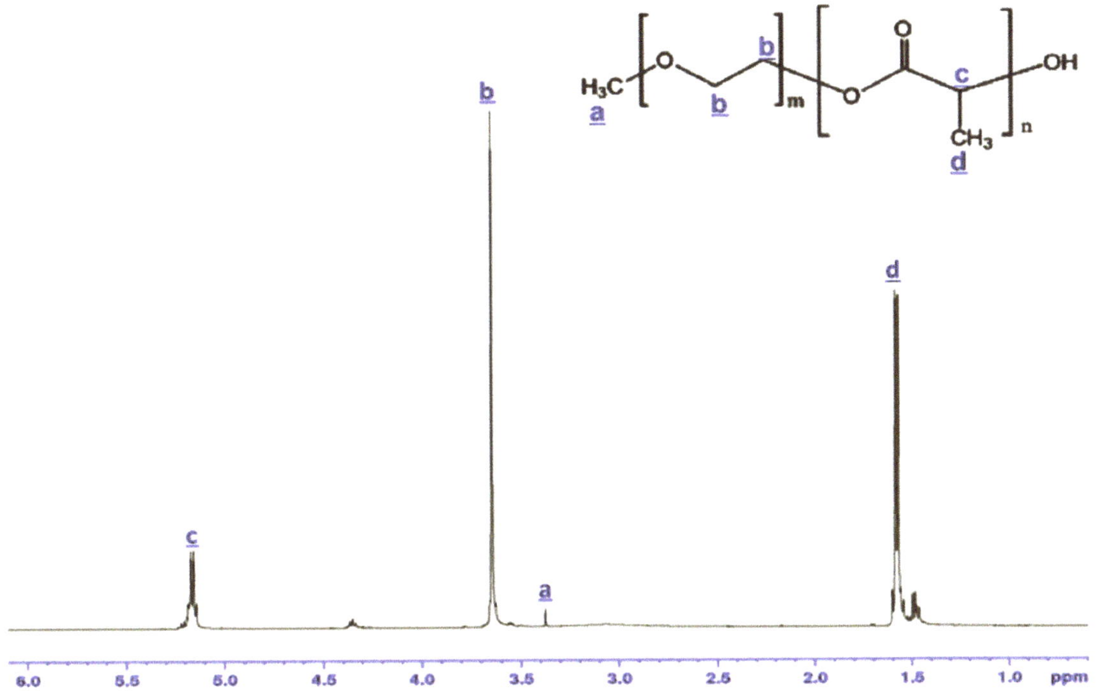

Figure 1. ^{1}H NMR spectra of the synthesized poly(ethylene glycol)-*b*-poly(L-lactide) block copolymer.

2.2. Size Distribution of Reverse Nanoparticles

The water-in-oil emulsion formulation was studied to assess the physicochemical equilibrium and suitable size distribution of the subsequent reverse nanoparticles (RNPs) in the presence of CHX-digluconate. Size distribution of RNPs that were assembled in 1,3-dimethyl-2-imidazolidinone (DMI) and N,N-dimethylacetoamide (DMA) had an average size diameter of 164 nm and a polydispersity index (PDI) of 0.33. These outcomes are means of three independent consecutive measurements.

The water-in-oil emulsion prepared with the organic solvents DMI and DMA, which density had been adjusted to 1.00 g/cm^3, was stable even after 24 h. There was no phase separation, and the size distribution of the RNPs as determined through DLS analysis remained roughly the same.

2.3. Size Distribution and Morphology of Trilayered Nanoparticles

The water-in-oil emulsion that contained RNPs was added to an aqueous solution containing the PEG-*b*-PLA block copolymer to create the trilayered nanoparticles (TNPs). Figure 2A shows the average size distribution of TNPs with one predominant peak at 295 nm that corresponded to the TNPs while the less intense peak at 105 nm could be related to the formation of BNPs as byproduct. This experiment was replicated four times (n = 4) and each time the DLS frequency spectra was evaluated.

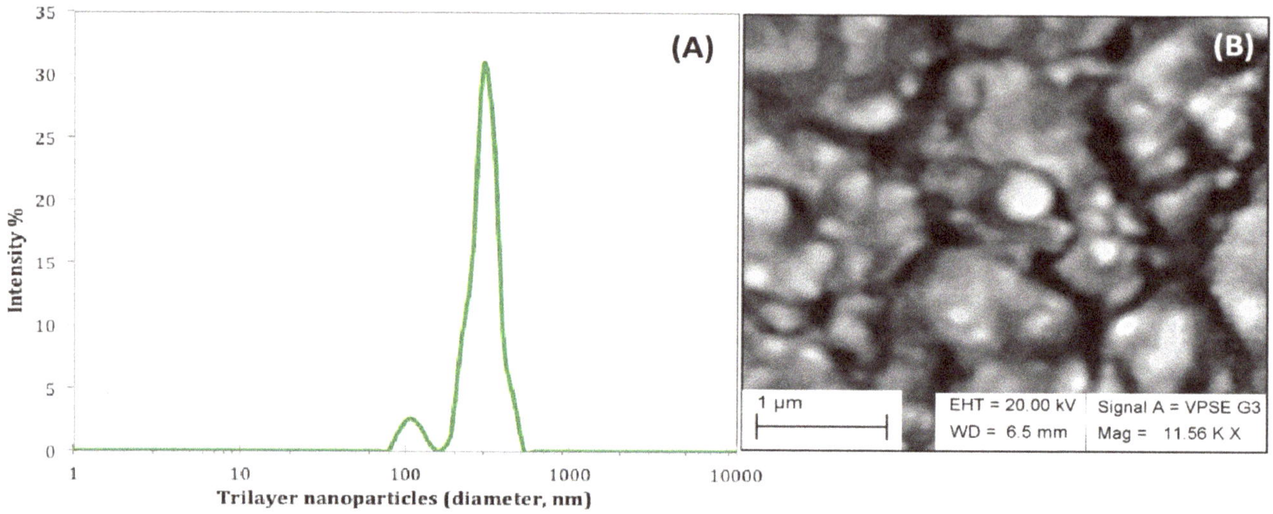

Figure 2. (**A**) Average DLS frequency distribution of trilayered nanoparticles (TNPs) presented in logarithmic scale as a function of intensity (n = 4), which encapsulated CHX-digluconate in the most inner core. (**B**) The SEM image shows TNPs after the freeze-drying process necessary to avoid diffusion of CHX and erosion of the polymeric nanoparticle. SEM imaging was done in variable pressure aperture.

The inner core of the conventional BNP is hydrophobic, while these TNPs contain a hydrophilic core that encapsulates CHX-digluconate, which is a hydrophilic drug. The shell of the TNP was composed of the overlapping regions of the block copolymer that corresponded to its hydrophobic part from PLA.

Energy dispersive X-ray spectroscopy (EDS) elemental analysis, in variable pressure (VP) mode, confirmed the presence of CHX-digluconate in the encapsulated nanoparticles by signal emission of chlorine (Cl) (Table 1).

Table 1. Energy dispersive X-ray spectroscopy (EDS) quantification analysis of selected element peaks.

Element	Intensity (counts/second)	Kα (KeV)	Concentration (weight %)
Carbon (C)	1910.74	0.277	37.24
Nitrogen (N)	13.61	0.392	1.44
Oxygen (O)	1884.44	0.525	60.05
Chlorine (Cl)	189.48	2.622	1.27

As with most investigative methodologies, it is frequently best to use a combination of procedures to characterize nanoparticles. 3D and 2D atomic force microscopy (AFM) imaging of TNPs that were purified through dialysis was also used to assess the morphological structure of TNPs (Figure 3). PeakForce^{TM} QNM (quantitative nanomechanics) data from AFM revealed information about sample surface profiles and particle analysis defined features of well-isolated nanoparticles. From this analysis, the average diameter range of TNPs was 140–245 nm, although there was also a significant number of BNPs in the diameter range of 40 to 100 nm. In general, scanning electron microscopy (SEM) images and AFM analyses presented here were consistent with DLS data.

Examination of the morphological mapping and quantitative measurements were made with section analysis and verified with particle analysis. Section analysis revealed information about sample surface contours and particle investigation demarcated structures of well-isolated particles or features of interest. From this study, the median diameter range of TNPs was 140–245 nm, nonetheless there was also a substantial number of other nanoparticles in the diameter range of 40 to 100 nm, which could be credited to the formation of BNPs as a byproduct. In general, SEM images and AFM analyses presented here were consistent with DLS data.

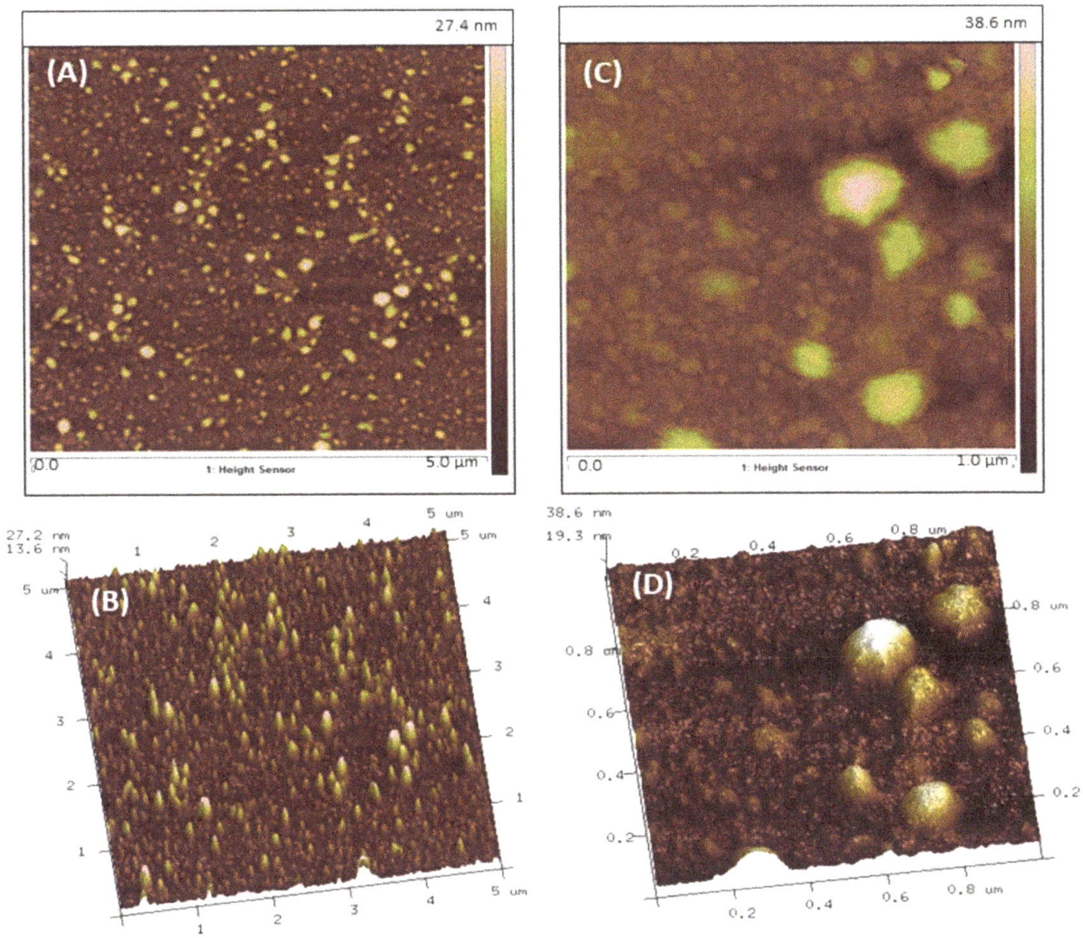

Figure 3. AFM analysis in air PeakForceTM QNM mode images of TNPs assembled from RNPs. (**A**) 2D (**B**) 3D topographic images of 5.0 × 5.0 µm scan. (**C**) 2D (**D**) 3D topographic images of 1.0 × 1.0 µm scan.

2.4. Nanoparticle Loading Efficiency

The self-assembly of TNPs proved to be a reproducible method to encapsulate CHX-digluconate for controlled release of CHX-digluconate. Investigation of the amount of drug encapsulated in TNPs was determined using UV-Vis spectroscopy at the wavelength at which CHX-digluconate has its maximum absorbance, λ_{max} = 281 nm. The solutions used to plot this calibration curve ranged from 0.064 mg/mL to 0.64 mg/mL, with a correlation coefficient R^2 = 0.995.

From the absorbance analyses of the CHX loaded TNPs at 281 nm and using Equations (1)–(3) (as described in Materials and Methods), the drug encapsulation efficiency (DEE) was calculated, in relation to the theoretical drug loading (TDL), and the experimental drug loading (EDL). The self-assembly method employed here allowed for a drug encapsulation efficiency (DEE) of 84.5%, with TDL of 3.8% and EDL of 3.2%. This was the result for a PEG-*b*-PLA to CHX-digluconate ratio of 4 to 1 to make RNPs. For the second polymeric layer that makes the TNPs the amount of PEG-*b*-PLA necessary was 2.5 times higher than the one used for RNPs.

2.5. Antimicrobial Effectiveness

The TNPs drug release was tested in vitro by submerging them in brain heart infusion (BHI) broth at 37 °C, to simulate the body's physiological temperature. CHX-digluconate TNPs were immersed in BHI for varied periods (1 day, 7 days, 14 days, and 21 days). Then these broths were inoculated with *E. faecalis* and their optical density (OD) data recorded over 17 h. This data was used to generate bacterial growth curves made by averaging triplicates from three trials together. Representative results from the bacterial proliferation assays are shown in Figure 4 for 1 day, 7 days, 14 days and 21 days.

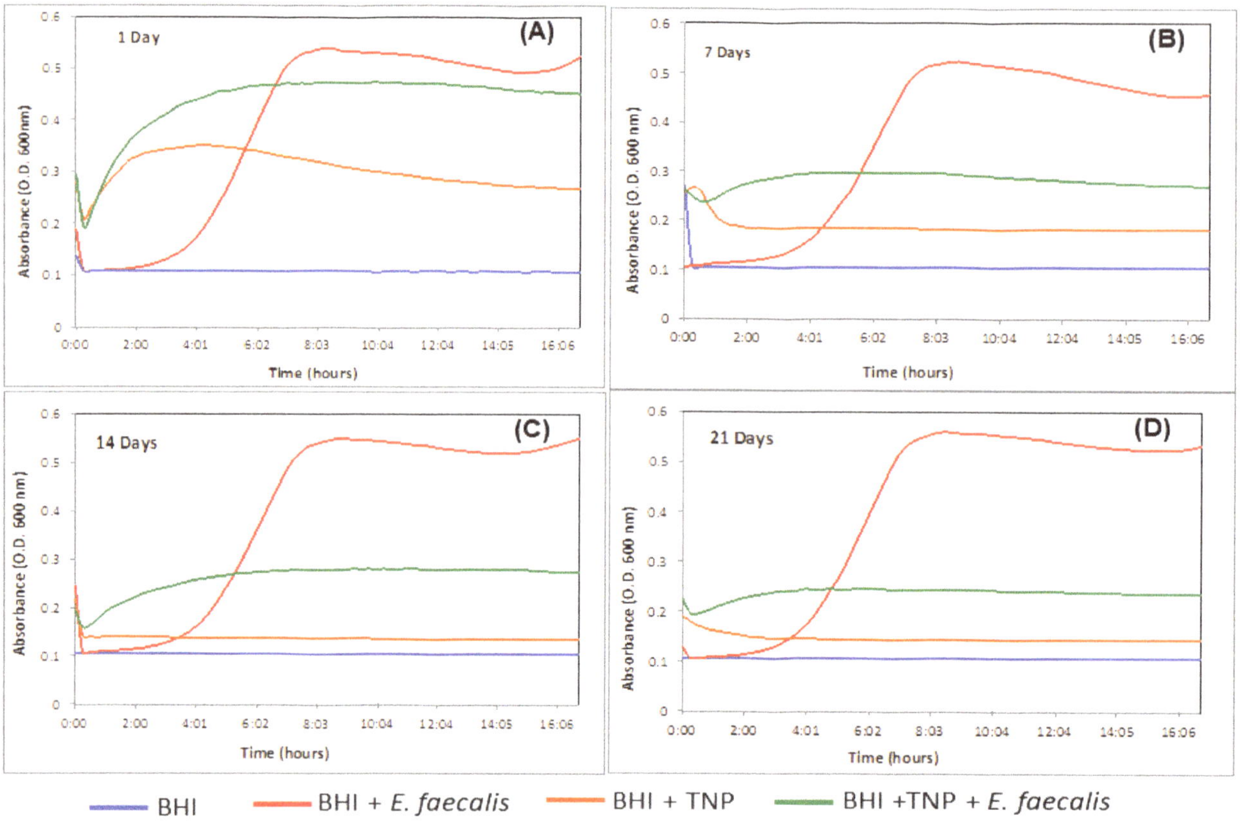

Figure 4. The effect CHX released from TNPs had on *E. faecalis*. TNPs were immersed in brain heart infusion (BHI) for (**A**) 1 day, (**B**) 7 days, (**C**) 14 days, and (**D**) 21 days, then tested against *E. faecalis*. Optical density (O.D.) measured at 600 nm. The OD data was used to generate bacterial growth curves made by averaging triplicates from three trials together, not including clear outliers obtained during the experiments.

The drug release profile showed a biphasic pattern with a rapid initial burst release followed by a sustained release of CHX-digluconate. After TNPs were incubated for 1 day there was a 14% bacterial inhibition, after 7 days of incubation 50% bacterial inhibition, after 14 days of incubation 63% bacterial inhibition, and 80% bacterial inhibition after 21 incubation days.

The OD data at the intermediate time period, when the control was entering the growth phase, was also analyzed using statistical comparisons. A one-way ANOVA was conducted at 95% significance level. When the growth curves of the broth that had contained the TNPs (BHI + TNP + *E. faecalis)* were compared to the control (BHI + *E. faecalis*), a significant difference was observed ($p \leq 0.05$). The results also indicated that the nanoparticle remained effective for the period investigated (up to 21 days).

3. Discussion

This work investigated the self-assembly, physicochemical characterization, and antimicrobial effectiveness of an advanced nanoparticle engineering technology to be delivered inside root canal systems. The aim of adapting a new controlled release nanoparticle system was to achieve sustained delivery of CHX-digluconate throughout the complex root canal for up to 21 days. The initial hypothesis was that nanoparticles self-assemble with a proper core/shell (PEG/PLA) ratio to improve CHX-digluconate encapsulation efficacy, with a narrow size distribution, and an efficient release profile of CHX-digluconate loaded polymeric nanoparticles. This TNP formulation improved the physicochemical equilibrium of the nanoparticles without the use of additional surfactants in the aqueous mixture solution.

The CHX-digluconate gel has been employed as an intracanal therapeutic drug. According to Gomes et al. (2013), it must remain inside the root canal system for at least 3 to 5 days [25]. Thus, it is important to provide sustained release of bactericidal for an extended period of time to improve root canal system disinfection. In vitro studies showed that 2% CHX gels may prevent *C. albicans* growth for 14 days, it may also diffuse through dentine and achieve the external root surface [26], and maintains its antimicrobial effect against *E. faecalis* for up to 12 weeks [27,28]. There is no consensus on the period that an intracanal medicament must remain inside the root canal system to achieve its maximum disinfection effect. However, it is important to develop alternatives to deliver the medicament and improve its diffusion through dentine tubules and the entire root canal system. To the best of the authors' knowledge, this is the first time that a nanoparticle system composed of TNP encapsulated with CHX-digluconate is designed for targeted drug delivery in the root canal system (Figure 5).

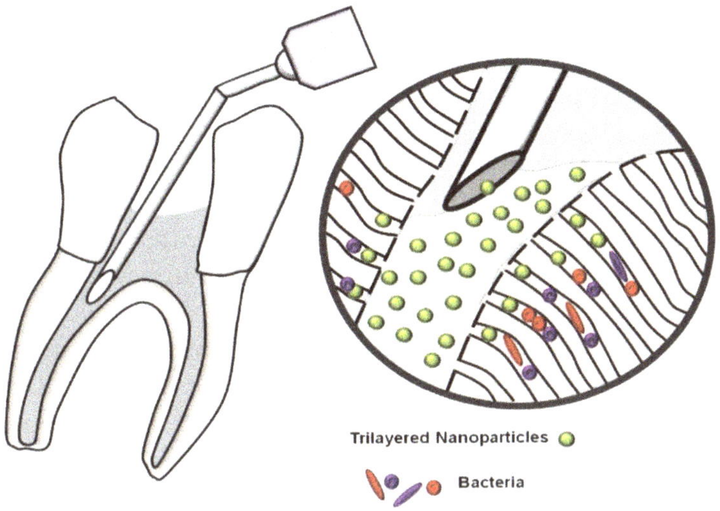

Figure 5. Schematics of the delivery of TNPs within dentinal tubules matrix.

The improved TNPs had a size range from 140–295 nm as determined by multiple characterization techniques. This is an important result because the goal was to obtain a size distribution that could penetrate the smallest dentinal tubules, for which size is reported to range from 500 nm to 1 μm [28]. The TNPs exhibited a steady CHX-digluconate profile and were suitable to be directly delivered deep into the complex matrix of dentinal tubules. Furthermore, investigation of the antimicrobial effectiveness of the CHX encapsulated TNPs experiments performed in bacterial broth demonstrated significant reduction in bacterial load up to 21 days, which supports the hypothesis that the system developed in this study will allow for continuous arrest of bacteria in a root canal anatomy. Earlier work by Haseeb and colleagues on BNPs demonstrated the effective encapsulation of CHX using the block copolymer PEG-*b*-PLA, which yielded nanoparticles with size range 300–500 nm in diameter [22]. On the other hand, the TNPs reproduced in this investigation were much smaller (140–295 nm) than their BNP counterparts, even with the same type of PEG-*b*-PLA block copolymer as starter material. A plausible explanation for the reduced size of the TNPs is the entangling of two critical polymeric chains, the PLA in the corona of the water-in-oil emulsion RNPs (emulsion-like loose nanoparticles), and the PLA chain that comes from the PEG-*b*-PLA block copolymer dissolved in an aqueous bulk solution [29]. This spontaneous self-assembly offers a moderately packed architecture because the hydrophobic polymeric chains of the corona (inner core) and the overlapping hydrophobic polymeric chains form a contracted shell.

A common problem observed during purification of nanoparticles is clogging of filter pores. This is due to the presence of polyvinyl alcohol (PVA), a surfactant commonly used in the self-assembly of nanoparticles to improve their equilibrium in solution and reduce aggregation [30]. Thus, enhancing the self-assembly of TNPs in the reduction or total absence of PVA was a central task in this study. The optimal polymer to drug ratio to form the RNPs was found to be 4 to 1. This ratio was optimal to self-assemble the right polymeric shell of the TNPs without the use of PVA in the bulk solution, since PVA hinders an exertive filtration of nanoparticles by settling them at the pores resulting in a "filter cake" that obstructs the filter. This optimization enabled the purification step of TNPs without affecting the stability of the TNPs. This was apparent by the results of DLS spectra in which a high intensity peak was observed at 295 nm. The lower intensity peak at 105 nm may be related to BNPs, a byproduct of the self-assembly process. Moreover, these two peaks continued to display the same constant values even after leaving the final TNPs solutions at a standstill for 24 h.

The satisfactory drug entrapment efficiency (DEE) of CHX-digluconate (84.5%) can be accredited to the high concentration of PEG-*b*-PLA in the bulk aqueous solution to which the RNPs were added dropwise. Within this highly concentrated solution the polymer precipitated fast enough on the surface of the RNPs, which locked the drug inside the core of the TNP preventing diffusion across the phase boundary [31]. Furthermore, this effective encapsulation of CHX-digluconate may avoid premature precipitation of the insoluble CHX base in the oral cavity as it comes in contact with chlorine ions from saliva [23,32] or from residual sodium hypochlorite. In addition, this may render adequate transport of CHX into deeper areas of the dentinal tubular matrix, to arrest the bacterial growth of different microorganisms that can penetrate inside dentin at different depths [33].

The nanotoxicity study on *E. faecalis* revealed an early drug burst release from the TNPs. This event correlates to a reduced bacterial growth observed at day 1, which was probably associated to a fraction of the drug that was adhered or weakly attached onto the surface of TNPs. The second phase of CHX-digluconate release between 7 days to 21 days was attributed to diffusion mechanisms. This diffusion is directed by chemical potential gradients arising from osmotic pressure. In addition to diffusion, CHX-digluconate could be released by erosion of the polymer matrix, which leads to pore formation in the TNP [34]. The slow drug release between 7 days and 14 days declined bacterial proliferation by an additional 13%. Drug release between 14 days and 21 days declined bacterial proliferation an additional 17%, which resulted in a total accumulated bacterial inhibition of approximately 80%. The early drug burst release from TNPs was slower when compared with the BNPs that were previously studied [22]. Moreover, the second phase release of the TNPs had a steadier profile than the BNPs. The steadier release observed from TNPs could be attributed to their relative packed architecture from the overlapping of hydrophobic polymeric chains on the shell, as explained above.

In the earlier study involving BNPs, it was proved that when PEG-*b*-PLA nanoparticles were self-assembled without the addition of CHX and submerged in *E. faecalis* they did not have any bacterial inhibition. This experiment certified that the self-assembly of nanoparticles did not introduce reactive oxygen species (ROS) that could be toxic to cells [22]. ROS are partially reduced metabolites of oxygen, including hydrogen peroxide and hydroxyl radical, a by-product from polymer degradation during sonication of the emulsion [35,36]. Wang and collaborators have observed this degradation, which can start taking place after 5 to 15 min of sonication depending on the polymer [36]. ROS cause oxidative stress in many pathological pathways making them toxic to cells [37]. During sonication, sonolytic degradation of PEG-*b*-PLA nanoparticles was avoided by only sonicating for 4 min the RNPs dispersion. In this way, the nanotoxicity study of the TNPs discussed above can be interpreted based only on the activity of CHX-digluconate release. Thus, the TNPs can be classified as safe and suitable systems for delivery of CHX-digluconate inside the dentinal matrix.

In summary, this study developed and characterized a nanoparticle structure for efficient encapsulation of CHX for targeted drug delivery inside the anatomical dentinal matrix to be used in disinfection of the root canal. Some of the limitations of the study involved determining how far

TNPs can penetrate throughout the different lengths dentinal tubules and what concentrations would cause too much adhesion of these TNPs to dentinal walls. A future study will discuss the design of a hydrogel matrix that would prevent TNPs from immediately adhering to the dentinal wall and aggregate. Additionally, experiments in vitro of the diffusion capabilities of these hydrogel-TNPs systems through the complex dentinal matrix may help clarify the actual depth of penetration and the fluid-flow mechanisms involved.

4. Materials and Methods

4.1. Materials

All chemicals were used as received from the manufacturers without any further purification, with the exception of tin(II) 2-ethylhexanoate, which was purified with high vacuum distillation. Poly(ethylene glycol) methyl ether [average molecular weight (MW) = 2000 g/mol], L-lactide, toluene, and pentane were all analytical grade and used to synthesize the block copolymer. Chlorhexidine digluconate (concentration 20% in H_2O, density 1.06 g/mL), dichloromethane (DCM), 1,3-dimethyl-2-imidazolidinone (DMI), and N,N-dimethylacetoamide (DMA) were used to prepare the trilayered nanoparticles. All chemicals were obtained from Sigma-Aldrich (St. Louis, MO, USA).

4.2. Polyethylene Glycol-block-Polylactic Acid (PEG-b-PLA) Synthesis

Poly(ethylene glycol)-*b*-poly(L-lactide) (PEG-*b*-PLA) was synthesized in house by ring-opening polymerization of L-lactide according to a previously reported method [38]. Briefly, 143 mg of poly(ethylene glycol) methyl ether (M_n = 2000 g/mol) and 1.03 g of L-lactide (Lactide-(3*S*)-*cis*-3,6-Dimethyl-1,4-dioxane-2,5-diene) were transferred to a Schlenk flask and stirred under vacuum for 1 h at 25 °C to remove moisture. Then the Schlenk flask was transferred to a nitrogen-filled box. 40 mg of tin(II) 2-ethylhexanoate (stannous octoate), as the catalyst in 0.5 mL of toluene, was added to the Schlenk flask. The flask was closed, taken out of the glove box, and heated in an oil bath at 110 °C overnight under continuous stirring to allow polymerization. The resulting polymer was precipitated in hexane and air-dried at room temperature to form a white powder.

The catalyst system delineated above was primarily chosen because of several advantages over other systems. Specifically, it is highly soluble in organic solvents and molten lactide in the bulk state, and it is stable during storage. The most significant advantage is that it is approved by the US Food and Drug Administration (FDA) for use in medical and food applications because it is biologically safe, although the mandate is dependent on empirical safety data [39].

4.3. Spectroscopy

^{1}H NMR spectra were recorded on a Bruker ADVANCE III 500 MHz, (Bruker, Santa Barbara, CA, USA), in 5 mm sample tubes at 298 K (digital resolution of ±0.01 ppm) in DMSO-d_6 using TMS as internal reference, with a spectrometer frequency for ^{1}H at 500.23 MHz. The number-average molecular weight of each chain on the block copolymer was determined by ^{1}H NMR. Sample temperature was kept constant for all measurements at 25 °C. The NMR peak of DMSO (δ = 2.54) was used as the reference in determining the chemical shifts of ^{1}H in PEG-*b*-PLA.

4.4. Reverse Nanoparticle Preparation

The first step to produce TNPs was to self-assemble RNPs. A water-in-oil emulsion was first prepared by sonicating for 4 min, in an ice bath. This emulsion was prepared as follows: a solution of 4 mL of 1,3-dimethyl-2-imidazolidinone (DMI) and N,N-dimethylacetoamide (DMA) mixed solvent (density adjusted to 1.00 g/cm^3) was mixed with PEG-*b*-PLA block copolymer (4 mg) and 50 µL of aqueous solution (2 w/w %) containing chlorhexidine digluconate (10.6 mg/mL). The resulting water-in-oil emulsion was vigorously stirred for 2 h before measuring the diameter of the resulting RNPs. Then this emulsion was used in the self-assembling of TNPs.

4.5. Trilayered Nanoparticle Preparation

The scheme process for TNPs is shown in Figure 6. The water-in-oil emulsion recovered from the reverse nanoparticles (RNP) was added dropwise to 35 mL of aqueous solution containing PEG-*b*-PLA block copolymer (0.3 mg/mL). After 24 h of gentle stirring, the solution containing TNPs was dialyzed against deionized water by means of a SnakeSkin™ Dialysis Tubing (molecular weight cut-off 3.5 KDa); Thermo Fisher Scientific Inc. Waltham, MA, USA). This step removed the residual organic solvents and unincorporated CHX digluconate.

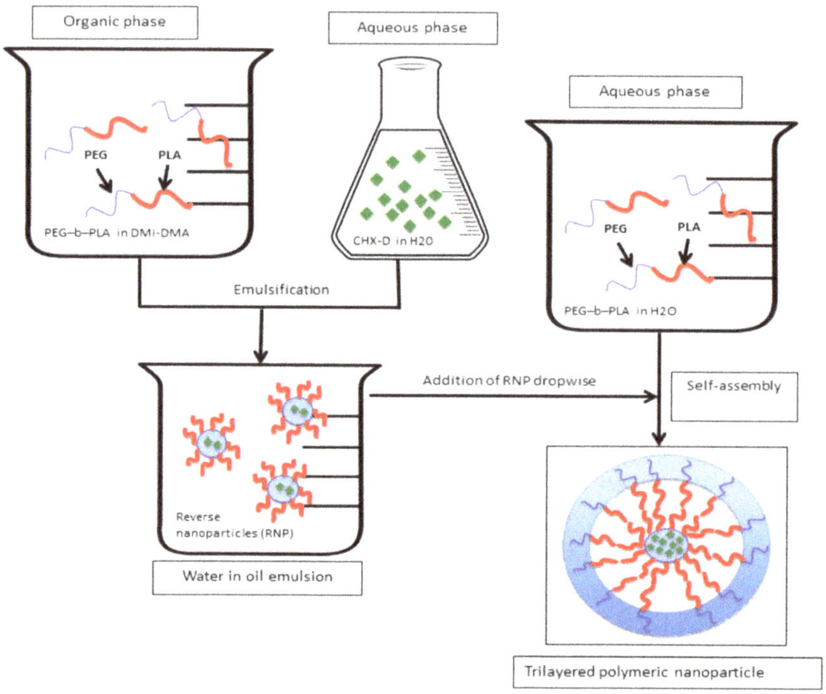

Figure 6. Schematic representation for assembling polymeric trilayered nanoparticles (TNP) with a hydrophilic core (chlorhexidine digluconate, a hydrophilic drug).

4.6. Nanoparticle Size Measurements

Nanoparticle size is an important parameter, as chlorhexidine has to be directly delivered into the dentinal tubules with size ranging from 500 nm to 1.3 μm. A particle size less than 500 nm is then ideal to allow transport of the nanoparticles through even the smallest dentinal tubules. Dynamic Light Scattering (DLS) was employed to measure both particle size and particle size distribution using a Zetasizer Nano ZS90 (Malvern Instruments Ltd., Malvern, UK).

4.7. Dynamic Light Scattering

The prepared TNPs were dispersed in deionized water while the RNPs were dispersed in DMI-DMA mixed solvent (density adjusted to 1.00 g/cm^3), then added to a quartz cuvette and analyzed by DLS (Zetasizer Nano ZS90, Malvern Instruments Ltd., Malvern, UK), to obtain their size distribution and polydispersity index (PDI). This experiment was replicated four times ($n = 4$) and each time the DLS frequency spectra was evaluated with the Zetasizer Nano ZS90 accompanying software.

4.8. Imaging

The evaluation of the TNPs' morphology and size were analyzed with two different techniques: (1) scanning electron microscopy (SEM, ZEISS EVO® LS-15, Cambridge, UK) using a variable pressure aperture, and (2) atomic force microscopy (AFM, Bruker, Bioscope Catalyst, Santa Barbara, CA, USA).

For SEM imaging, TNPs were first freeze dried then deposited onto a metallic 12-mm diameter stub. Copper sticky tape was used to reduce the build-up of electrons in the sample that can create unwanted image artifacts. The atomic material composition of the TNPs was measured with Energy Dispersive X-ray Spectroscopy (EDS, SEM-XRF, IXRF SYSTEMS Austin, TX, USA), which enabled detection of the individual elements of the nanoparticles.

For AFM analysis, CHX-encapsulated TNPs were dispersed in a hydrogel solution (1% Natrosol™ hydroxyethyl cellulose in water). A drop of solution containing nanoparticles was deposited on a glass slide and was allowed to dry forming a thin film. AFM analysis was performed using PeakForce™ quantitative nanomechanics (QNM) microscopy to map the morphology and quantitative measurement of material properties at a nanoscale level. For high-performance imaging and force control, specific probes, designed by Bruker SNL-10A, were selected. These probes had a spring constant of $k = 0.35$ N/m.

4.9. Drug Entrapment Efficiency Methodology

Drug entrapment efficiency (DEE) is defined as the percentage or fraction of the drug added in the process of nanoparticle synthesis that was successfully entrapped into the nanoparticle. The drug encapsulation efficiency (DEE) was calculated in relation to the theoretical drug loading (TDL), and the experimental drug loading (EDL) as described in Equations (1)–(3). The DEE of TNPs loaded with CHX-digluconate was calculated by constructing a calibration curve that relates CHX-digluconate wavelength at maximum absorbance to concentration. These absorbance measurements were collected using a UV-Vis spectrophotometry (Nanodrop 2000 spectrophotometer; Thermo Fisher Scientific, Waltham, MA, USA).

CHX-digluconate (Molecular Formula: $C_{22}H_{30}Cl_2N_{10}\cdot 2C_6H_{12}O_7$; Molecular Weight: 897.8 g/mol) is one of the salt forms of CHX that a solubility in water up to 50% (w/v) and other solvents at room temperature. The creation of a calibration plot of absorbance versus concentration was successfully created due to the high solubility of CHX-digluconate. The first step was to obtain the highest absorbance of CHX-digluconate in dimethyl sulfoxide (DMSO) at different concentrations. Several solutions, which concentrations ranged from 0.064 mg/mL to 0.64 mg/mL, were prepared. Then a calibration curve was plotted using the maximum absorbance wavelength (λ_{max}) and a linear fit calculated the absorbance as a function of CHX-digluconate concentration. The second step was to evaluate the assembled TNPs by dissolving them in 1 mL of DMSO then four different measurements ($n = 4$) of the absorbance at λ_{max} were taken to calculate the TNPs loading efficiency (Equations (1)–(3)). A PEG-*b*-PLA block copolymer curve was measured and evaluated to ensure that the polymer maximum absorbance (λ_{max}) did not overlap with the one from CHX-digluconate.

$$TDL = \frac{Weight\ of\ drug\ added\ (g)}{Weight\ of\ polymers\ and\ drug\ added\ (g)} \times 100\% \tag{1}$$

$$EDL = \frac{Weight\ of\ drug\ after\ freeze\ drying\ (g)}{Weight\ of\ polymers\ and\ drug\ after\ freeze\ drying\ (g)} \times 100\% \tag{2}$$

$$DEE = \frac{Experimental\ drug\ loading\ (EDL)}{Theoretical\ drug\ loading\ (TDL)} \times 100\% \tag{3}$$

4.10. Antimicrobial Effectiveness

Chlorhexidine-encapsulated TNPs were submerged in BHI (Brain Heart Infusion) broth at different time periods (1 day, 7 days, 14 days and 21 days). These time periods represent how long the nanoparticles would be dynamically active inside the complex dentinal matrix. The broth was then inoculated with *E. faecalis* at an initial optical density of 600 nm (OD600) of ~0.001.

The bacterial strain used in this study was the gram-positive bacterium *E. faecalis* (V583), which was isolated from the bloodstream of a hospitalized patient [40]. *E. faecalis* was selected for this proliferation assay because its pervasiveness in failed root canal treatments and chronic periodontitis [41].

First step: *E. faecalis* was cultured at 37 °C on 1.5% agar plates supplemented with BHI (Brain Heart Infusion) for 24 h. Second step: Preparation of the inocula for proliferation assays, an *E. faecalis* V583 colony from a freshly struck BHI agar plate was re-suspended in 10 mL. Step three: BHI broth was incubated for 24 h at 37 °C. Step four: 200 μL of the culture was aliquoted to inoculate the nanoparticles at the different time periods (1 day, 7 days, 14 days and 21 days). Step five: each TNP sample was inoculated in triplicate in a 96-well plate and incubated at 37 °C for 17 h. Three control trials were incubated in parallel as follows: Uninoculated BHI, BHI with TNPs and no *E. faecalis*, and BHI with *E. faecalis* and no TNPs. Step six: the OD600 was monitored with a Monochrometer-based Multi-Mode Microplate Reader (Synergy Mx, Winooksi, VT, USA) every 15 min during the 17 h incubation period. Step seven: The OD data was used to generate bacterial growth curves made by averaging triplicates from three trials together, not including clear outliers obtained during the experiments. The mean values of intermediate OD readings when the control broth was entering the growth phase were analyzed statistically with one-way ANOVA (analysis of variance) method at a 5% significance level. The OD readings of the broth that were inoculated with the TNPs were set side by side to the control sample to check if indeed the broth with CHX nanoparticles was the actual cause of delay in the bacterial growth phase.

5. Conclusions

The TNPs developed and investigated in this work presented a hydrophilic interior core that easily encapsulated CHX-digluconate. The TNPs had an adequate mean particle diameter to penetrate the anatomical structure of the dentinal matrix, thus presenting a potential methodology for local and sustained delivery of CHX. These also possessed good encapsulation efficiency, drug loading capacity, and showed steady inhibition of bacteria. The optimized TNPs had acceptable bioavailability against *E. faecalis*. There was an initial discharge of CHX-digluconate followed by a sustained release that was controlled by diffusion and degradation mechanism of the TNPs. These results established the potential application of TNPs for use in endodontic treatments as an intracanal regimen for better disinfection of the root canal system.

Acknowledgments: We thank the contributions of Sathyanarayanan Sridhar, in this study. We also thank the Department of Chemistry and Biochemistry at the University of Texas at Dallas for providing access to the NMR facilities (instrument grant NSF number CHE-1126177). The authors would like to thank the University of Texas at Dallas for providing resources for this research through startup funds (D. Rodrigues). M.C. Stefan gratefully acknowledges financial support from Welch Foundation (AT-1740), NSF (CHE-1609880), and NSF (che-1566059).

Author Contributions: G.Q., F.M. and D.C.R. conceived and designed the experiments; G.Q. performed the experiments; All authors discussed and analyzed the data; M.C.S., K.E.W and K.L.P. contributed with analysis tools; G.Q., F.M. and D.C.R. wrote the paper, D.C.R. secured funding for the research.

References

1. Margelos, J.; Eliades, G.; Verdelis, C.; Palaghias, G. Interaction of calcium hydroxide with zinc oxide-eugenol type sealers: A potential clinical problem. *J. Endod.* **1997**, *23*, 43–48. [CrossRef]
2. Shrestha, A.; Kishen, A. Antibacterial Nanoparticles in Endodontics: A Review. *J. Endod.* **2016**, *42*, 1417–1426. [CrossRef] [PubMed]
3. Langer, R.; Folkman, J. Polymers for the sustained release of proteins and other macromolecules. *Nature* **1976**, *263*, 797–800. [CrossRef] [PubMed]
4. Hoffman, A.S. The origins and evolution of "controlled" drug delivery systems. *J. Controll. Release* **2008**, *132*, 153–163. [CrossRef] [PubMed]
5. Cegnar, M.; Kos, J.; Kristl, J. Cystatin incorporated in poly (lactide-*co*-glycolide) nanoparticles: Development and fundamental studies on preservation of its activity. *Eur. J. Pharm. Sci.* **2004**, *22*, 357–364. [CrossRef] [PubMed]

6. Blanco, M.D.; Alonso, M.J. Development and characterization of protein-loaded poly (lactide-*co*-glycolide) nanospheres. *Eur. J. Pharm. Biopharm.* **1997**, *43*, 287–294. [CrossRef]
7. Redhead, H.M.; Davis, S.S.; Illum, L. Drug delivery in poly (lactide-*co*-glycolide) nanoparticles surface modified with poloxamer 407 and poloxamine 908: In vitro characterisation and in vivo evaluation. *J. Controll. Release* **2001**, *70*, 353–363. [CrossRef]
8. Barichello, J.M.; Morishita, M.; Takayama, K.; Nagai, T. Encapsulation of Hydrophilic and Lipophilic Drugs in PLGA Nanoparticles by the Nanoprecipitation Method. *Drug Dev. Ind. Pharm.* **1999**, *25*, 471–476. [CrossRef] [PubMed]
9. Perez, C.; Sanchez, A.; Putnam, D.; Ting, D.; Langer, R.; Alonso, M.J. Poly(lactic acid)-poly(ethylene glycol) nanoparticles as new carriers for the delivery of plasmid DNA. *J. Controll. Release* **2001**, *75*, 211–224. [CrossRef]
10. Elamanchili, P.; Diwan, M.; Cao, M.; Samuel, J. Characterization of poly (D,L-lactic-*co*-glycolic acid) based nanoparticulate system for enhanced delivery of antigens to dendritic cells. *Vaccine* **2004**, *22*, 2406–2412. [CrossRef] [PubMed]
11. Varoni, E.; Tarce, M.; Lodi, G.; Carrassi, A. Chlorhexidine (CHX) in dentistry: State of the art. *Minerva Stomatol.* **2012**, *61*, 399–419. [PubMed]
12. Puig Silla, M. Use of chlorhexidine varnishes in preventing and treating periodontal disease. A review of the literature. *Med. Oral Patol. Oral Cir. Bucal* **2008**, *13*, E257. [PubMed]
13. Jenkins, S.; Addy, M.; Wade, W. The mechanism of action of chlorhexidine. *J. Clin. Periodontol.* **1988**, *15*, 415–424. [CrossRef] [PubMed]
14. Segreto, V.A.; Collins, E.M.; Beiswanger, B.B.; Rosa, M.; Isaacs, R.L.; Lang, N.P.; Mallatt, M.E.; Meckel, A.H. A comparison of mouthrinses containing two concentrations of chlorhexidine. *J. Periodontal Res.* **1986**, *21*, 23–32. [CrossRef]
15. Gomes, B.; Souza, S.F.C.; Ferraz, C.C.R.; Teixeira, F.B.; Zaia, A.A.; Valdrighi, L.; Souza-Filho, F.J. Effectiveness of 2% chlorhexidine gel and calcium hydroxide against *Enterococcus faecalis* in bovine root dentine in vitro. *Int. Endod. J.* **2003**, *36*, 267–275. [CrossRef] [PubMed]
16. Rosenthal, S.; Spångberg, L.; Safavi, K. Chlorhexidine substantivity in root canal dentin. *Oral Surg. Oral Med. Oral Pathol. Oral Radiol. Endod.* **2004**, *98*, 488–492. [CrossRef] [PubMed]
17. Siqueira, J.F.; Paiva, S.S.M.; Rôças, I.N. Reduction in the Cultivable Bacterial Populations in Infected Root Canals by a Chlorhexidine-based Antimicrobial Protocol. *J. Endod.* **2007**, *33*, 541–547. [CrossRef] [PubMed]
18. Hans, M.L. *Synthesis, Characterization, and Application of Biodegradable Polymeric Prodrug Micelles for Long-Term Drug Delivery*; Drexel University: Philadelphia, PA, USA, 2005.
19. Domb, A.J.; Amselem, S.; Maniar, M.; Dumitriu, S. *Polymeric Biomaterials*; Marcel Dekker Inc.: New York, NY, USA, 1994.
20. Fulzele, S.V.; Satturwar, P.M.; Dorle, A.K. Novel biopolymers as implant matrix for the delivery of ciprofloxacin: Biocompatibility, degradation, and in vitro antibiotic release. *J. Pharm. Sci.* **2007**, *96*, 132–144. [CrossRef] [PubMed]
21. Yeo, Y.; Park, K. Control of encapsulation efficiency and initial burst in polymeric microparticle systems. *Arch. Pharm. Res.* **2004**, *27*, 1–12. [CrossRef] [PubMed]
22. Haseeb, R.; Lau, M.; Sheah, M.; Montagner, F.; Quiram, G.; Palmer, K.; Stefan, M.C.; Rodrigues, D.C. Synthesis and characterization of new chlorhexidine-containing nanoparticles for root canal disinfection. *Materials* **2016**, *9*, 452. [CrossRef] [PubMed]
23. Zeng, P.; Rao, A.; Wiedmann, T.S.; Bowles, W. Solubility properties of chlorhexidine salts. *Drug Dev. Ind. Pharm.* **2009**, *35*, 172–176. [CrossRef] [PubMed]
24. Richards, S.A.; Hollerton, J.C. *Essential Practical NMR for Organic Chemistry*; John Wiley & Sons: Hoboken, NJ, USA, 2010.
25. Gomes, B.P.F.A.; Vianna, M.E.; Zaia, A.A.; Almeida, J.F.A.; Souza-Filho, F.J.; Ferraz, C.C.R. Chlorhexidine in endodontics. *Braz. Dent. J.* **2013**, *24*, 89–102. [CrossRef] [PubMed]
26. Delgado, R.J.R.; Gasparoto, T.H.; Sipert, C.R.; Pinheiro, C.R.; de Moraes, I.G.; Garcia, R.B.; Duarte, M.A.H.; Bramante, C.M.; Torres, S.A.; Garlet, G.P.; et al. Antimicrobial activity of calcium hydroxide and chlorhexidine on intratubular Candida albicans. *Int. J. Oral Sci.* **2013**, *5*, 32–36. [CrossRef] [PubMed]

27. Gomes, B.P.F.A.; Montagner, F.; Berber, V.B.; Zaia, A.A.; Ferraz, C.C.R.; de Almeida, J.F.A.; Souza-Filho, F.J. Antimicrobial action of intracanal medicaments on the external root surface. *J. Dent.* **2009**, *37*, 76–81. [CrossRef] [PubMed]
28. Komabayashi, T.; Nonomura, G.; Watanabe, L.G.; Marshall, G.W.; Marshall, S.J. Dentin tubule numerical density variations below the CEJ. *J. Dent.* **2008**, *36*, 953–958. [CrossRef] [PubMed]
29. Uchida, Y.; Murakami, Y. Trilayered polymeric micelle: A newly developed macromolecular assembly that can incorporate hydrophilic compounds. *Colloids Surf. B Biointerfaces* **2010**, *79*, 198–204. [CrossRef] [PubMed]
30. Rawat, S.; Gupta, P.; Kumar, A.; Garg, P.; Suri, C.R.; Sahoo, D.K. Molecular mechanism of poly(vinyl alcohol) mediated prevention of aggregation and stabilization of insulin in nanoparticles. *Mol. Pharm.* **2015**, *12*, 1018–1030. [CrossRef] [PubMed]
31. Rafati, H.; Coombes, A.G.A.; Adler, J.; Holland, J.; Davis, S.S. Protein-loaded poly (DL-lactide-*co*-glycolide) microparticles for oral administration: Formulation, structural and release characteristics. *J. Controll. Release* **1997**, *43*, 89–102. [CrossRef]
32. Wu, M.; Dummer, P.M.H.; Wesselink, P.R. Consequences of and strategies to deal with residual post-treatment root canal infection. *Int. Endod. J.* **2006**, *39*, 343–356. [CrossRef] [PubMed]
33. Siqueira, J.F.; Magalhães, K.M.; Rôças, I.N. Bacterial Reduction in Infected Root Canals Treated With 2.5% NaOCl as an Irrigant and Calcium Hydroxide/Camphorated Paramonochlorophenol Paste as an Intracanal Dressing. *J. Endod.* **2007**, *33*, 667–672. [CrossRef] [PubMed]
34. Blasi, P.; D'Souza, S.S.; Selmin, F.; DeLuca, P.P. Plasticizing effect of water on poly (lactide-*co*-glycolide). *J. Controll. Release* **2005**, *108*, 1–9. [CrossRef] [PubMed]
35. Singh, R.P.; Ramarao, P. Accumulated polymer degradation products as effector molecules in cytotoxicity of polymeric nanoparticles. *Toxicol. Sci.* **2013**, *136*, 131–143. [CrossRef] [PubMed]
36. Wang, R.; Hughes, T.; Beck, S.; Vakil, S.; Li, S.; Pantano, P.; Draper, R.K. Generation of toxic degradation products by sonication of Pluronic® dispersants: Implications for nanotoxicity testing. *Nanotoxicology* **2013**, *7*, 1272–1281. [CrossRef] [PubMed]
37. Cabiscol, E.; Tamarit, J.; Ros, J. Oxidative stress in bacteria and protein damage by reactive oxygen species. *Int. Microbiol.* **2000**, *3*, 3–8. [CrossRef] [PubMed]
38. Carvalho, A.J.F. *Monomers, Polymers and Composites from Renewable Resources*; Elsevier: New York, NY, USA, 2008.
39. US Food and Drug Administration. *Code of Federal Regulations*; US Food and Drug Administration: Silver Spring, MD, USA, 2015; Chapter 1; Volume 177, p. 21.
40. Sahm, D.F.; Kissinger, J.; Gilmore, M.S.; Murray, P.R.; Mulder, R.; Solliday, J.; Clarke, B. In vitro susceptibility studies of vancomycin-resistant Enterococcus faecalis. *Antimicrob. Agents Chemother.* **1989**, *33*, 1588–1591. [CrossRef] [PubMed]
41. Wang, Q.-Q.; Zhang, C.-F.; Chu, C.-H.; Zhu, X.-F. Prevalence of Enterococcus faecalis in saliva and filled root canals of teeth associated with apical periodontitis. *Int. J. Oral Sci.* **2012**, *4*, 19–23. [CrossRef] [PubMed]

4

Rapidly-Dissolving Silver-Containing Bioactive Glasses for Cariostatic Applications

Omar Rodriguez [1,2], Adel Alhalawani [1,2], Saad Arshad [1,2] and Mark R. Towler [1,2,*]

1 Department of Mechanical & Industrial Engineering, Ryerson University, Toronto, ON M5B 2K3, Canada; omaralejandro.rodrig@ryerson.ca (O.R.); adel.alhalawani@ryerson.ca (A.A.); saad.arshad@ryerson.ca (S.A.)
2 Li Ka Shing Knowledge Institute, St. Michael's Hospital, Toronto, ON M5B 1W8, Canada
* Correspondence: mtowler@ryerson.ca

Abstract: A novel bioactive glass series containing incremental amounts of silver oxide was synthesized, ground down, and subsequently incorporated into a dentifrice for the purpose of reducing the incidence of dental caries and lesion formation. Three glasses were synthesized using the melt quench route: Si-Control ($70SiO_2–12CaO–3P_2O_5–15Na_2O$, mol %), Si-02 and Si-05, where 0.2 and 0.5 mol % Ag_2O were substituted, respectively, for SiO_2 in Si-Control. The glasses were then ground, sieved, characterized, and dissolved in Tris buffer solution (pH = 7.30) for 6, 12, and 24 h, with the pH of the resultant solution being recorded and the ions that were released into solution quantified. Samples of each glass were subsequently embedded into a non-fluoridated, commercially available toothpaste which was then used to brush resin-mounted lamb molars which, up to the point of testing, had been stored in a 1.0 M HCl solution. Knoop microhardness measurements of the molars were recorded before and after brushing to determine the presence of remineralization on the surface of the teeth (surface hardness loss of 37%, 35%, and 34% for Si-Control, Si-02 and Si-05, respectively, after 24 h). Four oral cavity bacterial strains were isolated through swabs of the inner cheek, gums, and teeth surfaces of three volunteers, and placed on agar discs. Of each glass, 0.5 g was placed onto the discs, and the resultant inhibition zones were measured after 6, 12, and 24 h. Si-05 performed better than Si-02 on two strains after 24 h, while exhibiting similar behavior for the remaining two strains after 24 h; the largest inhibition zone measured was 2.8 mm, for Si-05 after 12 h. Si-Control exhibited no antibacterial effect at any time point, providing evidence for the role of silver oxide as the antibacterial component of these glasses.

Keywords: bioactive glass; dental caries; remineralization; microhardness; cavity bacteria

---

1. Introduction

Dental caries, known as tooth decay, is among the most prevalent diseases worldwide [1]. It is caused by internal factors, such as saliva secretion and components, nutritional and hormonal status, microbial flora colonizing the teeth, and tooth surface morphology and external factors, such as oral hygiene, fluoride availability, and diet [2]. Dental caries causes pain, and may result in serious infection, hospitalization, and fatality under extreme circumstances [3]. Bacteria, such as *Streptococcus mutans*, exist within plaque buildup and process fermentable carbohydrates to produce weak acids [4]. These acids cause calcium, carbonate, and phosphate ions to leach out of the enamel and dentine phases of the tooth, weakening the mineral and resulting in decay [4,5]. This process can be reversed by buffering the oral environment and restoring it to its original pH; saliva being an effective natural buffer [1]. Demineralization and remineralization occur in a continuous cycle; if the pH is not restored or if the ions needed for remineralization are not available, demineralization dominates, resulting in lesions, and subsequently, cavities [6].

Dentifrices are used to impede the erosion of the tooth surface [7]. A dentifrice is a preparation that is generally used with a toothbrush in order to clean or polish teeth [8]. Modern dentifrices often claim various beneficial effects, including plaque removal, anti-caries, and anti-bacterial effects and remineralization [8]; the latter promoted by fluoride compounds, as well as strontium and potassium compounds [7,9]. Stannous fluoride (SnF_2), an ingredient in many toothpastes, can form complexes resistant to acid attack in vitro [10,11] as well as in situ [12], through the deposition of a tin-rich surface on the enamel [7]. Zinc fluoride (ZnF_2), another common ingredient in toothpaste, can provide the antibacterial action of zinc in addition to the cariostatic effect of fluoride [11,13].

Bioactive glasses can be formulated to deliver therapeutic ions that may bond with bone, initiate remineralization, and provide antibacterial effects [14–16]. 45S5 Bioglass® was the first inorganic material designed to bond with bone which did not form scar tissue upon implantation in rat femurs [14,17,18]. Bioactive glasses can be doped with ions such as strontium (Sr^{2+}) and fluoride (F^-), which release from the glass to promote remineralization upon degradation [19–21]. Antibacterial agents, such as silver and zinc, can also be incorporated into the glass phase [22,23]; their release minimizing further decay.

Incorporation of bioactive glasses into dentifrices has been reported in the literature, proving the efficacy of these glasses in occluding dentinal tubules to treat or prevent demineralization [24]. NovaMin™, a phosphosilicate-based bioactive glass, has been added to toothpaste, and has been shown to reduce hypersensitivity [25–27]. By embedding the glass in a dentifrice such as toothpaste, the dissolution of such glasses results in therapeutic ion release in the environment. This research evaluates the ability of silver-containing glasses, when embedded into a toothpaste, to reduce dental caries. A series of novel silver-containing bioactive glasses were synthesized, which were tailored to be a proactive solution to dental caries. Calcium and phosphorous are incorporated in order to increase remineralization effects, as both are key components of hydroxyapatite (HA); which chemically resembles the mineral component of dentine and enamel [28]. Silver is included in ionic form as it is antibacterial [29–33], even if the mechanism of action is not fully understood [34]. Several attempts to explain the antibacterial effect of silver have been developed [29,34]. Silver has been reported to inactivate metabolism and inhibit bacterial growth [35], uncouple the respiratory chain from phosphorylation [36], interfere with membrane permeability to protons and phosphate [37], and react with thiol groups of membrane-bound enzymes and proteins to inactivate bacteria [34]. It is observed that the most common site of action at low concentrations is the cytoplasmic membrane [38]. At higher concentrations, silver has been observed to interact with cytoplasmic components within the cell [34].

By firing a series of glasses, the effect of different loadings of silver incorporated, and subsequently released in ionic form from a dentifrice, on enamel remineralization and biofilm formation can be determined.

2. Results

2.1. Network Connectivity

Network connectivity of the three glasses were calculated using Equation (1), and results are shown in Table 1.

$$Network\ Connectivity = \frac{Bridging\ Oxygens - Nonbridging\ oxygens}{Total\ bridging\ species} \quad (1)$$

Table 1. Network connectivity for each composition (mol %) assuming silver is either a network modifier (NM) or network former (NF).

Glass	NM	NF
Si-Control	1.314	1.314
Si-02	1.309	1.315
Si-05	1.302	1.317

2.2. Glass Characterization

2.2.1. Particle Size Analysis (PSA)

Table 2 contains PSA results. The average particle diameter for all glasses was found to be approximately 4–5 μm. Also, from Table 2, it can be seen that the particle size for all glasses is comparable.

Table 2. Particle size analysis (PSA) results. All measurements are in micrometers (μm). d_{10}, d_{50}, and d_{90} indicate the 10%, 50%, and 90% diameter on the cumulative volume distribution, respectively.

Glass	d_{10}	d_{50}	d_{90}
Si-Control	2.29	4.22	9.31
Si-02	2.29	4.31	10.33
Si-05	2.38	5.11	12.73

2.2.2. X-ray Diffraction (XRD)

The XRD patterns of the formulated materials provided evidence that all glasses were amorphous. All patterns exhibited a broad hump centered at around 30° 2θ with no crystalline phases present in any of the spectra.

2.2.3. Differential Scanning Calorimetry (DSC)

Table 3 summarizes the glass transition (T_g) and crystallization (T_c) temperatures of the formulated glasses; a sample DSC trace for the Si-Control glass, is shown in Figure 1.

Table 3. Glass transition and crystallization temperatures of glass compositions. Variation was based on equipment accuracy of 2%.

Glass	T_g (°C)	T_c (°C)
Si-Control	610 ± 12	838 ± 17
Si-02	618 ± 12	848 ± 17
Si-05	620 ± 12	826 ± 17

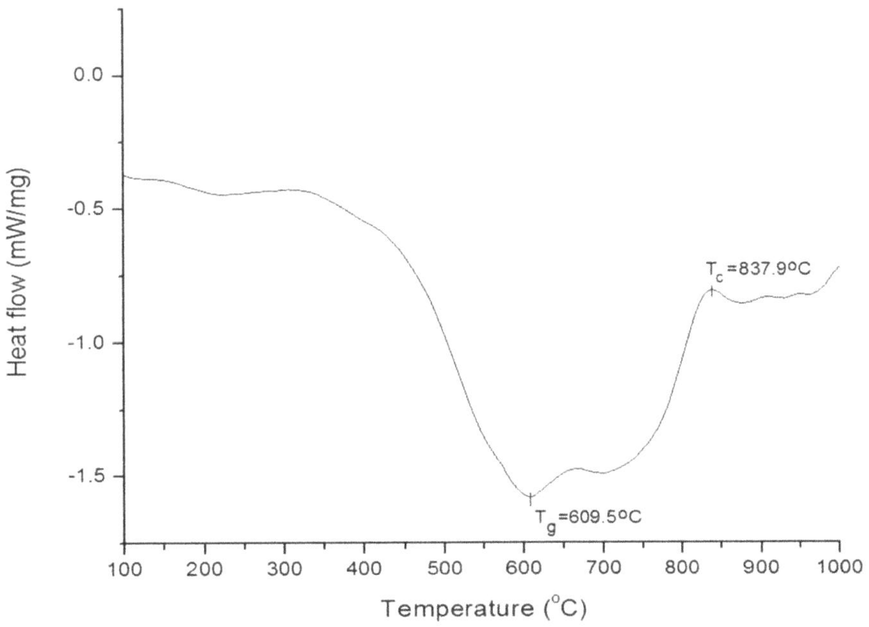

Figure 1. Sample DSC trace for Si-Control glass showing T_g and T_c.

2.2.4. Scanning Electron Microscopy–Energy Dispersive X-ray Spectroscopy (SEM–EDX)

SEM images are shown in Figure 2, for (a) Si-Control, (b) Si-02 and (c) Si-05.

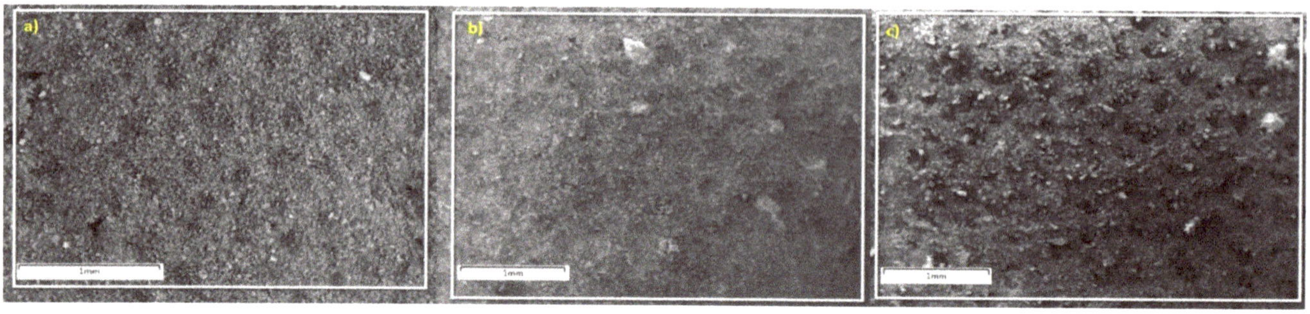

Figure 2. SEM photos of compositions: (**a**) Si-Control (**b**) Si-02 (**c**) Si-05.

EDX traces were taken at multiple sites to determine the composition of the glasses. As can be seen in Table 4, the glass compositions were close to the reagent amounts fired in the crucible.

Table 4. Average of wt % in compositions for each composition.

Element	Si-Control	Si-02	Si-05
O	50.6	54.8	54.7
Si	29.0	25.9	24.9
Na	10.3	10.3	10.6
Ca	7.60	6.60	6.77
P	2.50	2.03	2.03
Ag	0	0.3	0.97

2.3. Solubility Studies

2.3.1. pH Changes

Figure 3 summarizes the pH results. pH of the Tris buffer solution increased over time as the glass degraded. After 6 and 12 h, the mean pH of the Tris solution was the highest for Si-Control, but it was the lowest after 24 h; Si-02 and Si-05 glasses exhibited statistically-similar pH that was higher than the pH of Si-Control.

2.3.2. Ion Release Studies

Figure 4 summarizes the ion release data. Si-05 released more Ag^+ than Si-02. While all ion amounts increased over time, they did not increase linearly. Si-02, for example, exhibited a spike of $PO_4{}^{3-}$ release after 12 h of incubation, with the highest $PO_4{}^{3-}$ release compared to Si-Control and Si-05. Si-02 also experienced an increase after 12 h incubation in its Na^+ release. Ca^{2+} release exhibited more constant ion release rates for all compositions across all time spans.

2.4. Antibacterial Studies

Figure 5 presents the inhibition zones against oral bacteria colonies when exposed to the glass powders. As expected, Si-05 exhibited a larger inhibition zone against D2 and D3 strains after 24 h, with statistically similar inhibition zones measured for D1 and D3 strains after 24 h. Additionally, the inhibition zone increased over time for bacteria D2 and D3, whereas D1 and D4 experienced a dip in the inhibition zone from 12 h to 24 h. Furthermore, since the control glasses did not produce any inhibition zone at any time period, the effects of pH rise can be eliminated as a potential bactericidal effect.

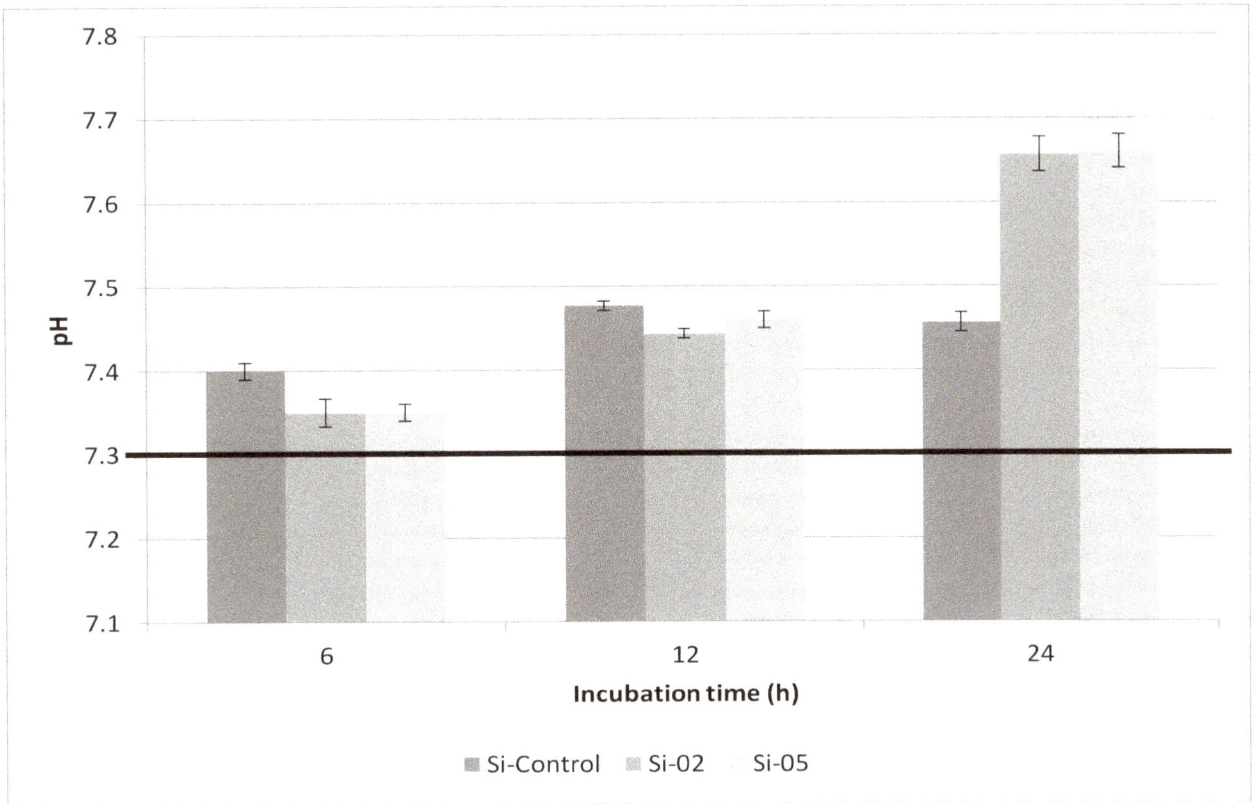

Figure 3. pH response of Tris buffer solution upon glass dissolution after 6, 12, and 24 h. Black horizontal bar represents the initial pH value of the Tris buffer solution before dissolution. Scatter bars indicate standard deviation from the mean.

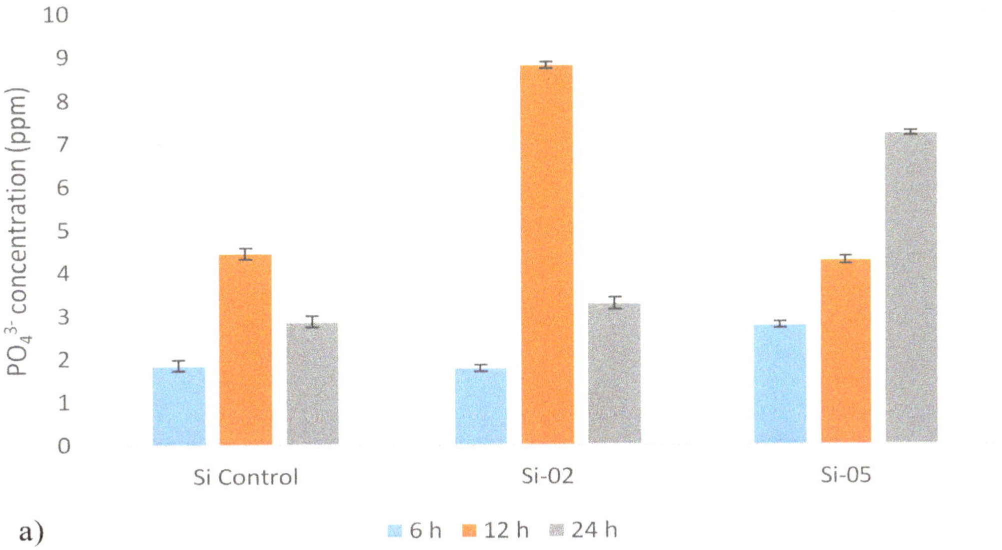

a)

Figure 4. *Cont.*

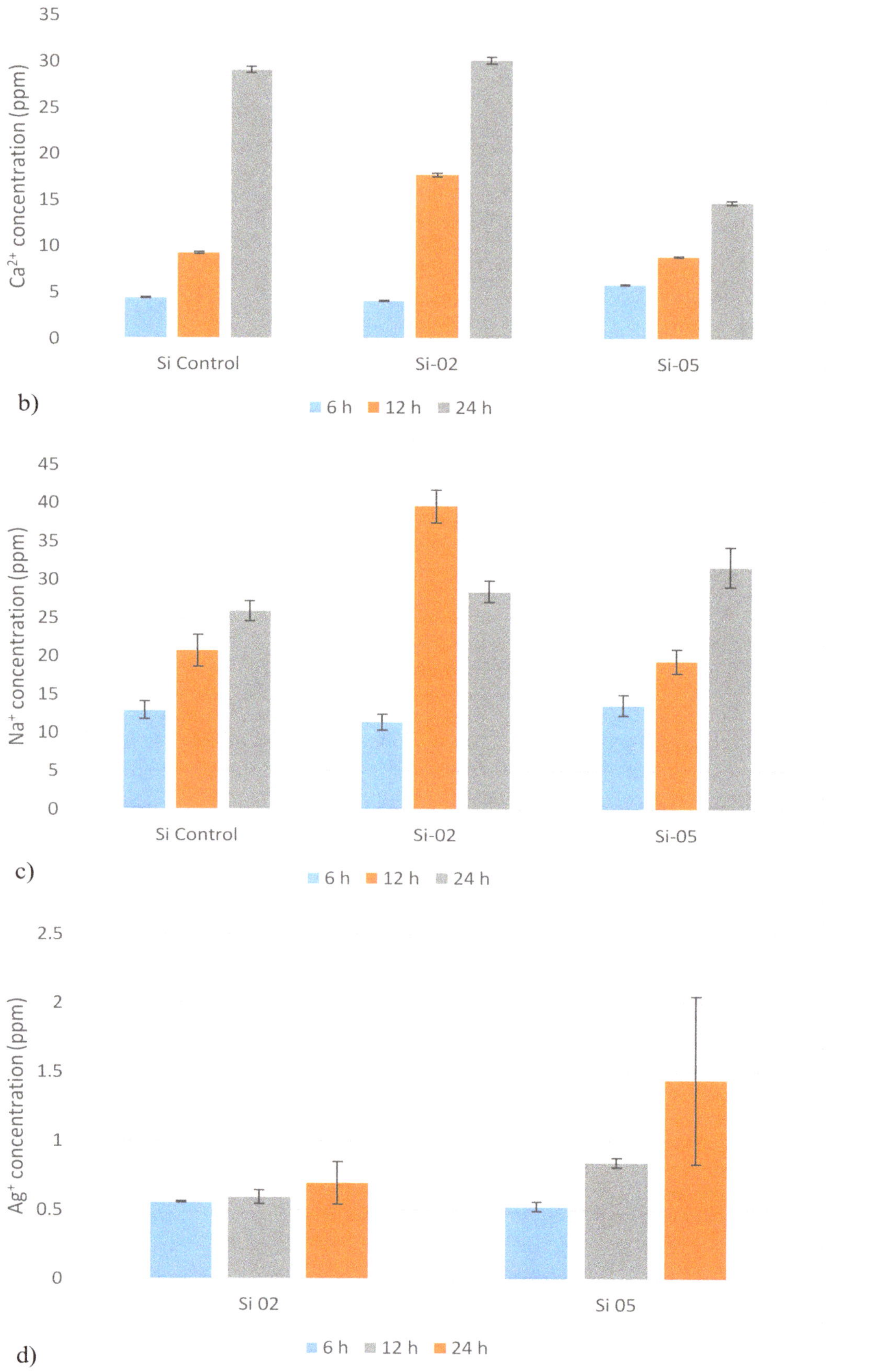

Figure 4. Ion release profiles for (**a**) PO_4^{3-}, (**b**) Ca^{2+}, (**c**) Na^+, and (**d**) Ag^+. Si-Control Ag^+ release has been omitted from (**d**) as no silver was present in the composition. Scatter bars indicate standard deviation from the mean.

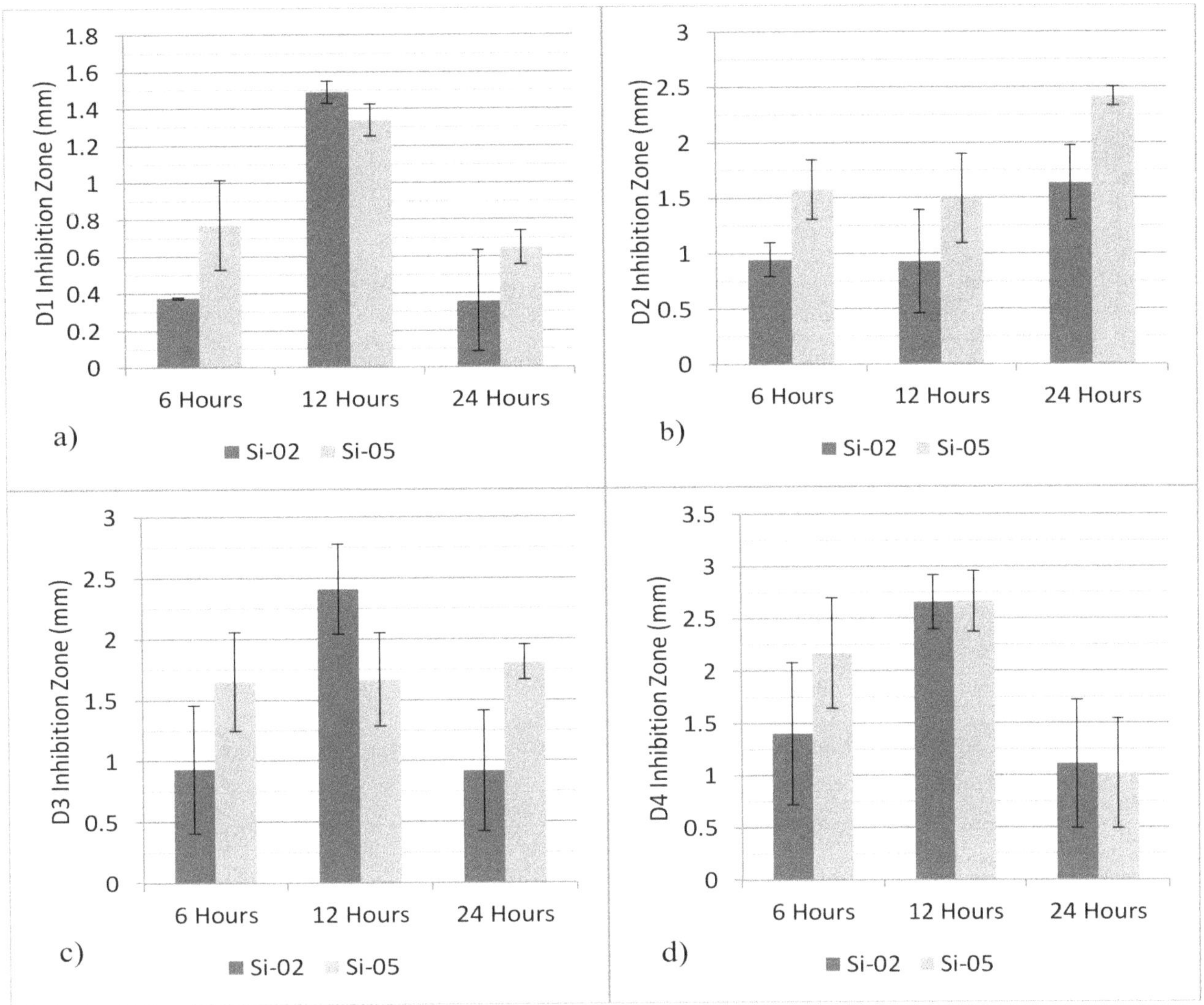

Figure 5. Inhibition zone against bacterial colony D1 (**a**), D2 (**b**), D3 (**c**) and D4 (**d**). The inhibition zone produced by glass powders against four bacterial isolate strains. Si-Control was excluded as it produced no inhibition zone throughout the time period measured. Scatter bars indicate standard deviation from the mean.

2.5. Toothpaste Remineralization Studies

Figure 6 shows the demineralization and remineralization of dentin molars as a result of their immersion in 1.0 M HCl for 12 h and their subsequent brushing with a glass-embedded toothpaste, respectively. The degree of mineralization was quantified through Knoop microhardness and control measurements were taken after the pucks were prepared and before they were subjected to an acid challenge, as well as before and after their dentifrice remineralization treatments.

The percentage of remineralization and demineralization are quantified through percentage hardness loss (%SHL) in Table 5. Percentage hard loss is also plotted against the concentration of Ca^{2+} released per glass, as shown in Figure 7.

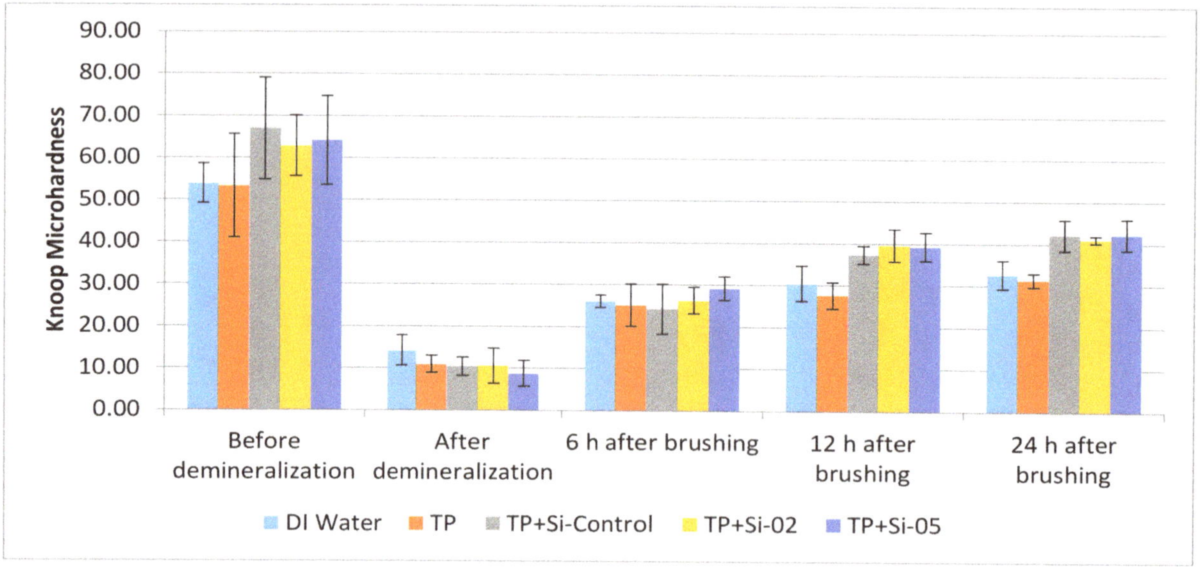

Figure 6. Knoop microhardness remineralization and demineralization on lamb molar dentin samples. All measurements are Knoop hardness (HK). DI is deionized water, TP is toothpaste. Scatter bars indicate standard deviation from the mean.

Table 5. Percent surface hardness loss (%SHL) for each stage of treatment as compared with baseline Knoop values.

Treatment	After Demineralization	6 h after Brushing	12 h after Brushing	24 h after Brushing
DI Water	73%	51%	43%	39%
TP	79%	52%	47%	39%
TP + Si-Control	84%	64%	43%	36%
TP + Si-02	83%	58%	37%	34%
TP + Si-05	86%	53%	37%	32%

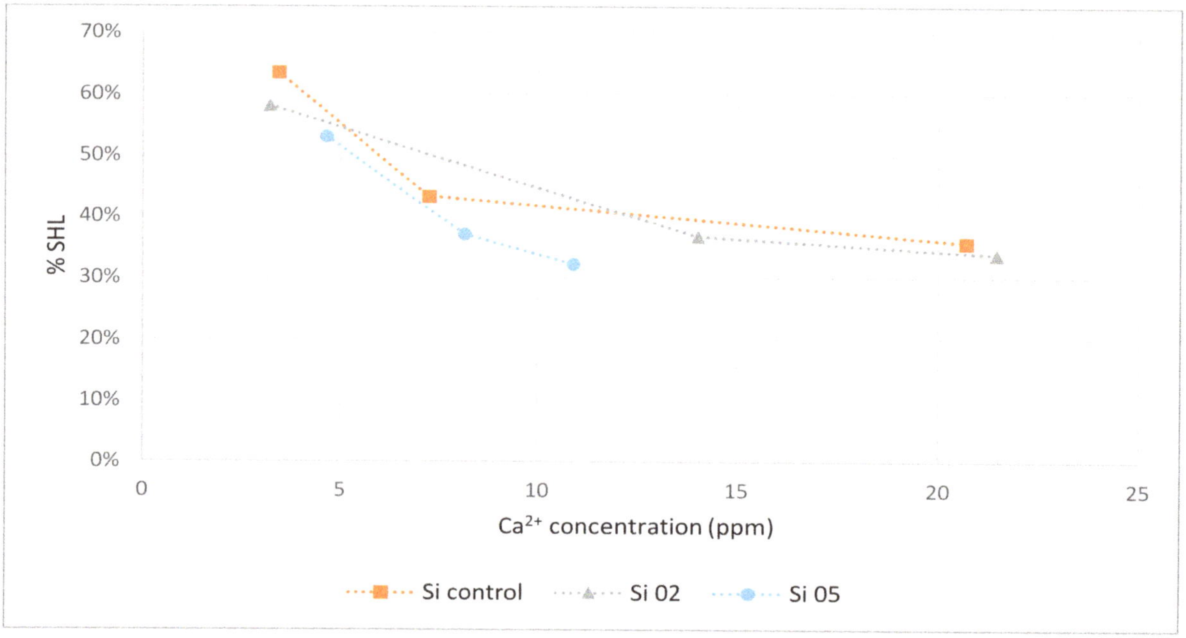

Figure 7. Knoop hardness as a function of Ca^{2+} release from Si-Control, Si-02 and Si-05 glasses.

3. Discussion

Bioactive glasses can be formulated to deliver therapeutic ions that may bond with bone, initiate remineralization, and provide antibacterial effects [14–16]. The delivery of ions depends, to a large extent, on the network connectivity of the bioactive material. In the formulated glasses, SiO_2 is a network former contributing two bridging oxygens, whereas P_2O_5, CaO, and Na_2O are network modifiers. Ag_2O, however, is a network intermediate. Ca^{2+} provides two non-bridging oxygens, while Na^+ provides one non-bridging oxygen per Na^+ ion. Recent work by Hill et al. has shown that P_2O_5 functions as an orthophosphate (Q^0) modifier, contributing three non-bridging oxygen per PO_4^{3-} ion [39,40]. However, since Ag^+ ions can function as a network former under certain circumstances, network connectivity has been calculated for the case of Ag^+ as a network modifier and as a network former.

Particle sizes were also evaluated. Ideally, the particle sizes are required to be below 20 μm as smaller particle sizes promote faster dissolution due to their greater specific surface area [41]. This allows for the particles to degrade faster, resulting in quicker release of therapeutic ions [42]. The average particle diameter for all glasses was found to be approximately 4–5 μm. This is close to the 3 μm particle size that Mneimne et al. indicate is favorable so that the glass may enter the dentinal tubules, and ultimately, reduce dentine hypersensitivity [43], and as these glasses were designed and proven to be degradable (Section 2.3, Solubility studies), the 4–5 μm diameter would reduce and fit without Mneimne et al.'s criteria. Precipitation of apatite inside the tubules would occlude them and decrease sensitivity. Results show that particle sizes for all glasses are comparable, which means that any changes observed in the glasses' behavior may be attributed to their different compositions and not to their particle size. SEM images confirmed that all compositions have similar particle sizes. However, morphology, on the small sample size examined, appeared different; Si-05 appears to be more granular and has sharper edges in its particles compared to the more homogeneous scans of Si-Control and Si-02.

DSC results show that T_g was not significantly affected by the inclusion of Ag_2O in the glass network, whereas an increase in T_c was first observed at 0.2 mol % Ag_2O, with a decrease below the T_c of the control glass for 0.5 mol % Ag_2O.

EDX traces confirm that all glass compositions were close to the reagent amounts fired in the crucible. This confirms that the glass thoroughly melted during the firing process, and an increase in silver content is also observed from Si-02 to Si-05.

Based on the pH results, it can be postulated that bioactive glasses can increase the pH of an aqueous solution, such as Tris buffer, upon dissolution. This facilitates apatite formation but can also cause a pH rise too great for the oral environment; an oral pH greater than 7.5 can irritate the oral mucous membranes [43,44]. The Tris buffers containing the Si-02 and Si-05 compositions exhibited a pH of 7.35 at 6 h, while the solution containing Si-Control shows a higher pH rise at 7.4. These values were not determined to be significantly different at $p < 0.05$. After 12 h, the pH responses of the solutions are 7.48, 7.44, and 7.46 for Si-Control, Si-02, and Si-05, respectively, indicating that the advantage gained by the early rise in pH of the Tris solution due to the control glass is lost over longer time frames. Indeed, by 24 h, solutions containing Si-02 and Si-05 both show a pH of 7.66 while the solution containing Si-Control shows a pH of 7.46. This compares favorably with other bioactive glasses in aqueous solution. Brauer et al. found the pH response of a simulated body fluid (SBF) solution containing fluoridated bioactive glass reached 7.6 after 24 h, but plateaued at 7.8 shortly afterward (from day 3 to the end of the experiment at 14 days) [44]. Tris buffer solutions containing Si-02 and Si-05 both reached the same pH after 24 h, 7.66, while the solution containing Si-Control did not show a significant pH rise from 7.48 after 12 h. Time frames greater than 24 h were not examined, as they were not deemed relevant to the application of toothpaste in the oral environment; it is unlikely that the ions deposited from the degrading glass powders would remain in the mouth after a day's consumption of liquids diluting the contents of the mouth.

These glasses were designed with rapid ion release in mind, and it was observed that, after 12 h, the release rate accelerated. Si-02 releases Ag^+, on average, 2.5 times faster after 12 h, while Si-05 releases Ag^+ on average 1.5 times faster after 12 h. The incorporation of silver into the network structure changes the more linear response of the control composition into an accelerating one, although with a slower initial response time. This is due to the complex nature of the network structure when silver is incorporated. As silver oxide is added at the expense of silica, a network modifier is added at the expense of a network former, which should increase bioactivity and solubility of the glass as bridging oxygens are being lost and replaced with non-bridging oxygens facilitating a greater release of cations, specifically sodium and calcium ions, which are basic [45–47], and will produce a pH rise. This would disrupt the dissolution mechanism and promote remineralization. However, the initial lag before the 12 h acceleration indicates that the cations are not exchanged as readily during the early stages of dissolution. The complex network may take longer to degrade, and favors dissolution of its formers more than its modifiers. This trend holds up when compared with the ion release profiles obtained in this study. The larger silver content yielded higher initial release volumes, but smaller release rates over time, leading to lower cumulative final release volumes. Interestingly, Si-Control displayed ion release volumes either between the two silver-containing compositions or closer to Si-02 ion profiles. Si-05 releases less silver ions initially, but greater quantities of all other ions when compared with Si-02 after 6 h, with the exception of sodium. However, over time, silver ion release rates increased rapidly for Si-05 while Si-02 released silver ions at a constant rate. Si-02 exhibited higher ion release volumes than Si-05 after 24 h for calcium. It was not possible to measure Silica release, but it may be useful in further explaining how the network degradation functioned as silica was the backbone of the network.

To measure the ion release kinetics of an alkali-silicate glass, the heterogeneous model was used [48,49], which assumes two stages in ionic release: first, the extraction of alkali and silica varies with the square root of time with the exchange of alkali with protons in solution dominating the glass dissolution, then, second, the ion extraction is linear with time. To confirm dissolution behavior under the heterogeneous model, the total silver ion concentration was graphed against the square root of the time, and a linear regression was employed. The correlation coefficient (R2) was above 0.95 for both Si-02 and Si-05 compositions, confirming the model. The network is expected to be complex, formed by a backbone of SiO_4 tetrahedra connected at the oxygen atoms to form a 3D network. However, the presence of alkali species breaks up the network continuity, hence increasing dissolution, as oxygen atoms no longer bridge to the next tetrahedra, but to an alkali ion instead. As silver ions were added at the expense of silica ions, this would further reduce the network connectivity as network formers were replaced with network modifiers. Ion release rates should be seen to be higher in Si-05 than Si-02, as well as being higher in Si-02 than Si-Control. While this was observed over short time periods, with the exception of silver ion release, longer dissolution time periods favored Si-02.

PO_4^{3-} and Na^+ release from Si-02 behaved differently to Ca^{2+} and Ag^+ release as it reached a peak around 12 h and then diminished after 24 h. The decrease of PO_4^{3-} and Na^+ over longer time periods is assumed to be due to a measurement error. This conclusion is based on the fact that phosphorous content is low (3 mol %), and is not expected to release around 9 ppm after 12 h. This will be further investigated in future studies which would focus on pH and ion release of these materials when matured in deionized water, simulated body fluid, and Tris buffer.

The inhibition zones against oral bacteria show that Si-05 exhibits a larger inhibition zone against D2 and D3 strains after 24 h, with statistically similar inhibition zones measured for D1 and D3 strains after 24 h. Additionally, the inhibition zone increased over time for bacteria D2 and D3, whereas D1 and D4 experienced a dip in the inhibition zone from 12 h to 24 h. Furthermore, since the control glasses did not produce any inhibition zone at any time period, the effects of pH rise can be eliminated as a potential bactericidal effect. Antibacterial studies were singularly affected by Ag^+ release as all agar discs were stored under similar conditions, and Si-Control exhibited no antibacterial response. It is therefore possible to eliminate pH as a bactericidal factor, since all compositions are known to cause similar pH rises. Referring to bacterial testing results, across all time frames and all bacterial strains, Si-05 outperformed Si-02 in its bactericidal efficacy, which further indicates that silver is the lone bactericidal agent. Silver is known to have wide ranging antibacterial properties; it is believed that DNA stops being able to replicate and proteins become inactive after contact with Ag^+ [49]; additionally, positively charged silver ions induce an antibacterial effect through electrostatic attraction between negative charged cell membrane of the microorganism and the silver ions [50].

Demineralization and remineralization results show that the glass compositions were more effective than the controls, with the highest microhardness after 24 h belonging to toothpaste (TP) + Si-05 followed by TP + Si-Control, TP + Si-02, deionized (DI) water, and finally, TP. However, when taking into account the initial demineralization effects, TP+Si-Control, TP + Si-02 and TP + Si-05 had similar remineralization percentages. Additionally, the response was higher than just the dentifrice treatment alone, indicating that the glass had a positive effect to the mineralization treatments.

Referring to demineralization and remineralization results, all three glasses significantly remineralized enamel after 24 h compared to the demineralized samples. As Si-02 released the greatest amount of calcium and phosphorous after 12 h (17.7 ppm and 8.79 ppm, respectively), samples treated with Si-02 should have exhibited the greatest degree of remineralization at that time frame, which is consistent with the results; from 12 h to 24 h, remineralization of the teeth treated with the toothpaste embedded with Si-02 decreased from 37 to 34% surface hardness loss (%SHL). This study shows that higher Ca^{2+} release resulted in a low %SHL (which is inversely proportional to the % remineralization). There was an upper limit to the amount of remineralization possible after demineralization observed in this experiment after 24 h, which is approximately 34%SHL. To compare, a toothpaste containing 1100 ppm fluoride exhibited a maximum of 38%SHL after four 7-day phases of demineralization/remineralization cycles [51]. Percentage hardness losses for enamel treated with over the counter bleaching agents and then stored in artificial saliva range from 12–40%, according to Zantner et al. [52], while a study by Chen et al. [53] found an 18–32%SHL for enamel treated with fluoridated bleaching agents followed by buffer saline solution. The upper limit can be explained by calcium and phosphorous uptake into the enamel being limited by the concentration of the ions available as the remineralization process requires an excess of calcium and phosphate ions in order to take place [54]: remineralization is hindered by insufficient Ca^{2+} and PO_4^{3-} in the media. Therefore, there may simply not be enough calcium or phosphorous to repair the lesions and form HA. It is also possible that apatite crystals precipitated over the surface level of the pucks, preventing the penetration of glass deeper into the lesions and remineralization the bulk of the material. However, it is also possible that the reason the teeth did not fully remineralize is due to damage caused by stress propagation to the underlying dentin and cementum during the sample preparation process (grinding and mounting), as well as the resin holding the teeth [55]. Since all compositions had the same amount of calcium and phosphorous, all pucks restored with the glass-loaded dentifrices are expected to reach a similar remineralizing point. While the dentifrice alone was effective at remineralizing the dentine (39 %SHL), the glass loading did increase the remineralization slightly, with a percent difference of 14% between the average glass remineralization and the toothpaste surface hardness loss. However, the difference was not statistically significant at the $p < 0.05$ level.

4. Materials and Methods

4.1. Glass Synthesis

4.1.1. Glass Fabrication

Three SiO_2–CaO–P_2O_5–Na_2O_5–Ag_2O glasses were synthesized in a series with silver oxide content increased at the expense of silica (Table 6); the quantity of each reagent was selected such that the ratio of calcium to phosphorus (Ca/P) is close to that in the enamel phase of tooth (Ca/P = 1.7) [56] and such that silver oxide is sufficient to be incorporated into the glass network. The glasses were prepared by weighing out appropriate amounts of analytical grade reagents (Fisher Scientific, Ottawa, ON, Canada & Sigma-Aldrich, Oakville, ON, Canada) and firing in a platinum crucible at 1600 °C for 1 h. The melt was subsequently shock-quenched in water, and the resulting glass frit retrieved and dried (24 h, 37 °C). The dried glass was placed in a 50 mL grinding jar and positioned in a Retsch PM100 Planetary Ball Mill (Retsch GmbH, Haan, Germany). Distilled water (25 mL) was added to the grinding jar along with eight 10 mm Ø grinding balls. The remainder of the volume was filled with glass. The jar was placed inside of the mill and allowed to grind at 550 revolutions per minute (RPM) for 15 min. The solution was then removed and placed in a Buchner funnel with a #1 size 9 cm Ø filter paper and a vacuum pressure of about 300–350 mmHg was maintained overnight until the powder was dry. The powder was then scraped off the filter paper and sieved through a 20 μm sieve.

Table 6. Silica glass series formulations (mol %).

Glass	SiO_2	CaO	P_2O_5	Na_2O	Ag_2O
Si-Control	70	12	3	15	0
Si-02	69.8	12	3	15	0.2
Si-05	69.5	12	3	15	0.5

4.1.2. Network Connectivity

Network connectivity (NC) is a measure of the average number of bridging oxygens on each [SiO_4] tetrahedron [57], which can be used to predict the bioactivity of bioactive glass materials. Generally, the bioactivity increases as NC decreases. NC was calculated using Equation (1). The network formers are assumed to be SiO_2 and the network modifiers, CaO, Na_2O, and P_2O_5. Ag_2O generally behaves as a network modifier but can change its role to that of a network former [58]. This usually occurs if Ag_2O is present in high concentrations, or if metallic silver particles form during glass synthesis. Both cases of silver behaving as a modifier or as a former were considered.

4.2. Glass Characterization

4.2.1. Particle Size Analysis (PSA)

A Microtrac S3500 Particle Size Analyzer (Microtrac Inc., Montgomeryville, PA, USA) was used to collect particle size information about the glass powders. Three powder samples per glass were evaluated in the range of 2–60 μm. Results were analyzed by Multisizer software (Version 4, Beckham Coulter, Mississauga, ON, Canada), with means and standard deviations based on counting statistics of 30,000 particles per measurement.

4.2.2. X-ray Diffraction (XRD)

X-ray diffraction (XRD) was performed to confirm that all glass samples were amorphous. Ground samples were placed on a glass slide and inserted into an X'Pert PRO PANanlytical XRD machine (PANanlytic Inc., St Laurent, QC, Canada). Samples were adhered to glass slides and placed inside the machine. Samples were analyzed over the range of $20° \leq 2\theta \leq 80°$, with a step size of 0.05° and a step time of 1.00 s. The generator was set to 40 mA, 45 kV, using a CuKα (1.54 Å) anode.

4.2.3. Differential Scanning Calorimetry (DSC)

Differential scanning calorimetry (DSC) was performed on a NETZSCH STA 449 F3 Jupiter (NETZSCH-Geratebau GmbH, Germany), with an accuracy of 2%, using sapphire crucibles. The analysis was performed for one sample per glass (n = 1) from 20 °C to 1000 °C with a step size of 20 °C/min to measure the glass transition (T_g) and crystallization temperatures (T_c). For the purpose of this work, T_g was chosen as the endset of the inflection in heat flow.

4.2.4. Scanning Electron Microscopy–Energy Dispersive X-ray Spectroscopy (SEM–EDX)

Ground glass samples were placed on a stage using two-sided tape, and excess powder was shaken off. The stage was then placed inside of a JEOL JSM-6380LV scanning electron microscope (JEOL Ltd., Tokyo, Japan). EDX spectra were also collected using a beam energy of 20 kV in order to determine the elements present in the glass. Three different sites were examined and averaged in order to limit the impact of localized testing.

4.3. Solubility Studies

A buffer solution was prepared by mixing 15.09 g of Tris (hydroxymethyl) aminomethane in 800 mL of deionized water and adding 44.2 mL of 1 M hydrochloric acid (HCl). The volume was then filled to 2 L using deionized water, and a pH of 7.30 was maintained by adding HCl and testing with a pH meter. The solution was then left at 37 °C overnight. Of each glass powder, 75 mg was added, along with 50 mL of Tris solution in Nalgene plastic bottles. The bottles were then placed in an incubator at 37 °C for 6, 12, and 24 h. The bottles were removed, and the solutions were run through a filter paper to remove undissolved glass. The fluid, meanwhile, was collected and tested for pH and ion release.

4.3.1. pH Change

After 6, 12, and 24 h of incubation of glass powder samples (0.5 g) in Tris buffer solution, the pH of the solution was measured using an Omega PHH222 pH meter (Omega, Laval, QC, Canada) and compared to the initial pH value of the Tris buffer solution to determine how pH varied in the presence of the glass powder.

4.3.2. Ion Release Studies

The collected fluid from the Tris buffer solubility test was evaluated for the presence of silver, calcium, sodium, and phosphate ions (Ag^+, Ca^{2+}, Na^+, and PO_4^{3-}, respectively) using atomic absorption spectroscopy (AAS, PinAAcle 500 Flame Atomic Absorption Spectrometer (PerkinElmer, Waltham, MA, USA) equipped with a nitrous oxide (N_2O)/acetylene flame. Calibration standard solutions were prepared for each ion by mixing their corresponding AAS standard (Sigma-Aldrich, Oakville, ON, Canada) in deionized water. AAS standards of 1000 ppm were diluted to 0.10 ppm, 0.50 ppm, 1.0 ppm, 5.0 ppm, 10.0 ppm, and 20.0 ppm. Deionized water was also kept for testing as a blank (0.00 ppm). Each sample was tested three times.

4.4. Antibacterial Studies

Oral cavity bacteria were collected by swabbing the teeth, gums, and tongues of three volunteers (all male, healthy, and ages 25, 25, and 24 years old) at Ryerson University (Toronto, ON, Canada). The swabs were then placed in nutrient broth and allowed to grow for 3 days, after which they were inoculated onto strep agar plates, and left to grow for a further 3 days. Four colonies of interest, such as those exhibiting satellitism or microcolonies, were then extracted and suspended in broth again for another three days; these colonies are expected to be formed of *Staphylococcus*, *Streptococcus*, and *Lactobacillus* genus bacteria, typically found in healthy mouths [59]. These isolates were then streaked across agar plates with glass powder. These agar plates were divided into three sections, and 0.5 g of each glass composition measured out in Eppendorf tubes were placed in each third. After 6, 12, and 24 h, the inhibition zone was measured for each composition by comparing the dark, inoculated spaces against the lighter, inhibited spaces, and measuring using a caliper. The difference in the diameters of the inhibited zone and the glass deposit was measured.

4.5. Toothpaste Remineralization Studies

Fifteen lamb molars were obtained from a local butcher, and their buccal surfaces ground with 600 grit sandpaper on a water-cooled disc grinder. The molars were then mounted, three per puck, in cold-curing resin, with the buccal surfaces facing upward. The resin was then ground down with 400, 600, and 1200 grit sandpaper, successively, on a water-cooled bench disc grinder (Buehler Ltd., Lake Bluff, IL, USA). The microhardness of the buccal surfaces were determined using an HM-114 Mitutoyo Testing Machine (Mitutoyo, Mississauga, ON, Canada) equipped with a Knoop indenter. The test was performed by loading the samples with a force of 1 kgf (9.81 N) for 10 s and measuring the size of the indentation using SEM images. All five pucks were then submerged in 1.0 M HCl for 12 h at 37 °C to simulate demineralization. The pucks were then retested for their microhardness, and SEM images of the buccal surfaces were captured. Subsequently, three of the pucks were randomly selected for remineralization through brushing with a glass-embedded toothpaste (1g toothpaste with 0.5 g of glass) while two pucks were selected for control. One control involved brushing employing a glass-free dentifrice (1 g), while the other involved brushing with deionized water. All pucks were brushed for 1 min and only once. After remineralization, microhardness testing was performed again at 6, 12, and 24 h, and SEM images were recorded using a JSM-6380LV SEM (JEOL Ltd., Tokyo, Japan). The pucks are shown in Figure 8.

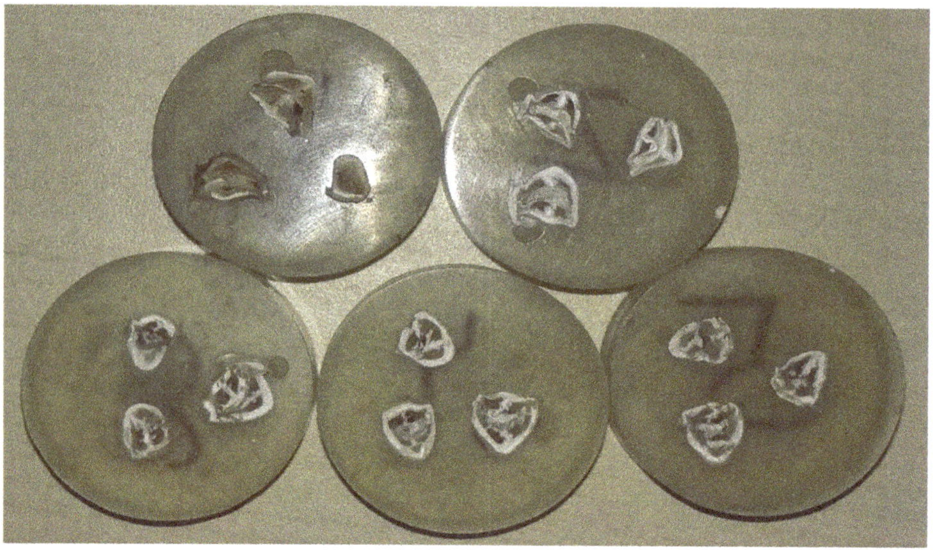

Figure 8. Dental pucks mounted in resin and with their buccal surfaces exposed. Picture was taken after they were brushed.

The degree of remineralization was quantified by the percentage of surface hardness loss (%SHL), a standard metric commonly used to describe mineral loss during dissolution as a function of microhardness [60]. A lower %SHL is desirable, as it indicates less mineral loss. %SHL can be calculated using Equation (2).

$$\%SHL = \frac{Baseline\ Hardness - Treated\ Hardness}{Baseline\ Hardness} \times 100\% \qquad (2)$$

4.6. Statistical Analysis

Non-parametric Kruskal–Wallis H Test was used to analyze the data. The Mann–Whitney U test was used to compare the relative means and to report the statistically significant differences when $p \leq 0.05$. Statistical analysis was performed on all groups where $n \geq 3$. Statistical analysis was performed using SPSS software (IBM SPSS statistics 21, IBM Corp., Armonk, NY, USA).

5. Conclusions

Three glass compositions were synthesized and evaluated to determine effectiveness as anti-caries components when incorporated into dentifrices. The glasses were characterized and tested for their antibacterial properties as well as their enamel remineralization capability.

- The addition of 0.2 and 0.5 mol % silver oxide to a SiO_2–CaO–P_2O_5–Na_2O glass composition at the expense of silica did not cause the glasses to crystallize when fired through the melt-quench method.
- The glasses caused a pH response in Tris buffer solution, raising pH from 7.3 to approximately 7.6. This is invaluable as remineralization and demineralization are pH dependent processes. An acidic environment will promote demineralization, while a more alkaline environment will be more conducive to remineralization. However, an excessive increase in oral pH, typically over 7.5, can cause irritation.
- Ion release profiles were found to be dependent on time and silver content. The network structure of the glass is complex and glass dissolution follows the heterogeneous model, meaning the release of silver occurs in two phases; the first involving alkali ions being replaced with hydronium ions, which varies with the square root of time, while the second is the dissolution of the network, which varies linearly with time.
- Si-05 glass exhibited a stronger antibacterial effect than the Si-02 glass, while Si-Control exhibited no antibacterial effect. This stronger antibacterial response was due to the silver content in each composition; while pH changes are caused by all glasses, Si-Control contains no silver. It can be said then that Ag^+ is the sole bactericidal factor in the glasses.
- All glasses remineralized lamb dental enamel when incorporated into a dentifrice that the molars were exposed to post a standard in vitro demineralization process. This remineralization effect was more potent than the toothpaste alone, which itself is more effective than deionized water. All compositions contain the same amount of calcium and phosphorous. As these are the constituent elements in HA, it is believed that Ca^{2+} and PO_4^{3-} cause the remineralization effect. This section is not mandatory, but can be added to the manuscript if the discussion is unusually long or complex.

Limitations:

- The proposed formulations for the glasses involved higher mole percentages of silver oxide than those synthesized; however, it was determined, upon firing such glasses, that in order for the glass to fully incorporate the silver oxide in its structure, the amount of silver oxide had to be reduced to a maximum of 0.5 mol % Ag_2O.
- The amount of silicon ions released after incubating the glass samples was not measured; in future works, silicon ion release is necessary, as this may be useful to explain how the glass network degradation functioned as silica was the backbone the here-in proposed silver-containing glasses.
- Incubation studies in SBF should be performed to evaluate the deposition of calcium phosphate (CaP) on the teeth surface.
- The ion release studies performed in this study show some unexpected results particularly for PO_4^{3-} and Na^+. The non-linear results obtained for Si-02 samples could be due to machine error. Another study will be performed to provide further insight into the ion release of the formulated materials when matured in de-ionized water, SBF and Tris buffer solutions.

Acknowledgments: The authors would like to thank the Discovery program of the National Sciences and Engineering Research Council (NSERC) for funding this element of Towler's research programme and financing Mr. Arshad's stipend.

Author Contributions: Mark R. Towler and Saad Arshad conceived and designed the experiments; Saad Arshad performed the experiments; Saad Arshad, Omar Rodriguez and Adel Alhalawani analyzed the data; Saad Arshad, Omar Rodriguez and Adel Alhalawani wrote the paper.

References

1. Selwitz, R.H.; Ismail, A.I.; Pitts, N.B. Dental caries. *Lancet* **2007**, *369*, 51–59. [CrossRef]
2. Lenander-Lumikari, M.; Loimaranta, V. Saliva and Dental Caries. *Adv. Dent. Res.* **2000**, *14*, 40–47. [CrossRef] [PubMed]
3. Casamassimo, P.S.; Thikkurissy, S.; Edelstein, B.L.; Maiorini, E. Beyond the dmft: The human and economic cost of early childhood caries. *J. Am. Dent. Assoc.* **2009**, *140*, 650–657. [CrossRef] [PubMed]
4. Marsh, P.D. Dental plaque as a biofilm: The significance of pH in health and caries. *Compend. Contin. Educ. Dent.* **2009**, *30*, 76–78, 80, 83–87; quiz 88, 90. [CrossRef] [PubMed]
5. Featherstone, J.D.B. Dental caries: A dynamic disease process. *Aust. Dent. J.* **2008**, *53*, 286–291. [CrossRef] [PubMed]
6. Hamba, H.; Nikaido, T.; Inoue, G.; Sadr, A.; Tagami, J. Effects of CPP-ACP with sodium fluoride on inhibition of bovine enamel demineralization: A quantitative assessment using micro-computed tomography. *J. Dent.* **2011**, *39*, 405–413. [CrossRef] [PubMed]
7. Hooper, S.; Seong, J.; Macdonald, E.; Claydon, N.; Hellin, N.; Barker, M.L.; He, T.; West, N.X. A randomised in situ trial, measuring the anti-erosive properties of a stannous-containing sodium fluoride dentifrice compared with a sodium fluoride/potassium nitrate dentifrice. *Int. Dent. J.* **2014**, *64* (Suppl. 1), 35–42. [CrossRef] [PubMed]
8. Valkenburg, C.; Slot, D.E.; Bakker, E.W.P.; Van der Weijden, F.A. Does dentifrice use help to remove plaque? A systematic review. *J. Clin. Periodontol.* **2016**, *43*, 1050–1058. [CrossRef] [PubMed]
9. Karim, B.F.A.; Gillam, D.G. The Efficacy of Strontium and Potassium Toothpastes in Treating Dentine Hypersensitivity: A Systematic Review. *Int. J. Dent.* **2013**, *2013*, 573258. [CrossRef] [PubMed]
10. Babcock, F.D.; King, J.C.; Jordan, T.H. The reaction of stannous fluoride and hydroxyapatite. *J. Dent. Res.* **1978**, *57*, 933–938. [CrossRef] [PubMed]
11. Schlueter, N.; Duran, A.; Klimek, J.; Ganss, C. Investigation of the effect of various fluoride compounds and preparations thereof on erosive tissue loss in enamel in vitro. *Caries Res.* **2009**, *43*, 10–16. [CrossRef] [PubMed]
12. Ganss, C.; Neutard, L.; von Hinckeldey, J.; Klimek, J.; Schlueter, N. Efficacy of a tin/fluoride rinse: A randomized in situ trial on erosion. *J. Dent. Res.* **2010**, *89*, 1214–1218. [CrossRef] [PubMed]
13. Lynch, R.J.M.; Churchley, D.; Butler, A.; Kearns, S.; Thomas, G.V.; Badrock, T.C.; Cooper, L.; Higham, S.M. Effects of zinc and fluoride on the remineralisation of artificial carious lesions under simulated plaque fluid conditions. *Caries Res.* **2011**, *45*, 313–322. [CrossRef] [PubMed]
14. Hench, L.L.; Splinter, R.J.; Allen, W.C.; Greenlee, T.K. Bonding mechanisms at the interface of ceramic prosthetic materials. *J. Biomed. Mater. Res.* **1971**, *5*, 117–141. [CrossRef]
15. Prabhakar, A.R.; Kumar, S.C. Antibacterial effect of bioactive glass in combination with powdered enamel and dentin. *Indian J. Dent. Res.* **2010**, *21*, 30–34. [CrossRef] [PubMed]
16. Alhalawani, A.M.; Mehrvar, C.; Stone, W.; Waldman, S.D.; Towler, M.R. A novel tantalum-containing bioglass. Part II. Development of a bioadhesive for sternal fixation and repair. *Mater. Sci. Eng. C* **2017**, *71*. [CrossRef] [PubMed]
17. Hench, L.L. Chronology of Bioactive Glass Development and Clinical Applications. *New J. Glas. Ceram.* **2013**, *3*, 67–73. [CrossRef]
18. Greenlee, T.K.; Beckham, C.A.; Crebo, A.R.; Malmorg, J.C. Glass ceramic bone implants. A light microscopic study. *J. Biomed. Mater. Res.* **1972**, *6*, 235–244. [CrossRef] [PubMed]
19. Curzon, M.E. The relation between caries prevalence and strontium concentrations in drinking water, plaque, and surface enamel. *J. Dent. Res.* **1985**, *64*, 1386–1388. [CrossRef] [PubMed]
20. Thuy, T.T.; Nakagaki, H.; Kato, K.; Hung, P.A.; Inukai, J.; Tsuboi, S.; Nakagaki, H.; Hirose, M.N.; Igarashi, S.; Robinson, C. Effect of strontium in combination with fluoride on enamel remineralization in vitro. *Arch. Oral Biol.* **2008**, *53*, 1017–1022. [CrossRef] [PubMed]
21. Mavbogobdato, T. The Preventive Role of Fluorine Against Caries. *J. Dent. Res.* **1951**, *30*, 225–228. [CrossRef] [PubMed]
22. Besinis, A.; De Peralta, T.; Handy, R.D. The antibacterial effects of silver, titanium dioxide and silica dioxide nanoparticles compared to the dental disinfectant chlorhexidine on Streptococcus mutans using a suite of bioassays. *Nanotoxicology* **2014**, *8*, 1–16. [CrossRef] [PubMed]

23. Mohammed, N.R.; Mneimne, M.; Hill, R.G.; Al-Jawad, M.; Lynch, R.J.M.; Anderson, P. Physical chemical effects of zinc on in vitro enamel demineralization. *J. Dent.* **2014**, *42*, 1096–1104. [CrossRef] [PubMed]
24. Kanwal, N.; Brauer, D.S.; Earl, J.; Wilson, R.M.; Karpukhina, N.; Hill, R.G. In-vitro apatite formation capacity of a bioactive glass-containing toothpaste. *J. Dent.* **2018**, *68*, 51–58. [CrossRef] [PubMed]
25. Macon, A.; Valliant, E.; Earl, J.; Jones, J. Bioactivity of toothpaste containing bioactive glass in remineralizing media: Effect of fluoride release from the enzymatic cleavage of monofluorophosphate. *Biomed. Glas.* **2015**, *1*, 41–50.
26. Gendreau, L.; Barlow, A.P.S.; Mason, S.C. Overview of the clinical evidence for the use of NovaMin in providing relief from the pain of dentin hypersensitivity. *J. Clin. Dent.* **2011**, *22*, 90–95. [PubMed]
27. Du Min, Q.; Bian, Z.; Jiang, H.; Greenspan, D.C.; Burwell, A.K.; Zhong, J.; Tai, B.J. Clinical evaluation of a dentifrice containing calcium sodium phosphosilicate (novamin) for the treatment of dentin hypersensitivity. *Am. J. Dent.* **2008**, *21*, 210–214. [PubMed]
28. Gjorgievska, E.S.; Nicholson, J.W.; Slipper, I.J.; Stevanovic, M.M. Remineralization of demineralized enamel by toothpastes: A scanning electron microscopy, energy dispersive X-ray analysis, and three-dimensional stereo-micrographic study. *Microsc. Microanal.* **2013**, *19*, 587–595. [CrossRef] [PubMed]
29. Kim, J.S.; Kuk, E.; Yu, K.N.; Kim, J.-H.; Park, S.J.; Lee, H.J.; Kim, S.H.; Park, Y.K.; Park, Y.H.; Hwang, C.-Y.; et al. Corrigendum to "Antimicrobial effects of silver nanoparticles" [*Nanomed Nanotechnol Biol Med.* 2007;1:95-101]. *Nanomed. Nanotechnol. Biol. Med.* **2014**, *10*, e1119. [CrossRef]
30. Kwakye-Awuah, B.; Williams, C.; Kenward, M.A.; Radecka, I. Antimicrobial action and efficiency of silver-loaded zeolite X. *J. Appl. Microbiol.* **2008**, *104*, 1516–1524. [CrossRef] [PubMed]
31. Mijnendonckx, K.; Leys, N.; Mahillon, J.; Silver, S.; Van Houdt, R. Antimicrobial silver: Uses, toxicity and potential for resistance. *Biometals* **2013**, *26*, 609–621. [CrossRef] [PubMed]
32. Payami, R.; Ghorbanpour, M.; Parchehbaf Jadid, A. Antibacterial silver-doped bioactive silica gel production using molten salt method. *J. Nanostructure Chem.* **2016**, *6*, 215–221. [CrossRef]
33. Valappil, S.P.; Knowles, J.C.; Wilson, M. Effect of Silver-Doped Phosphate-Based Glasses on Bacterial Biofilm Growth. *Appl. Environ. Microbiol.* **2008**, *74*, 5228–5230. [CrossRef] [PubMed]
34. Feng, Q.L.; Wu, J.; Chen, G.Q.; Cui, F.Z.; Kim, T.N.; Kim, J.O. A mechanistic study of the antibacterial effect of silver ions on *Escherichia coli* and *Staphylococcus aureus*. *J. Biomed. Mater. Res.* **2000**, *52*, 662–668. [CrossRef]
35. Kim, T.N.; Feng, Q.L.; Kim, J.O.; Wu, J.; Wang, H.; Chen, G.C.; Cui, F.Z. Antimicrobial effects of metal ions (Ag^+, Cu^{2+}, Zn^{2+}) in hydroxyapatite. *J. Mater. Sci. Mater. Med.* **1998**, *9*, 129–134. [CrossRef] [PubMed]
36. Holt, K.B.; Bard, A.J. Interaction of Silver(I) Ions with the Respiratory Chain of *Escherichia coli*: An Electrochemical and Scanning Electrochemical Microscopy Study of the Antimicrobial Mechanism of Micromolar Ag^+. *Biochemistry* **2005**, *44*, 13214–13223. [CrossRef] [PubMed]
37. Lok, C.-N.; Ho, C.-M.; Chen, R.; He, Q.-Y.; Yu, W.-Y.; Sun, H.; Tam, P.K.-H.; Chiu, J.-F.; Che, C.-M. Proteomic Analysis of the Mode of Antibacterial Action of Silver Nanoparticles. *J. Proteome Res.* **2006**, *5*. [CrossRef] [PubMed]
38. Schreurs, W.J.; Rosenberg, H. Effect of silver ions on transport and retention of phosphate by *Escherichia coli*. *J. Bacteriol.* **1982**, *152*, 7–13. [PubMed]
39. Hill, R.G.; Brauer, D.S. Predicting the bioactivity of glasses using the network connectivity or split network models. *J. Non. Cryst. Solids* **2011**, *357*, 3884–3887. [CrossRef]
40. O'Donnell, M.D.; Watts, S.J.; Law, R.V.; Hill, R.G. Effect of P2O5 content in two series of soda lime phosphosilicate glasses on structure and properties—Part II: Physical properties. *J. Non. Cryst. Solids* **2008**, *354*, 3561–3566. [CrossRef]
41. Young, R.A. Implications of atomic substitutions and other structural details in apatites. *J. Dent. Res.* **1974**, *53*, 193–203. [CrossRef] [PubMed]
42. Deliormanlı, A.M. Size-dependent degradation and bioactivity of borate bioactive glass. *Ceram. Int.* **2013**, *39*, 8087–8095. [CrossRef]
43. Mneimne, M.; Hill, R.G.; Bushby, A.J.; Brauer, D.S. High phosphate content significantly increases apatite formation of fluoride-containing bioactive glasses. *Acta Biomater.* **2011**, *7*, 1827–1834. [CrossRef] [PubMed]
44. Brauer, D.S.; Mneimne, M.; Hill, R.G. Fluoride-containing bioactive glasses: Fluoride loss during melting and ion release in tris buffer solution. *J. Non. Cryst. Solids* **2011**, *357*, 3328–3333. [CrossRef]
45. O'Donnell, M.D.; Watts, S.J.; Hill, R.G.; Law, R.V. The effect of phosphate content on the bioactivity of soda-lime-phosphosilicate glasses. *J. Mater. Sci. Mater. Med.* **2009**, *20*, 1611–1618. [CrossRef] [PubMed]

46. Alhalawani, A.M.F.; Towler, M.R. The effect of $ZnO \leftrightarrow Ta_2O_5$ substitution on the structural and thermal properties of SiO_2-ZnO-SrO-CaO-P_2O_5 glasses. *Mater. Charact.* **2016**, *114*, 218–224. [CrossRef]
47. Alhalawani, A.M.F.; Towler, M.R. A novel tantalum-containing bioglass. Part I. Structure and solubility. *Mater. Sci. Eng. C* **2017**, *72*, 202–211. [CrossRef] [PubMed]
48. Cerruti, M.G.; Greenspan, D.; Powers, K. An analytical model for the dissolution of different particle size samples of Bioglass®in TRIS-buffered solution. *Biomaterials* **2005**, *26*, 4903–4911. [CrossRef] [PubMed]
49. El-Kady, A.M.; Ali, A.F.; Rizk, R.A.; Ahmed, M.M. Synthesis, characterization and microbiological response of silver doped bioactive glass nanoparticles. *Ceram. Int.* **2012**, *38*, 177–188. [CrossRef]
50. Kim, J.S.; Kuk, E.; Yu, K.N.; Kim, J.-H.; Park, S.J.; Lee, H.J.; Kim, S.H.; Park, Y.K.; Park, Y.H.; Hwang, C.-Y.; et al. Antimicrobial effects of silver nanoparticles. *Nanomed. Nanotechnol. Biol. Med.* **2007**, *3*, 95–101. [CrossRef] [PubMed]
51. Vale, G.C.; Tabchoury, C.P.M.; Del Bel Cury, A.A.; Tenuta, L.M.A.; ten Cate, J.M.; Cury, J.A. APF and dentifrice effect on root dentin demineralization and biofilm. *J. Dent. Res.* **2011**, *90*, 77–81. [CrossRef] [PubMed]
52. Zantner, C.; Beheim-Schwarzbach, N.; Neumann, K.; Kielbassa, A.M. Surface microhardness of enamel after different home bleaching procedures. *Dent. Mater.* **2007**, *23*, 243–250. [CrossRef] [PubMed]
53. Chen, H.-P.; Chang, C.-H.; Liu, J.-K.; Chuang, S.-F.; Yang, J.-Y. Effect of fluoride containing bleaching agents on enamel surface properties. *J. Dent.* **2008**, *36*, 718–725. [CrossRef] [PubMed]
54. Buzalaf, M.A.R.; Hannas, A.R.; Magalhaes, A.C.; Rios, D.; Honorio, H.M.; Delbem, A.C.B. pH-cycling models for in vitro evaluation of the efficacy of fluoridated dentifrices for caries control: Strengths and limitations. *J. Appl. Oral Sci.* **2010**, *18*, 316–334. [CrossRef] [PubMed]
55. Yap, A.U.; Lye, K.W.; Sau, C.W. Surface characteristics of tooth-colored restoratives polished utilizing different polishing systems. *Oper. Dent.* **1997**, *22*, 260–265. [PubMed]
56. Arends, J.; Ten Cate, J.M. Tooth enamel remineralization. *J. Cryst. Growth* **1981**, *53*, 135–147. [CrossRef]
57. Hill, R. An alternative view of the degradation of bioglass. *J. Mater. Sci. Lett.* **1996**, *15*, 1122–1125. [CrossRef]
58. Baltzer, N.; Copponnex, T. *Precious Metals for Biomedical Applications*, 1st ed.; Elsevier: Amsterdam, The Netherlands, 2014.
59. Avila, M.; Ojcius, D.M.; Yilmaz, O. The oral microbiota: Living with a permanent guest. *DNA Cell Biol.* **2009**, *28*, 405–411. [CrossRef] [PubMed]
60. De Sousa Barbosa, R.P.; Pereira-Cenci, T.; da Silva, W.M.; Coelho-de-Souza, F.H.; Demarco, F.F.; Cenci, M.S. Effect of cariogenic biofilm challenge on the surface hardness of direct restorative materials in situ. *J. Dent.* **2012**, *40*, 359–363. [CrossRef] [PubMed]

5

Antimicrobial Monomers for Polymeric Dental Restoratives: Cytotoxicity and Physicochemical Properties

Diane R. Bienek *, Stanislav A. Frukhtbeyn, Anthony A. Giuseppetti, Ugochukwu C. Okeke and Drago Skrtic

Volpe Research Center, ADA Foundation, Gaithersburg, MD 20899, USA; stanislav.frukhtbeyn@nist.gov (S.A.F.); anthony.giuseppetti@nist.gov (A.A.G.); ugochukwu.okeke@nist.gov (U.C.O.); drago.skrtic@nist.gov (D.S.)
* Correspondence: bienekd@ada.org

Abstract: A trend for the next generation of polymeric dental restoratives is to incorporate multifunctional capabilities to regulate microbial growth and remineralize tooth surfaces. Polymerizable 2-(methacryloyloxy)-*N*-(2-(methacryloyloxy)ethyl)-*N*,*N*-dimethylethan-1-aminium bromide (IDMA1) and *N*,*N*′-([1,1′-biphenyl]-2,2′-diylbis(methylene))bis(2-(methacryloyloxy)-*N*,*N*-dimethylethan-1-aminium) bromide (IDMA2), intended for utilization in bi-functional antimicrobial and remineralizing composites, were synthesized, purified with an ethanol-diethyl ether-hexane solvent system, and validated by nuclear magnetic resonance (^{1}H and ^{13}C NMR) spectroscopy, mass spectrometry, and Fourier-transform infrared spectroscopy. When incorporated into light-curable urethane dimethacrylate (UDMA)/polyethylene glycol-extended UDMA (PEG-U)/ethyl 2-(hydroxymethyl)acrylate (EHMA) (assigned UPE) resins, IDMAs did not affect the overall resins' hydrophilicity/hydrophobicity balance (water contact angle: 60.8–65.5°). The attained degrees of vinyl conversion (DVC) were consistently higher in both IDMA-containing copolymers and their amorphous calcium phosphate (ACP) composites (up to 5% and 20%, respectively) reaching 92.5% in IDMA2 formulations. Notably, these high DVCs values were attained without an excessive increase in polymerization stress. The observed reduction in biaxial flexure strength of UPE-IDMA ACP composites should not prevent further evaluation of these materials as multifunctional Class V restoratives. In direct contact with human gingival fibroblasts, at biologically relevant concentrations, IDMAs did not adversely affect cell viability or their metabolic activity. Ion release from the composites was indicative of their strong remineralization potential. The above, early-phase biocompatibility and physicochemical tests justify further evaluation of these experimental materials to identify formulation(s) suitable for clinical testing. Successful completion is expected to yield a new class of restoratives with well-controlled bio-function, which will physicochemically, mechanically, and biologically outperform the conventional Class V restoratives.

Keywords: dental materials; amorphous calcium phosphate; antimicrobial methacrylate monomers; antimicrobial and remineralizing composites

---

1. Introduction

Most contemporary dental restoratives recover a tooth's anatomy and function, and yield good aesthetics [1,2]. These materials depend on adhesive systems of largely similar chemical composition, but with lower filler content as means of bonding to tooth structure. While concerns exist about their mechanical properties and abrasion resistance, their major disadvantage is the compromised bonding integrity that leads to the gaps at the adhesive/tooth interface, bacterial microleakage, and secondary caries. The bioactivity of the restoratives typically stems from the release of remineralizing ions (fluoride, calcium (Ca), and phosphate (PO_4)), or their combination [3–6]. Our group has been on the forefront of the research on polymeric, amorphous calcium phosphate (ACP)-based materials for over two decades. Building on systematic structure-composition-property relationship studies [7,8], we have designed remineralizing polymeric composites that release Ca and PO_4 ions in a sustainable manner and efficiently restore tooth mineral lost to decay [9,10]. While protecting from demineralization and regenerating mineral lost to caries, these restoratives do not guard against the ingression and accumulation of microorganisms at the restoration site. Therefore, recurrent dental caries remains a critical issue, even with the new(est) generation of dental restoratives. Adding antimicrobial (AM) functionality to these materials is seen as one of the enduring challenges, aimed at reducing the need for repetitive clinical intervention. Quaternary ammonium methacrylates, known for their AM action against both Gram-positive and Gram-negative bacteria, are typically utilized to impart AM activity to polymeric dental materials. They are, however, quite toxic due to the various biological effects of the quaternary ammonium "head" and its metabolism [11,12]. Multiple studies have indicated that quaternary ammonium compounds destroy cell membrane integrity and eventually lead to cell death [13–15]. Their AM action reportedly depends on the type of counter-ion [11], pendant active groups [16], molecular weight, and length of the alkyl chains [17]. So far, these structure/performance studies have not been successfully implemented to yield dental restorative(s) with sustained AM action [11,16–20]. Initially, most attention has been given to methacryloyloxydodecyl pyrimidinium bromide and its copolymer [1,21–23]. However, the composites with methacryloyloxydodecyl pyrimidinium bromide show poor color stability; thus, their use is limited to areas where aesthetics is not an issue. Among various quaternary ammonium compounds proposed for utility in bonding agents [24,25] and dental resin composites [26–28], ionic dimethacrylates were identified as viable candidates for offsetting concerns related to quaternary ammonium methacrylates. Dr. Xu's group has been active in integrating quaternary ammonium dimethacrylates (QADMs) alone or in combination with nanosilver (nAg) and/or nano-ACP (nACP) into resins, based on conventional monomers (Table 1). While collectively these recent studies indicate the potential of using QADMs as AM agents in dental materials, there are still knowledge gaps and deficiencies regarding: (1) optimization of the resin composition; (2) purity and structural characterization of the synthesized agent; and (3) in vitro cytotoxicity evaluations with biologically relevant QADMs concentrations.

In this study, we synthesized, purified, and characterized 2-(methacryloyloxy)-*N*-(2-(methacryloyloxy) ethyl)-*N*,*N*-dimethylethan-1-aminium bromide (IDMA1) and *N*,*N*′-([1,1′-biphenyl]-2,2′-diylbis (methylene))bis(2-(methacryloyloxy)-*N*,*N*-dimethylethan-1-aminium) bromide (IDMA2). Next, we assessed in vitro cytotoxicity of IDMAs using a standard direct contact method. We incorporated IDMA1 or IDMA2 into light-curable urethane dimethacrylate (UDMA), polyethylene glycol-extended UDMA (PEG-U)/ethyl 2-(hydroxymethyl)acrylate (EHMA) resins (designated UPE resin) and assessed IDMAs effect on resins' hydrophobic/hydrophilic balance. IDMA/UPE copolymers were assessed for degree of vinyl conversion (DVC) and biaxial flexural strength (BFS). Furthermore, we synthesized and validated ACP filler, homogenized it by milling and incorporated it into UDMA-based resins. The ensuing composites were evaluated for DVC, mechanical strength, and remineralizing potential. The underlying hypotheses were that: (1) IDMAs will have no detrimental effect on physicochemical and/or mechanical properties of copolymers; and (2) reduced DVC and/or mechanical stability of ACP/UPE-IDMA composites will be compensated by their remineralizing potential.

Table 1. Antimicrobial efficacy expressed as n-fold decrease in biofilm formation of experimental QADM-based dental materials.

Ref.	Dental Material	Experimental Groups	Fold Decrease [1]
[28]	**Composite** BisGMA-TEGDMA	Control: Commercial composite	
		20% nACP + 6% QADM (aged 1 day)	1.36
		20% nACP + 0.1% nAg (aged 1 day)	1.75
		20% nACP + 6% QADM + 0.1% nAg (aged 1 day)	2.69
[29]	**Composite** BisGMA-TEGDMA	Control: Composite (no fluoride)	
		19.5% nACP	1.25
		19.5% nACP + 7% QADM	1.73
		19.5% nACP + 0.028% nAg	1.98
		19.5% nACP + 7% QADM + 0.028% nAg	3.00
[24]	**Primer/adhesive** Primer: HEMA-acrylic/itaconic acids Adhesive: BisGMA-HEMA	Primer control + Adhesive control	
		Primer w/10% QADM + Adhesive w/10% QADM	1.65
		Primer w/0.05% nAg + Adhesive w/0.05% nAg	2.38
[25]	**Primer/adhesive** Primer: PMGDM-HEMA Adhesive: BisGMA-TEGDMA	Primer control + Adhesive control	
		Primer w/0.1% nAg + Adhesive control	2.70
		Primer w/0.1% nAg + Adhesive w/0.1% nAg, 10% QADM	2.86
		Primer w/0.1% nAg + Adhesive w/0.1% nAg, 10% QADM, 10% nACP	3.07
		Primer w/0.1% nAg + Adhesive w/0.1% nAg, 10% QADM, 20% nACP	2.98
		Primer w/0.1% nAg + Adhesive w/0.1% nAg, 10% QADM, 30% nACP	4.57
		Primer w/0.1% nAg + Adhesive w/0.1% nAg, 10% QADM, 40% nACP	5.11

[1] indicates n-fold decrease in metabolic activity (mean absorbance of control/mean absorbance of experimental group) of bacterial biofilms. Mean absorbance data extracted from published figures.

2. Results

2.1. IDMAs: Structural Validation

Assigned structures of IDMAs were verified by nuclear magnetic resonance (NMR), mass spectrometry (MS), and Fourier-transform infrared spectroscopy (FTIR). ^{1}H NMR and ^{13}C NMR spectra of IDMA1 and IDMA2 are shown in Figures 1 and 2, respectively with the accompanying assignments of chemical shifts to their structures (Tables 2 and 3).

FTIR spectra of IDMA1 and IDMA2 are shown in Figure 3. Both IDMA1 and IDMA2 are hygroscopic and gain moisture when stored in the open. Their hygroscopicity is verified by a broad peak at ~3400–3300 cm^{-1} in their FTIR spectra. Generally, the hygroscopic nature of quaternary ammonium salts have been demonstrated by X-ray crystallography and is attributed to hydrogen bonding between water molecules and quaternary ammonium's bromide ion (Br$\cdots$H–O–H) [30].

Table 2. Assignments of ^{13}C and ^{1}H NMR chemical shifts of IDMA1.

Atom #	^{13}C Chemical Shift, ppm	^{1}H Chemical Shift, ppm	# H's	Signal Splitting
1	18.2	1.95	6	singlet
2	135.0		0	
3	127.4	5.67, 6.15	2, 2	singlets
4	166.2		0	
5	58.2	4.71	4	multiplet
6	63.6	4.31	4	multiplet
7, 8	52.5	3.63	6	singlet

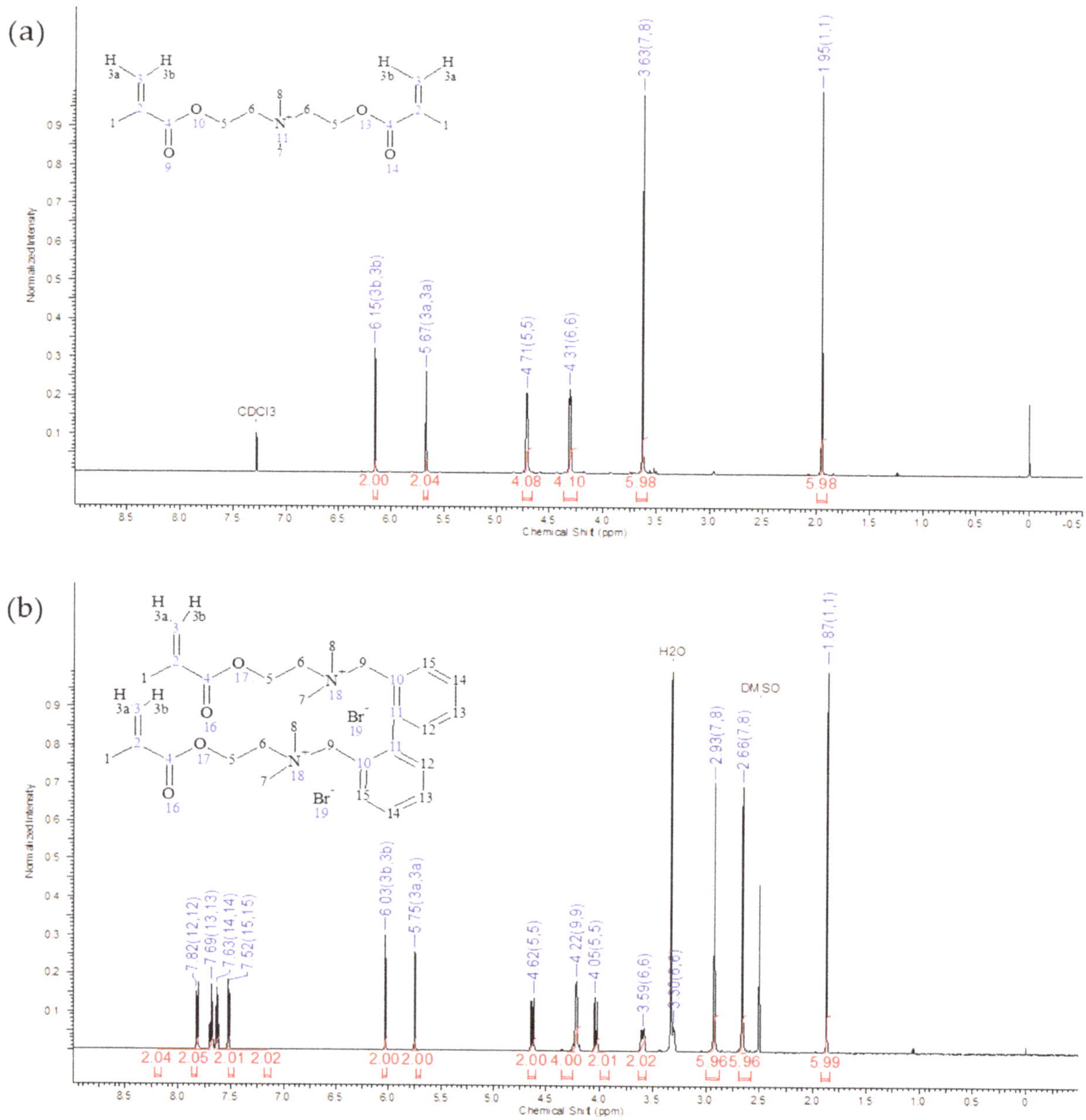

Figure 1. Typical ^{1}H NMR spectrum of (**a**) IDMA1 and (**b**) of IDMA2.

Table 3. Assignments of ^{13}C and ^{1}H NMR chemical shifts of IDMA2.

Atom #	^{13}C Chemical Shift, ppm	^{1}H Chemical Shift, ppm	# H's	Signal Splitting
1	17.9	1.87	6	singlet
2	135.3		0	
3	126.7	5.75, 6.03	2, 2	singlets
4	165.6		0	
5	64.7	4.04, 4.63	2, 2	doublets
6	62.2	3.30, 3.59	2, 2	multiplets
7, 8	49.9, 50.0	2.66, 2.93	6, 6	singlets
9	57.6	4.22	4	broad
10	141.8		0	
11	125.1		0	
12	135.1	7.82	2	multiplet
13	131.0	7.69	2	triplet
14	128.4	7.63	2	triplet
15	132.8	7.52	2	multiplet

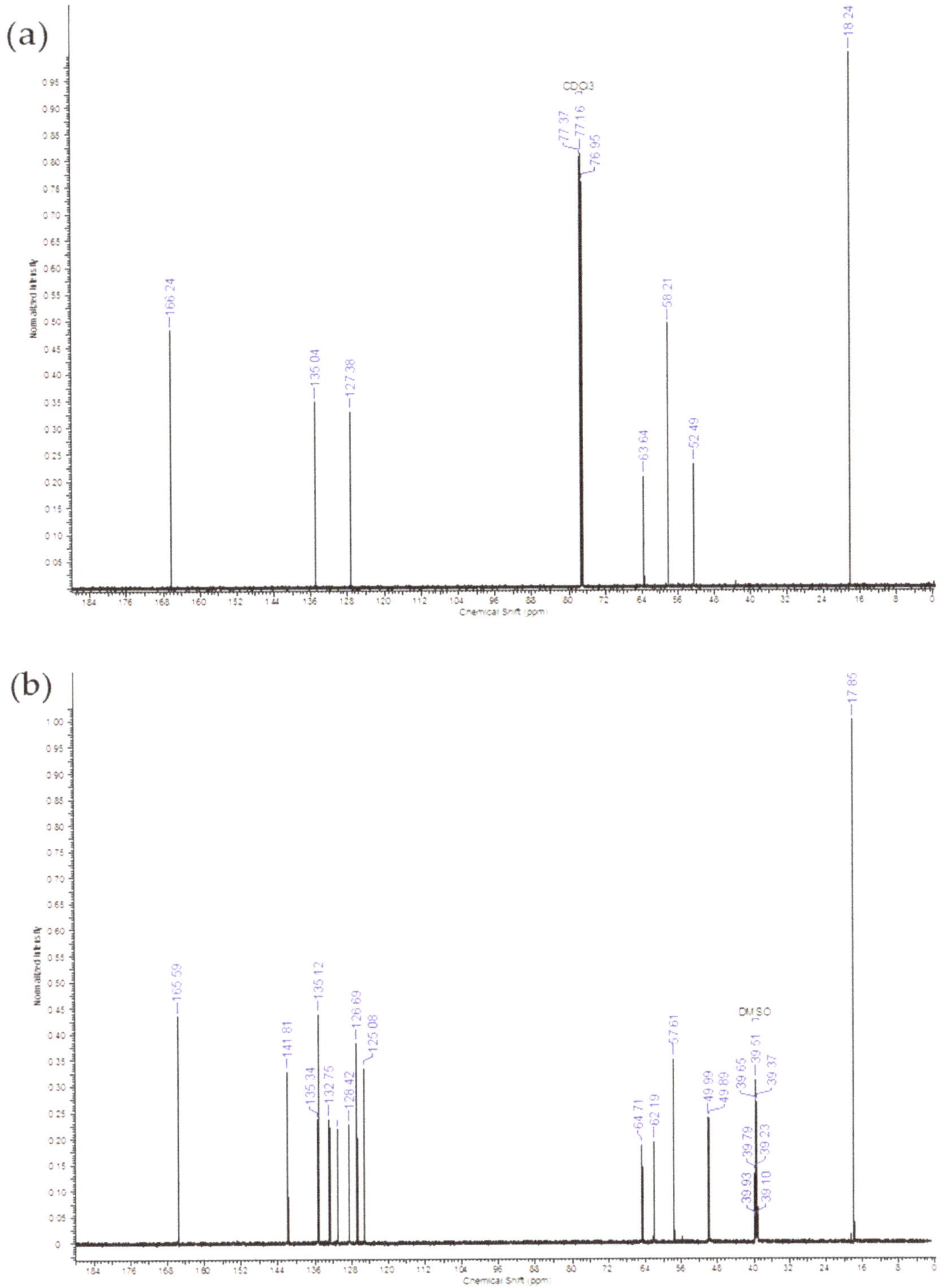

Figure 2. Typical ^{13}C NMR spectrum of (**a**) IDMA1 and (**b**) of IDMA2.

MS of IDMA1 ($C_{14}H_{24}NO_4Br$) generated prominent peaks at m/z 270.35 ($C_{14}H_{24}NO_4^+$, calculated m/z 270.17) and at m/z 113.06 ($C_6H_9O_2^+$, calculated m/z 113.06). MS of IDMA2 ($C_{30}H_{42}N_2O_4Br_2$) yielded prominent peaks at m/z 573.55/575.58, ($C_{30}H_{42}N_2O_4Br^+$, calculated m/z 573.23/575.23); 416.33/418.29 ($C_{22}H_{27}NO_2Br^+$, calculated m/z 416.12/418.12); 179.18 ($C_{22}H_{34}N_2O_2^{+2}$, calculated m/z 179.13); 113.07 ($C_6H_9O_2^+$, calculated m/z 113.07) (data not shown).

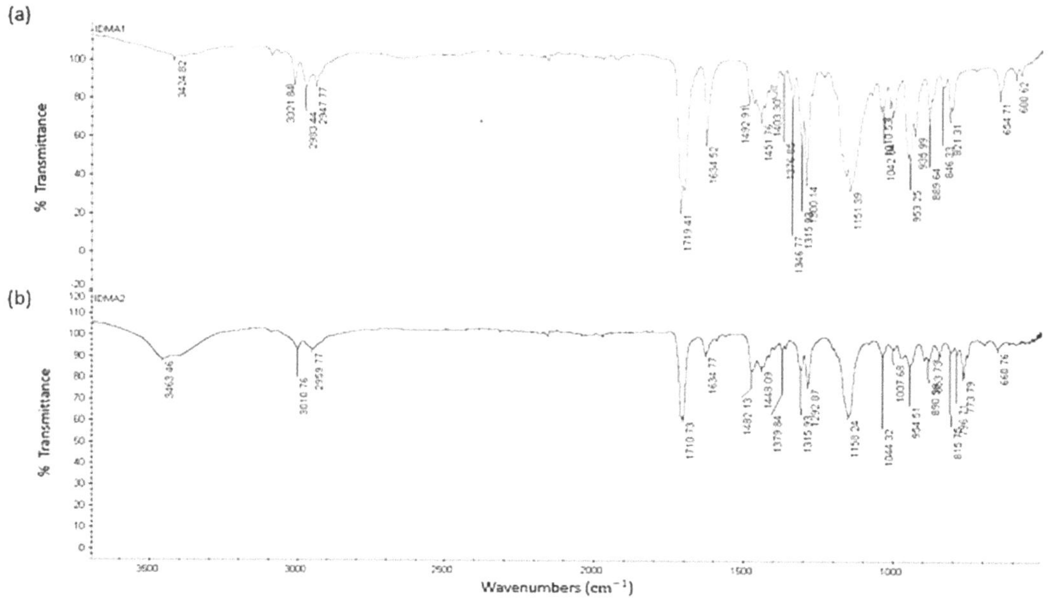

Figure 3. Typical FTIR spectrum of (**a**) IDMA1 and (**b**) of IDMA2.

2.2. *IDMAs: Biocompatibility*

2.2.1. Cellular Metabolic Activity

To determine the cytotoxic potential of QADMs targeted for dental restorations, human gingival fibroblasts (HGFs) were exposed to two-fold serial dilutions of IDMA1 (≤10.66 mmol/L). No statistical differences were observed when considering the main effect of IDMA1 concentration on the metabolic activity of HGFs (Figure 4a). However, time of IDMA1 exposure exerted a significant ($p \leq 0.05$) main effect on cellular metabolic activity. When comparing the effect of time, without regard to concentration, the cellular metabolic activity was consistently lower (~13% difference of means) after 72 h of exposure.

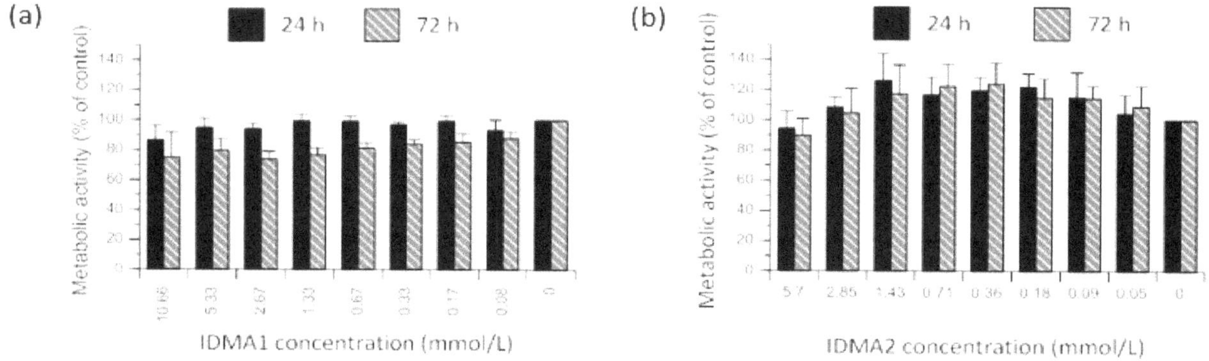

Figure 4. Percent control value of metabolic activity of HGF cells exposed for 24 h or 72 h to two-fold serial dilutions of (**a**) IDMA1 (≤10.66 mmol/L) or (**b**) IDMA2 (≤5.7 mmol/L). Data represent mean ± standard error of the mean (SEM) for five or more independent replicates tested in triplicate.

IDMA2 concentration (≤5.7 mmol/L) did not exert a significant main effect on HGF metabolic activity (Figure 4b). Further, cellular metabolic activity was not statistically affected by the time of IDMA2 exposure (up to 72 h).

For the testing of both IDMAs, negligible optical density values were observed in control wells, containing no cells. Controls (with or without cells) in which the tetrazolium compound was omitted resulted in low optical densities. Positive controls, containing non-exposed cells were not significantly different from cells that were previously stained with ethidium homodimer-1 and calcein (data not shown).

2.2.2. Cellular Viability

As with cell metabolic activity profiles, viability data indicated an overall insignificant effect of IDMA1 concentration (Figure 5a,b). Cell viability was 5.5% lower (difference of means without regard to concentration) between the time points. Although this comparison was insignificant, a trend for decreased viability was observed at higher concentrations after 72 h exposure.

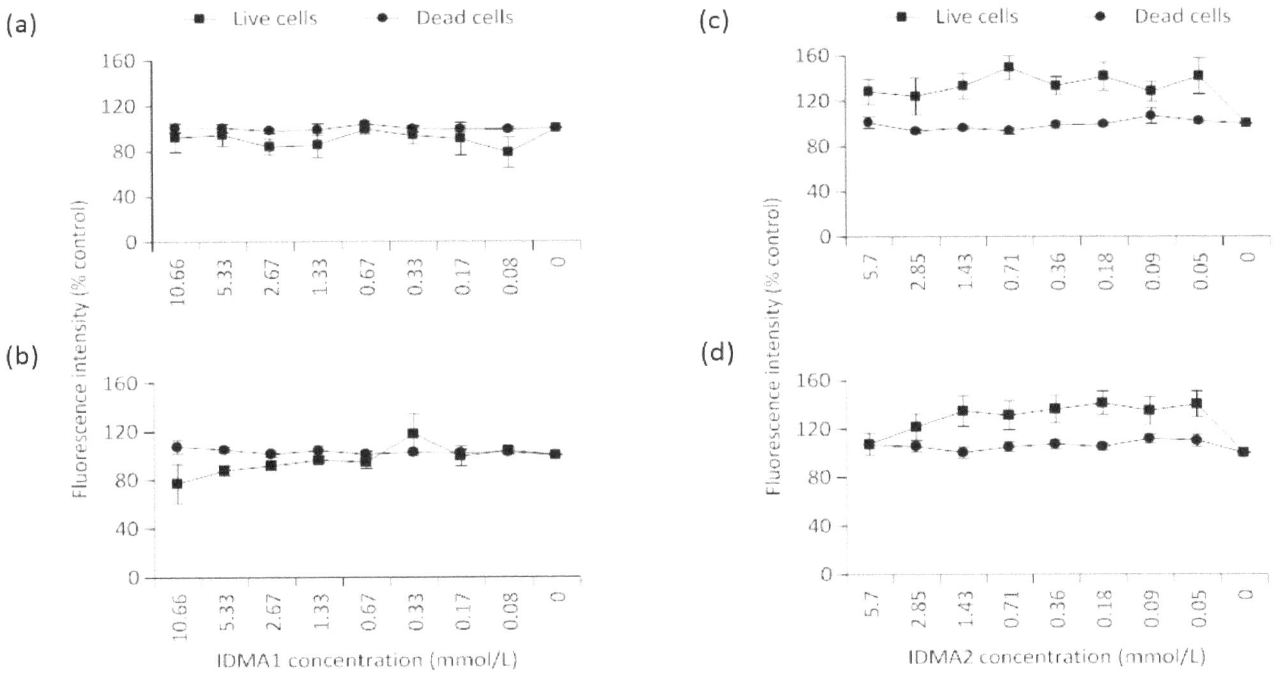

Figure 5. Percent control value of viability of HGF cells exposed to two-fold serial dilutions of IDMA1 (≤10.66 mmol/L) for (**a**) 24 h or (**b**) 72 h to two-fold serial dilutions of IDMA1. Percent control value of viability of HGF cells exposed for (**c**) 24 h or (**d**) 72 h to two-fold serial dilutions of IDMA2 (≤5.70 mmol/L). Data represent mean ± SEM for five independent replicates tested in triplicate.

When comparing IDMA2 concentrations within a given time point, no statistical differences were observed when the number of viable cells were compared (Figure 5c,d). Likewise, IDMA2 concentrations did not significantly affect the number of dead cells. A statistical main effect ($p \leq 0.05$) of time was observed in the number of dead cells (i.e., nearly a 7% increase in the difference of means).

2.3. ACP Filler Remineralizing Ability

Milled ACP utilized to fabricate ACP/UPE-IDMA composites had a median dimeter (d_m) of 2.73 ± 0.17 μm, which represents a 45% reduction compared to as-made ACP (d_m = 4.93 ± 0.52 μm). The particle size distribution (PSD) range (submicron to 70 μm) apparently was not affected by milling (data not shown). X-ray diffraction (XRD) spectrum of ACP showed two diffuse broad bands ((24–36) and (40–55) 2θ degrees); patterns typical for calcium phosphates with low crystallinity. Corresponding FTIR spectra exhibited two wide bands typical for PO_4 stretching and PO_4 bending in the region of 1200–900 cm^{-1} and 630–500 cm^{-1}, respectively. Typical morphology (scanning electron microscopy data), results of PSD analysis, and structural verification by FTIR and XRD are presented in Figure 6.

Kinetic profiles of Ca and phosphorus (P) release from milled-ACP UPE composites (Figure 7) revealed that within 4 months of aqueous immersion, a plateau (maximum) ion concentration had not been reached. The supersaturation conditions (SR >> 1) attained at any given time point were notably above the minimum necessary for the apatite re-deposition. It is particularly significant that the attained solution Ca/P ratio (average 1.66 ± 0.03) is practically identical to the apatite's theoretical Ca/P value of 1.66, meaning that solution conditions created by composite's immersion are highly conducive to apatite formation.

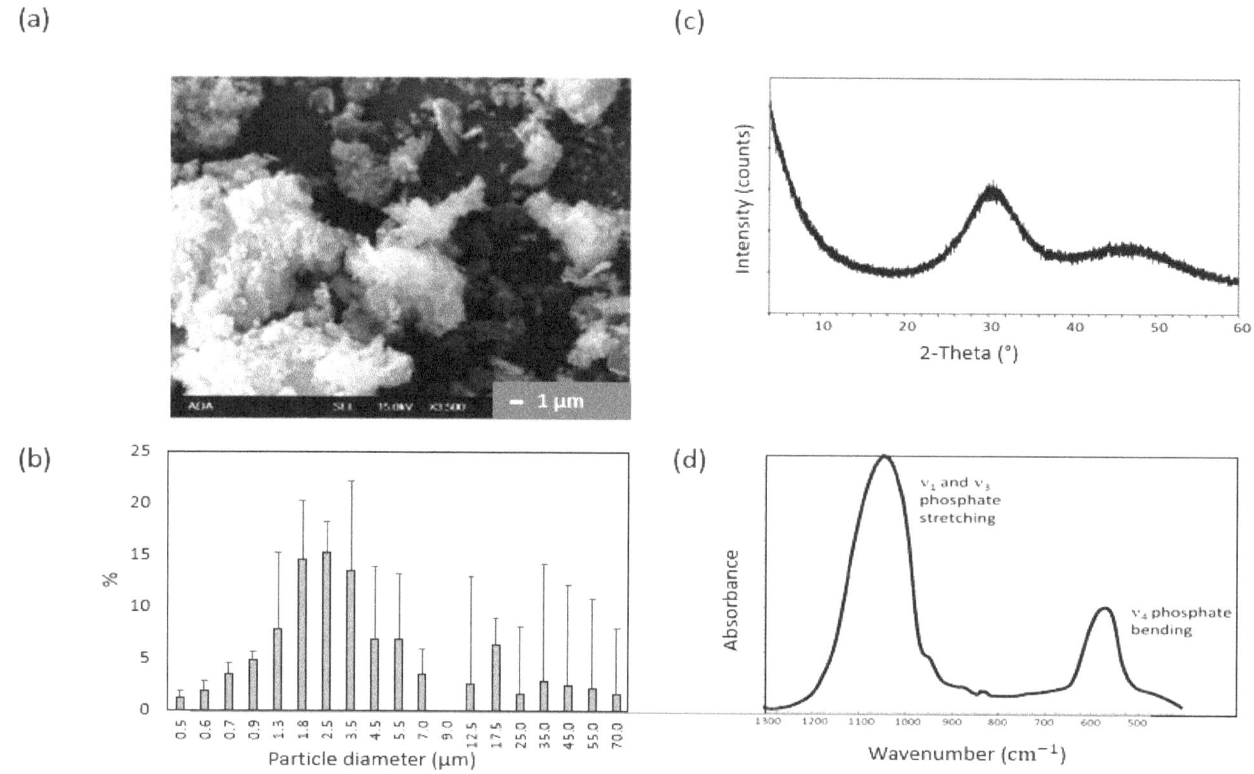

Figure 6. Validation of synthesized ACP. (**a**) Morphology of ACP particles under scanning electron microscopy (×3500 magnification); (**b**) Differential particle size distribution (mean values ± SD, $n = 2$); (**c**) XRD pattern; (**d**) FTIR spectrum of milled ACP utilized to fabricate ACP/UPE-IDMA composites.

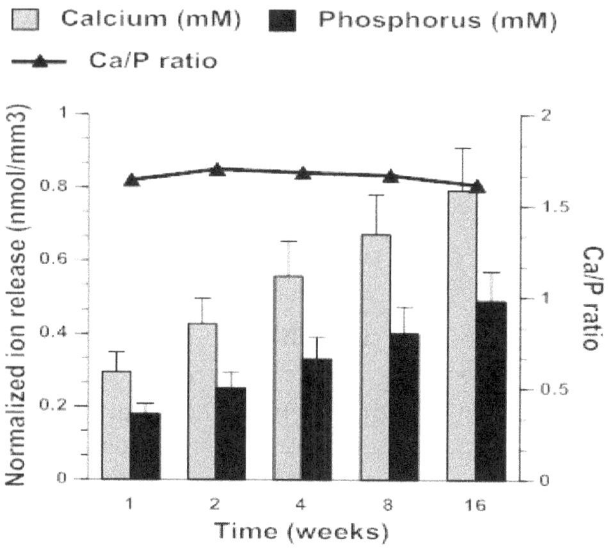

Figure 7. Kinetics of ion release from ACP UPE composites upon prolonged aqueous immersion. Indicated are mean values ± SD of triplicate measurements.

2.4. Preliminary Physicochemical Evaluation of Resins and Composites

Hydrophobic/hydrophilic balance of UPE resins (average contact angle 60.8 ± 5.1°) was not affected significantly by either the type or the concentration of IDMA monomer included in the matrix (average contact angle 64.4 ± 5.1°) (Figure 8).

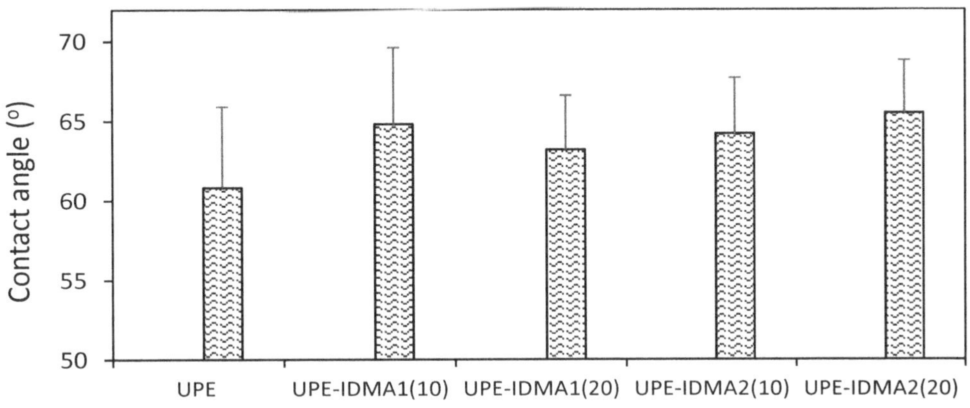

Figure 8. Changes in the overall hydrophilicity/hydrophobicity of the resins upon introduction of IDMAs (at 10 and 20 mass %) into UPE formulation. Indicated values represent mean ± SD for four replicate measurements.

DVC results (Figure 9) revealed that in both copolymer and composite series, significant differences ($p \leq 0.001$) existed between no IDMA, IDMA1, and IDMA2 formulations. The post-hoc multiple pair comparisons indicated that the observed up to 5% and 20% (copolymer and composite series, respectively) increases in DVC of IDMA-containing formulations are significant ($p \leq 0.001$). It is noteworthy that the high DVC values (85.5–92.7%) attained in the experimental ACP UPE-IDMA composites were, generally, not accompanied with the excessive polymerization stress (Figure 10). Notably, in IDMA2 composites that reached the highest level of vinyl conversion, the measured polymerization stress was almost 40% lower than in IDMA1 composites.

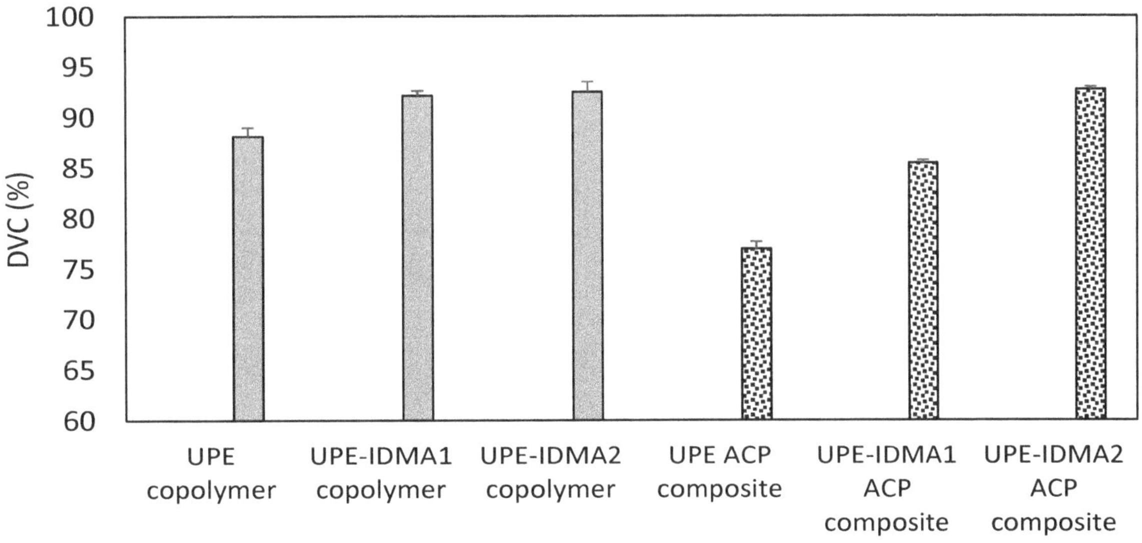

Figure 9. DVC attained in copolymers (near infra-red measurements; 24 h post cure) and the corresponding ACP composites; 15 min post-cure (curing conditions: 40 s, 500 mW/cm^2). Shown are mean values ± SD for three replicate measurements.

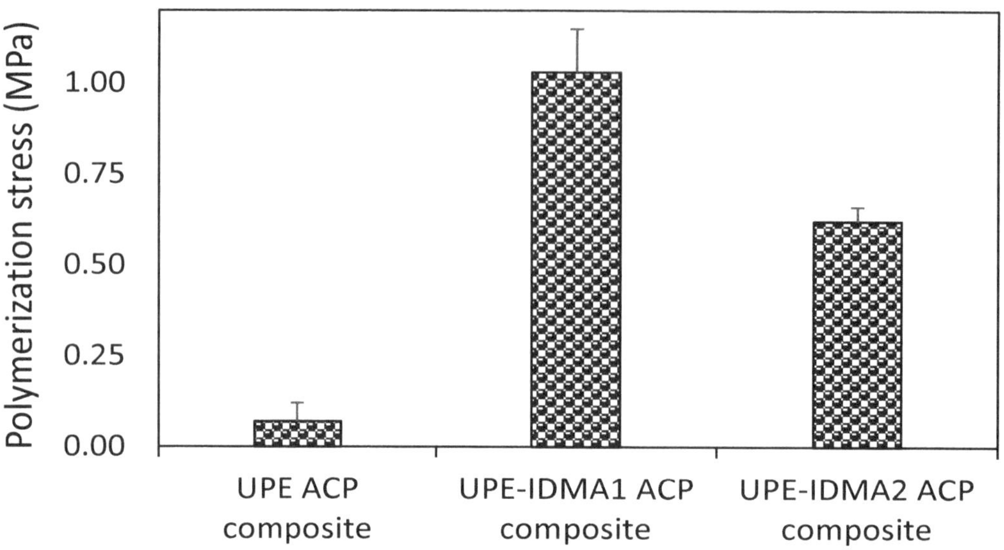

Figure 10. Polymerization stress (mean values ± SD for three replicate measurements) developed in ACP composite specimens 15 min after photo irradiation.

The results of biaxial flexural strength (BFS) testing of copolymer and composite specimens are summarized in Figure 11. Introducing IDMA monomers did not affect the BFS of copolymers (average 181.5 ± 12.6 MPa). Incorporation of ACP filler, however, resulted in 60% reduction in the BFS of composites (on average 72.2 ± 16.5 MPa).

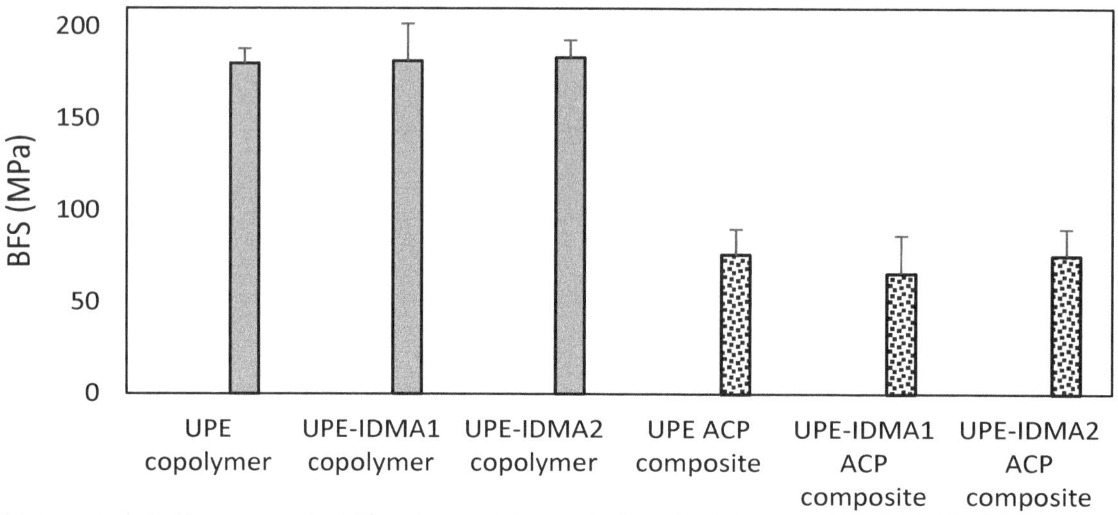

Figure 11. BFS of copolymers and composites. Indicated are mean values ± SD for $n = 5$ (copolymer group) and $n = 4$ (composite group).

3. Discussion

Any AM agent's biocompatibility is likely to be compromised by the presence of significant amounts of impurities, unreacted reagents, and/or residual solvents in the material. Therefore, the ability to purify crude IDMAs with an ethanol-diethyl ether-hexane solvent system, developed as a part of this study, is essential to minimize the potential toxicity of an AM agent towards host cells. The synthetic/purification approach that has yielded high purity (≥97%) IDMAs has strong potential to be extended to design a new generation of monomers with improved resin miscibility (AM_{misc}), adhesiveness to teeth (AM_{adh}) and coupling with the remineralizing ACP filler (AM_{cpl}). A successful fabrication of high-purity AM_{misc}, AM_{adh}, and AM_{cpl} monomers, anticipated in near future, will enable us to clearly delineate the ability of these new agents to cross-link with UDMA-based resins, while safeguarding their AM function and maintaining satisfactory mechanical performance of antimicrobial and remineralizing (AMRE) composites.

Although AM QADMs have received considerable attention for use in dental restoratives, the reports on their biocompatibility are generally scarce. Biocompatibility screenings of AM agents are commonly performed in direct contact with polymer, rather than by exposing cells to AM concentrations corresponding to their predicted levels in the oral milieu. The first published IDMA1 cytotoxicity study involved a conventional polymer matrix and mouse macrophage-like cells (RAW 264.7) [26]. Polymers containing 10 mass % IDMA1 reduced cell density without affecting their viability. At IDMA contents >10 mass %, both cell density and viability were reduced. Evaluation of the residual cells, remaining after polymer disk removal, led to the conclusion that leachables did not affect RAW 264.7 cells. Another study employing HGFs [24] found the eluent toxicity of bonding agent containing QADM equaled no-QADM controls. In both of the above studies, the leached extract was not characterized and QADM (IDMA1) concentrations were not determined. Our group considered the in vitro cytotoxicity of an AM agent, at biologically pertinent levels and in direct contact with relevant cells, as the crucial prognosticator for material(s) development and justification for further exploration. We have initially evaluated IDMA1 and IDMA2 employing mouse subcutaneous connective tissue fibroblasts [31] and found no adverse effect on cell viability or their metabolic activity at biologically relevant concentrations. In this study, we report no toxicity at biologically relevant concentrations of both IDMA1 and IDMA2 towards HGFs. The tested concentrations of IDMA1 and IDMA2 were calculated based on the accelerated leachability data reported for UDMA/PEG-U/2-hydroxyethyl methacrylate (HEMA) copolymers and their ACP composites [8]. It is reasonable to expect that, due to the high DVCs attained in our experimental formulations, the concentration of IDMA1 or IDMA2 leaching from the cured materials will not exceed leachability of small molecular weight and highly diffusive HEMA from UDMA/PEG-U/HEMA formulations. A quantitative leachability study of UPE-IDMA resins and composites will be executed in the near future to confirm our hypothesis. In a later phase of AMRE composite development, the bio-evaluation tests will be expanded to include genotoxicity, immunotoxicity, and inflammation studies.

UPE-IDMA copolymers attained DVCs (92.1–92.5%) that significantly exceeded DVC values of the 2,2-bis[p-(2-hydroxy-3-methacryloxypropoxy)phenyl]propane (Bis-GMA)/triethylene glycol dimethacrylate (TEGDMA)/IDMA counterparts (67.9–70.7%) [26]. Such high DVC values are likely due to a delayed vitrification point incited by the inclusion of PEG-U, EHMA, and IDMA into resin and the resulting reduction in the fraction of the base monomer (UDMA) in the formulation. These DVCs suggest that chain mobility of a cross-linked polymer is small and that the pathways for unreacted monomers to leach-out are limited. These experimental findings are in line with the results of our earlier structure/composition property studies indicating the improved DVCs were achieved by substituting a more flexible aliphatic UDMA/PEG-U mixture for rigid, aromatic base monomer Bis-GMA and replacing TEGDMA with diluent monomers, such as HEMA or EHMA [32–34]. It is particularly important that the elevated DVC in these systems was not accompanied with excessive polymerization stress. Moreover, in UPE-IDMA2 ACP composites, compared to the IDMA1 counterparts, higher DVC were attained while generating less stress. This phenomenon could be explained by the fact that during the curing process, not all the polymerization shrinkage is transformed into stress but is rather compensated by polymer reorganization. Internal rotation around the central biphenyl bond [35,36] of IDMA2 may allow it to assume multiple conformations, ranging from a planar to a "twisted" form, which may be conducive to such polymer rearrangement to dissipate some of the polymerization-generated stress. It is noteworthy that stresses generated in UPE-IDMA ACP composites (0.6–1.0 MPa), while exceeding the values seen in no-IDMA UPE ACP counterparts, remained well below the polymerization stress levels reported for UDMA/PEG-U/HEMA ACP composites (3.3–4.5 MPa) [37].

Results of UPE-IDMA1 and UPE-IDMA2 resin wettability testing (average contact angle 64.4°) correlated well with the upper thresholds of contact angles reported for commercial resin-based composites (range 31.5–64.5°) [38]. High contact angle values generally imply lower water sorption associated with lesser tooth staining, plaque accumulation, and pathogen adhesion and proliferation. Since, collectively, these factors lower the risk of secondary caries development [39], lesser risk should be associated with the use of restoratives based on the proposed formulations.

Typically, in composites utilizing the reinforcing fillers, a positive correlation exists between the high DVCs and mechanical/chemical stability and the composites longevity [40]. This relationship does not, however, apply to UPE-IDMA ACP composites for a simple reason—the remineralizing ACP filler has no reinforcing ability. The observed reduction in BFS in going from copolymers to ACP composites (60.0% in this study) appears to be marginally lower than the reduction in BFS reported for ACP filled Bis-GMA-based (63.2% reduction) [41], ACP filled EBPADMA-based (69.5% reduction) [41] and ACP filled UDMA-based (69.9% reduction) [7] composites compared to the corresponding copolymers. These consistently lower BFS values seen in ACP composites, regardless of the actual resin matrix, suggest that ACP/resin interlocking is inadequate to achieve better mechanical properties. Consequently, ACP composites' restorative potential should be restricted to dental applications where high mechanical strength is not the main requirement. Class V restorations, for which our experimental material is ultimately intended for, are an example of such applications. Therefore, the observed reduction in BFS of composites vs. copolymers in our experimental systems should not prevent further exploration of UPE-IDMA resins for intended AMRE application. This unwelcomed effect could possibly be ameliorated by introducing, in addition to the remineralizing ACP filler, reinforcing zirconia and silica particles, and/or mixture of silica plus barium silicate glass during AMRE composite fabrication.

The ion release data, recalculated in terms of solution supersaturation with respect to apatite and/or enamel, confirmed the potential of UPE-IDMA ACP composites to regenerate tooth mineral. This finding supports our previous findings [7] that the compositional changes in the resin phase of ACP bioactive composites do not compromise their remineralizing ability. Efficacy of ACP remineralizing composites has so far been documented in two in vitro studies involving bovine [9] and human teeth [10]. To overcome a significant gap that typically exists between the in vitro and in vivo evaluations, testing of the prototype AMRE materials should involve their testing in preclinical settings.

In conclusion, IDMAs of enhanced purity exhibited minimal or no cytotoxicity towards host cells. Their incorporation into UDMA-based matrices did not alter the resins' hydrophobic/hydrophilic balance while improving degree of vinyl conversion and even, in IDMA2 systems, reducing polymerization-generated stress. The ensuing ACP/UDMA-based composites displayed strong remineralizing potential. The observed reduction in BFS of ACP composites should not compromise their intended utilization as AMRE restoratives for Class V caries. The preliminary biological and physicochemical assessments of UDMA/PEG-U/EHMA copolymers and their ACP composites validate their further exploration.

4. Materials and Methods

4.1. Materials

IDMAs: 2-(*N*,*N*-dimethylamino)ethyl methacrylate (DMAEMA), 2-bromoethyl methacrylate (BEMA), and 2,2′-bis(bromomethyl)-1,1′-biphenyl (bBrMbP), polymerization inhibitor butylated hydroxytoluene, and the solvents (absolute ethanol, chloroform ($CHCl_3$), deuterated chloroform ($CDCl_3$), deuterated dimethyl sulfoxide (DMSO-d_6), hexane, and diethyl ether) used for IDMA syntheses and their purification were purchased from Sigma-Aldrich Co., St. Louis, MO, USA.

Biocompatibility: Immortalized human gingival fibroblasts (HGF) and PriGrow III medium were purchased from Applied Biological Materials, Inc. (Richmond, BC, Cananda). Fetal bovine serum was obtained from American Type Culture Collection (Manassas, VA, USA). The LIVE/DEAD® Viability/Cytotoxicity Kit and Dulbecco's phosphate-buffered saline were acquired from Life Technologies, Corp., Grand Island, NY, USA. Methanol (meeting ACS specifications) was purchased from Sigma-Aldrich Co. The CellTiter 96® AQueous One Solution Cell Proliferation Assay was obtained from Promega (Madison, WI, USA).

Resins: UDMA and PEG-U were donated by Esstech, Essington, PA. EHMA, camphorquinone (CQ), and ethyl-4-*N*,*N*-dimethylamino benzoate (4EDMAB) were purchased from Sigma-Aldrich Co.

ACP: $Ca(NO_3)_2$, Na_2HPO_4, $Na_2P_2O_7$ and $ZrOCl_2$ (ACP synthesis), 1-propanol (composite preparations), and NaCl, NaOH, and 4-(2-hydroxyethyl)piperazine-1-ethanesulfonic acid (HEPES) (ion release experiments) were acquired from Sigma-Aldrich Co.

All reagents/solvents were used as received.

4.2. IDMAs: Syntheses and Purification

For IDMA1 synthesis, DMAEMA (10 mmol), BEMA (10 mmol), BHT (1 mmol), and $CHCl_3$ were mixed in a reaction vessel equipped with a reflux column. Reaction mixture was heated (55–60 °C) for 24 h and then washed with hexane. IDMA2 was synthesized by reacting DMAEMA (10 mmol) and bBrMbP (5 mmol) under conditions similar to those employed in IDMA1 synthesis. Crude IDMAs were purified by a multi-step process, using an ethanol-diethyl ether-hexane solvent system. Purified IDMA2 was freeze-dried overnight and the remaining impurities were washed away with $CHCl_3$.

The yield of purified product of IDMA1 and IDMA2 was 25.6% and 79.5%, respectively of their theoretic value.

4.3. IDMAs: Structural Verification

The anticipated IDMAs' structures were confirmed by ^{1}H and ^{13}C NMR, and MS. NMR spectral data (^{1}H, ^{13}C NMR, and HSQC) were interpreted to assign the C and H chemical shifts to their structure.

NMR: Spectra were obtained using a Bruker Avance 2 (600 MHz) spectrometer equipped with a Broadband Observe room temperature probe. Samples were run using $CDCl_3$ and DMSO as solvents and tetramethylsilane (TMS) as an internal standard. Concentrations of the samples analyzed varied, but were generally within 0.1–0.5 M. HSQC was employed for spectra signal assignation.

MS: Mass spectroscope (Quattro Micro, Waters Corp., Millford, MA, USA) was operated in the positive ionization mode. Three kV potential was applied to the electrospray ionization needle and the de-solvation temperature was set at 250 °C. Nitrogen flow and sample injection rates were 500 L/h and 10 μL/min, respectively.

FTIR spectroscopy: FTIR spectra of IDMAs were recorded using a deuterated triglycine sulfate room temperature detector in the spectral range of 4000–500 cm^{-1} (Nexus 670 ThermoNicolet, Nicolet Instrument Corporation, Madison, WI, USA). The samples were measured on a diamond attenuated total reflection cell.

4.4. Biocompatibility Tests

Cell maintenance: Cells were maintained in PriGrow III Medium supplemented with 10% fetal bovine serum (37 °C, 5% CO_2 environment). To initiate experiments, cells were obtained from a subconfluent culture. An improved Neubauer hemocytometer using trypan blue staining and bright field microscopy was utilized to determine cell viability. A Falcon™ 96-well, black/clear, flat-bottomed, tissue culture treated plate (Corning, Inc., Big Flats, NY, USA) were seeded with 10,000 viable cells/well.

Leachability constraints: The cells were exposed to two-fold serial dilutions of IDMAs after 48 h incubation. Concentrations ($\leq$10.66 mmol/L for IDMA1 or $\leq$5.70 mmol/L for IDMA2) were used to approximate the maximum possible exposure, assuming 7% mass fraction in the composite with $\leq$2% leaching. An accelerated ACP UDMA/PEG-U/HEMA leachability study [8] was used to establish these experimental values. Negative control wells were without the dental monomers and/or cells. Cultures were assessed for viability and metabolic activity after 24 h and 72 h exposure. Experiments were performed on five independent occasions with triplicate wells on each plate.

Cell viability: After monomer exposure, cells were washed with Dulbecco's phosphate-buffered saline (without calcium chloride and magnesium chloride). Cells were then incubated for 20 min at room temperature with ethidium homodimer-1 (1 μM) and calcein acetoxymethyl ester (0.658 μM) (optimal stain concentrations were pre-determined by serial dilution). Fluorescence of ethidium homodimer-1 (excitation 530 nm, emission 645 nm) and calcein (excitation 485 nm, emission 530 nm) was assessed with a Spectra Max M5 plate reader (Molecular Devices, Corp., Sunnyvale, CA, USA). Assay controls included live and 70% methanol-treated cells that were subjected to ethidium homodimer-1 and/or calcein acetoxymethyl ester. These control values were used to estimate the percentage of live and dead cells, according to the manufacturer's instructions. In these calculations, the value associated with the live cells stained with calcein acetoxymethyl ester becomes mathematically influential. Consequently, inter-assay control limits were set for these wells (value of each triplicate well needed to be within 20% of their mean).

Cellular metabolic activity: The CellTiter 96® AQueous One Solution Cell Proliferation Assay is a colorimetric method based on the reduction of tetrazolium salt by metabolically intact cells to produce a formazan product. As with other tetrazolium salt assays, it is believed that most of this reduction occurs outside the mitochondrial inner membrane [42].

After assessing cellular viability, the metabolic activity of the cells was estimated using the CellTiter 96® AQueous One Solution Reagent. Specifically, the supernatant was removed and each well received 200 μL culture medium and 40 μL CellTiter 96® AQueous One Solution Reagent. Subsequently, plates were incubated at 37 °C in a 5% CO_2 environment for 40 min. An Epoch microplate spectrophotometer (BioTek Instruments, Inc., Winooski, VT, USA) set at 490 nm was used to determine optical densities. The optical densities were transformed into the percent increase or decrease of that observed in the control group (no monomer) to normalize assay responses. Wells that only contained an equal volume of culture medium served as controls.

4.5. Resin Formulation and Evaluation

UPE resins were formulated from the commercially available UDMA (50.91 mass %), PEG-U (18.18 mass %), EHMA (30.91 mass %) and a conventional visible light initiator system employing CQ (0.2 mass %) and 4EDMAB (0.8 mass %) [8]. Chosen 2.8:1.0:1.7 UDMA:PEG-U:EHMA mass ratio represents the average for the UDMA-based ternary formulations so far explored by our research team. IDMAs were blended into UDMA-based resins at 10 or 20 wt %. These concentrations were chosen based on the previously reported findings [26] that 10 wt % IDMA1 in Bis-GMA/TEGDMA polymers significantly reduced bacterial attachment while 30 wt % IDMA1 did not further reduce bacterial coverage, while diminishing macrophage density and activity. After combining the monomers, their mixture was magnetically stirred (38 rad/s) at room temperature until achieving uniform consistency.

Homogenized resin was pipetted into stainless steel molds (for contact angle evaluation; 13 mm diameter, 1.4 mm height) or hollow glass beams (DVC: 1.9 × 1.9 × 25 mm). Each side of the mold was covered sequentially with Mylar film and a glass slide and the assembly was clamped. Copolymerization was initiated by irradiating specimens for 120 s on each side (Triad 2000, Dentsply International, York, PA, USA). After curing, copolymer samples were de-molded and kept in the dark, under vacuum, for ≥24 h.

Changes in water contact angle (sessile drop technique), an indication of resin's hydrophobicity/ hydrophilicity upon introduction of IDMAs were measured by a drop shape analyzer DSA-100 (Krüss, Matthews, NC, USA; $n = 4$/experimental group).

DVC of UPE-IDMA copolymer specimens was determined by NIR spectroscopic method that monitors the reduction in C=C absorption at 6165 cm^{-1} in the overtone region. By maintaining a constant specimen thickness, a need to use an invariant absorption band as an internal standard has been circumvented. The NIR spectra (n = 3/group) were collected before cure and 24 h post-cure. The DVC was calculated according to the following formula:

$$DVC\ (\%) = (1 - Area_{polymer}/Area_{monomer}) \times 100 \quad (1)$$

where $Area_{polymer}$ and $Area_{monomer}$ represent the areas of 6165 cm^{-1} =C–H bond after and before curing, respectively.

The BFS of copolymer specimens (n = 5/group) was determined using a piston-on-three-ball loading cell with computer-controlled Universal Testing Machine (Instron 5500R; Instron Corp., Canton, MA, USA) supported by Testworks4 software. The BFS values were calculated according to the ASTM F394-78 specification. The same methodology was applied to measure BFS of ACP composite specimens.

4.6. Remineralizing ACP Composites

4.6.1. ACP Filler: Synthesis and Characterization

ACP was synthesized employing our well-established protocols [32–34]. It precipitated instantaneously in a closed system at 22 °C upon rapidly mixing equal volumes of an 800 mmol/L $Ca(NO_3)_2$ solution and a 536 mmol/L Na_2HPO_4 solution that contained a molar fraction of 2% $Na_4P_2O_7$ (to prevent premature ACP conversion to hydroxyapatite). The suspension was filtered, the solid phase washed subsequently with ice-cold ammoniated water and acetone, and then lyophilized. Amorphousness of the filler was validated by FTIR and X-ray diffraction (XRD; Rigaku X-ray diffractometer, Rigaku/USA Inc., Danvers, MA, USA). Particle size distribution (PSD; SA-CP3 analyzer, Shimadzu Scientific Instruments Inc., Columbia, MD, USA) was assessed before (as-made ACP) and after milling (5 g of ACP in 15 g of 1-propanol; 2 h at 200 rpm, Pulverisette 7 ball mill (Fritsch, Germany). To avoid exposure to humidity, ACP was kept under vacuum (2.7 kPa) until used in composite preparation.

4.6.2. Fabrication of ACP Composites

ACP was dispersed in 1-propanol, sonicated 1 h in a water bath, and mixed with the appropriate amount of UPE or UPE-IDMA resin to yield composite of homogeneous appearance containing 60 mass % resin and 40 mass % filler. Solvent was evaporated at 22 °C, under vacuum (overnight) and continuous magnetic stirring. The composite paste was then tightly packed into stainless steel molds (13 mm diameter, 1.4 mm height). Both sides of the mold were covered sequentially with Mylar film and a glass slide. The assembly was clamped and each side irradiated for 120 s with visible light (Triad 2000, Dentsply International, York, PA, USA). After curing, samples were de-molded and kept in the dark, under vacuum, for $\geq$24 h before testing. More detailed descriptions of composite fabrication have been reported [32–34].

4.6.3. Ion Release as Predictor of Remineralization Potential of ACP Composites

The ion release experiments were based on thermodynamic tenets, which have been previously used to indicate a composites potential for mineral repair [9,10]. For experiments (n = 5/group), composite disk specimens were individually immersed in 90 mL of HEPES-buffered (7.4 pH) 0.13 M NaCl solution. Immersing solutions were replaced with fresh buffers at 1, 2, 4, 8, and 16 weeks. Solution Ca and P concentrations were determined by atomic emission spectroscopy (AES; Prodigy High Dispersion ICP, Teledyne Leeman Labs, Hudson, NH, USA). The AES data were used to calculate the solutions' thermodynamic stability (Chemist Application version 1.0.1.0; Micromath Research, St. Louis, MO) and their supersaturation (supersaturation index, that relates the ion activity product defined as $[Ca]^{10}[PO_4]^6[OH]^2$ and hydroxyapatite's or enamel's solubility product) [41].

4.6.4. Simultaneous Assessment of Polymerization Stress and DVC

Simultaneous real-time measurements of polymerization stress and DVC of UPE-IDMA ACP composites employed the cantilever beam-based tensometer coupled with an in situ NIR spectrometer [43]. The synchronized stress/DVC data were collected for 15 min at clinically-relevant instrumental compliance of 0.33 µm/N. The 2.5 mm sample diameter and 2 mm sample height corresponded to a C-factor (ratio of bonded/unbonded area) of 0.625 [44,45]. Specimens, placed between two flat methacrylate-silane treated quartz rods (to promote specimen/rod adhesion), were cured (LZ1-10DB0, Mouser Electronics, Mansfield, TX, USA) for 40 s at 500 mW/cm^2 light intensity. The axial stress due to the specimen's shrinkage upon polymerization caused a deflection of the beam. This deflection, recorded by a displacement sensor, was used to quantify the polymerization stress. To determine the DVC (Equation (1)), NIR signal was guided through the sides of the specimen via optical fiber cable.

4.7. Statistical Analyses

Analysis of variance (ANOVA) was used to analyze experimental data as a function of material makeup, storage/exposure time or any other relevant factor included in the experimental design. When overall statistically significant effects were found with ANOVA, multiple comparisons (2-sided, $\alpha = 0.05$) were used to determine significant differences between groups (SigmaPlot™ 11.0; Systat® Software, Inc., San Jose, CA, USA or Excel2016, Microsoft Corp. (Redmond, WA, USA). Excel2016 or DeltaGraph6 for Windows® (Red Rock Software, Inc., Salt Lake City, UT, USA) were used to create graphics.

Acknowledgments: Described work was supported by the ADA, ADA Foundation, and a grant from the National Institute of Dental and Craniofacial Research (R01-DE26122-02). Authors gratefully acknowledge donation of monomers from Esstech, Essington, PA, USA. Special thanks to Richard M. Pires, Montgomery College, Germantown, MD for aiding the interpretation of mass spectroscopy data.

Author Contributions: S.A.F. conceptualized monomer synthesis and purification, fabrication of resins and composites and their physicochemical and mechanical evaluation. U.C.O. was instrumental in monomer characterization and together with A.A.G., contributed to physicochemical and mechanical testing of copolymers and composites. D.R.B. conceptualized and A.A.G. performed cytotoxicity experiments. D.R.B. and D.S. performed literature compilation and statistical data interpretation. All authors contributed to the preparation of this manuscript.

Disclaimer: Certain commercial materials and equipment are identified in this article to specify the experimental procedure. In no instance does such identification imply recommendation or endorsement by the ADA Foundation or that the material or equipment identified is necessarily the best available for the purpose.

Abbreviations

List of Acronyms

ACP	amorphous calcium phosphate
ADA	American Dental Association
AM	antimicrobial
AM_{adh}	antimicrobial monomer with improved adhesiveness
AM_{cpl}	antimicrobial monomer with improved coupling to filler
AM_{misc}	antimicrobial monomer with improved miscibility
AMRE	antimicrobial and remineralizing
ANOVA	analysis of variance
BEMA	2-bromoethyl methacrylate
BFS	biaxial flexural strength
Bis-GMA	2,2-bis[p-(2-hydroxy-3-methacryloxypropoxy)phenyl]propane
Ca	calcium
CQ	camphorquinone
d_m	median diameter

DVC	degree of vinyl conversion
4EDMAB	ethyl-4-*N*,*N*-dimethylamino benzoate
EHMA	ethyl 2-(hydroxymethyl)acrylate
FTIR	Fourier-transform infrared spectroscopy
HEMA	2-hydroxyethyl methacrylate
HGF	human gingival fibroblast
HSQC	heteronuclear single quantum coherence
IDMA1	2-(methacryloyloxy)-*N*-(2-(methacryloyloxy)ethyl)-*N*,*N*-dimethylethan-1-aminium bromide
IDMA2	*N*,*N*′-([1,1′-biphenyl]-2,2′-diylbis(methylene))bis(2-(methacryloyloxy)-*N*,*N*-dimethylethan-1-aminium) bromide
MS	mass spectroscopy
n	number of specimens (or repetitive experiments)
NIR	near infra-red
NMR	nuclear magnetic resonance
P	phosphorus
PEG-U	poly(ethylene glycol) extended urethane dimethacrylate
pH	-log (molar concentration of hydrogen ions)
PO_4	phosphate
PSD	particle size distribution
QADM	quaternary ammonium dimethacrylates
SD	standard deviation
SEM	standard error of the mean
TEGDMA	triethylene glycol dimethacrylate
UDMA	urethane dimethacrylate
UPE	UDMA/PEG-U/EHMA resin
XRD	X-ray diffraction

References

1. Imazato, S. Antibacterial properties of resin composites and dentin bonding systems. *Dent. Mater.* **2003**, *19*, 449–457. [CrossRef]
2. Imazato, S. Bio-active restorative materials with antibacterial effects: New dimension of innovation in restorative dentistry. *Dent. Mater. J.* **2009**, *28*, 11–19. [CrossRef] [PubMed]
3. Cochrane, N.J.; Cai, F.; Huq, N.L.; Burrow, M.F.; Reynolds, E.C. New approaches to enhanced remineralization of tooth enamel. *J. Dent. Res.* **2010**, *89*, 1187–1197. [CrossRef] [PubMed]
4. Mickenautsch, S.; Mount, G.; Yengopal, V. Therapeutic effect of glass-ionomers: An overview of evidence. *Aust. Dent. J.* **2011**, *56*, 10–15. [CrossRef] [PubMed]
5. Rodrigues, J.A.; Lussi, A.; Seemann, R.; Neuhaus, K.W. Prevention of crown and root caries in adults. *Periodontology 2000* **2011**, *55*, 231–249. [CrossRef] [PubMed]
6. Skrtic, D.; Antonucci, J.M. Dental composites: Bioactive polymeric amorphous calcium phosphate-based. In *Encyclopedia of Biomedical Polymers and Polymeric Biomaterials*; Taylor and Francis: New York, NY, USA, 2015; pp. 2443–2462.
7. Antonucci, J.M.; Skrtic, D. Fine-tuning of polymeric resins and their interfaces with amorphous calcium phosphate. A strategy for designing effective remineralizing dental composites. *Polymers* **2010**, *2*, 378–392. [CrossRef] [PubMed]
8. Skrtic, D.; Antonucci, J.M. Bioactive polymeric composites for tooth mineral regeneration: Physicochemical and cellular aspects. *J. Funct. Biomat.* **2011**, *2*, 271–307. [CrossRef] [PubMed]
9. Skrtic, D.; Hailer, A.W.; Takagi, S.; Antonucci, J.M.; Eanes, E.D. Quantitative assessment of the efficacy of amorphous calcium phosphate/methacrylate composites in remineralizing caries-like lesions artificially produced in bovine enamel. *J. Dent. Res.* **1996**, *75*, 1679–1686. [CrossRef] [PubMed]
10. Langhorst, S.E.; O'Donnell, J.N.; Skrtic, D. In vitro remineralization of enamel by polymeric amorphous calcium phosphate composite: Quantitative microradiographic study. *Dent. Mater.* **2009**, *25*, 884–891. [CrossRef] [PubMed]

11. Chen, C.Z.; Beck-Tan, N.C.; Dhurjati, P.; van Dyk, T.K.; LaRossa, R.A.; Cooper, S.L. Quaternary ammonium functionalized poly (propylene imine) dendrimers as effective antimicrobials: Structure–activity studies. *Biomacromolecules* **2000**, *1*, 473–480. [CrossRef] [PubMed]
12. Murata, H.; Koepsel, R.R.; Matyjaszewski, K.; Russell, A.J. Permanent, non-leaching antibacterial surface—2: How high density cationic surfaces kill bacterial cells. *Biomaterials* **2007**, *28*, 4870–4879. [CrossRef] [PubMed]
13. Gottenbos, B.; van der Mei, H.C.; Klatter, F.; Nieuwenhuis, P.; Busscher, H.J. In vitro and in vivo antimicrobial activity of covalently coupled quaternary ammonium silane coatings on silicone rubber. *Biomaterials* **2002**, *23*, 1417–1423. [CrossRef]
14. Lee, S.B.; Koepsel, R.R.; Morley, S.W.; Matyjaszewski, K.; Sun, Y.; Russell, A.J. Permanent, nonleaching antibacterial surfaces. 1. Synthesis by atom transfer radical polymerization. *Biomacromolecules* **2004**, *5*, 877–882. [CrossRef] [PubMed]
15. Lu, G.; Wu, D.; Fu, R. Studies on the synthesis and antibacterial activities of polymeric quaternary ammonium salts from dimethylaminoethyl methacrylate. *React. Funct. Polym.* **2007**, *67*, 355–366. [CrossRef]
16. Ikeda, T.; Hirayama, H.; Yamaguchi, H.; Tazuke, S.; Watanabe, M. Polycationic biocides with pendant active groups: Molecular weight dependence of antibacterial activity. *Antimicrob. Agents Chemother.* **1986**, *30*, 132–136. [CrossRef] [PubMed]
17. Ikeda, T.; Yamaguchi, H.; Tazuke, S. Molecular weight dependence of antibacterial activity in cationic disinfectants. *J. Bioact. Compat. Polym.* **1990**, *5*, 31–41. [CrossRef]
18. Kenawy, E.-R.; Worley, S.; Broughton, R. The chemistry and applications of antimicrobial polymers: A state-of-the-art review. *Biomacromolecules* **2007**, *8*, 1359–1384. [CrossRef] [PubMed]
19. Nonaka, T.; Hua, L.; Ogata, T.; Kurihara, S. Synthesis of water-soluble thermosensitive polymers having phosphonium groups from methacryloyloxyethyl trialkyl phosphonium chlorides–*N*-isopropylacrylamide copolymers and their functions. *J. Appl. Polym. Sci.* **2003**, *87*, 386–393. [CrossRef]
20. Thebault, P.; Taffin de Givenchy, E.; Levy, R.; Vandenberghe, Y.; Guittard, F.; Geribaldi, S. Preparation and antimicrobial behaviour of quaternary ammonium thiol derivatives able to be grafted on metal surfaces. *Eur. J. Med. Chem.* **2009**, *44*, 717–724. [CrossRef] [PubMed]
21. Ebi, N.; Imazato, S.; Noiri, Y.; Ebisu, S. Inhibitory effects of resin composite containing bactericide-immobilized filler on plaque accumulation. *Dent. Mater.* **2001**, *17*, 485–491. [CrossRef]
22. Imazato, S.; Tarumi, H.; Kato, S.; Ebisu, S. Water sorption and colour stability of composites containing the antibacterial monomer MDPB. *J. Dent.* **1999**, *27*, 279–283. [CrossRef]
23. Thome, T.; Mayer, M.P.; Imazato, S.; Geraldo-Martins, V.R.; Marques, M.M. In vitro analysis of inhibitory effects of the antibacterial monomer MDPB-containing restorations on the progression of secondary root caries. *J. Dent.* **2009**, *37*, 705–711. [CrossRef] [PubMed]
24. Li, F.; Weir, M.D.; Chen, J.; Xu, H.H. Comparison of quaternary ammonium-containing with nano-silver-containing adhesive in antibacterial properties and cytotoxicity. *Dent. Mater.* **2013**, *29*, 450–461. [CrossRef] [PubMed]
25. Melo, M.A.; Guedes, S.F.; Xu, H.H.; Rodrigues, L.K. Nanotechnology-based restorative materials for dental caries management. *Trends Biotechnol.* **2013**, *31*, 459–467. [CrossRef] [PubMed]
26. Antonucci, J.M.; Zeiger, D.N.; Tang, K.; Lin-Gibson, S.; Fowler, B.O.; Lin, N.J. Synthesis and characterization of dimethacrylates containing quaternary ammonium functionalities for dental applications. *Dent. Mater.* **2012**, *28*, 219–228. [CrossRef] [PubMed]
27. Cheng, L.; Zhang, K.; Weir, M.D.; Melo, M.A.; Zhou, X.; Xu, H.H. Nanotechnology strategies for antibacterial and remineralizing composites and adhesives to tackle dental caries. *Nanomedicine* **2015**, *10*, 627–641. [CrossRef] [PubMed]
28. Cheng, L.; Zhang, K.; Zhou, C.C.; Weir, M.D.; Zhou, X.D.; Xu, H.H. One-year water-ageing of calcium phosphate composite containing nano-silver and quaternary ammonium to inhibit biofilms. *Int. J. Oral Sci.* **2016**, *8*, 172–181. [CrossRef] [PubMed]
29. Cheng, L.; Weir, M.D.; Xu, H.H.; Antonucci, J.M.; Kraigsley, A.M.; Lin, N.J.; Lin-Gibson, S.; Zhou, X. Antibacterial amorphous calcium phosphate nanocomposites with a quaternary ammonium dimethacrylate and silver nanoparticles. *Dent. Mater.* **2012**, *28*, 561–572. [CrossRef] [PubMed]
30. Winstead, A.; Hart, K.; Hijji, Y.M.; Jasinski, J.P.; Butcher, R.J. 1-(5-Carboxy-pent-yl)-2,3,3-trimethyl-3*H*-indol-1-ium bromide monohydrate. *Acta Crystallogr. E* **2009**, *66*, o171–o172. [CrossRef] [PubMed]

31. Bienek, D.R.; Frukhtbeyn, S.A.; Giuseppetti, A.A.; Okeke, U.C.; Pires, R.M.; Antonucci, J.M.; Skrtic, D. Physiochemical characterization and biocompatibility of ionic dimethacrylates for dental restorations. *Adv. Mater. Sci. Eng.* **2018**, submitted.
32. Antonucci, J.M.; Fowler, B.O.; Weir, M.D.; Skrtic, D.; Stansbury, J.W. Effect of ethyl-alpha-hydroxymethylacrylate on selected properties of copolymers and ACP resin composites. *J. Mater. Sci. Mater. Med.* **2008**, *19*, 3263–3271. [CrossRef] [PubMed]
33. Antonucci, J.M.; Skrtic, D. Bioactive and biocompatible polymeric composites based on amorphous calcium phosphate. In *Integrated Biomaterials for Medical Applications*; Ramalingam, M., Tiwari, A., Ramakrishna, S., Kobayashi, H., Eds.; Scrivener Publishing: Salem, MA, USA, 2012; pp. 67–119.
34. Skrtic, D.; Antonucci, J.M. Dental composites based on amorphous calcium phosphate—Resin composition/physicochemical properties study. *J. Biomater. Appl.* **2007**, *21*, 375–393. [CrossRef] [PubMed]
35. Akiyama, M.; Watanabe, T.; Kakihana, M. Internal rotation of biphenyl in solution studied by IR and NMR spectra. *J. Phys. Chem.* **1986**, *90*, 1752–1755. [CrossRef]
36. Mazzanti, A.; Lunazzi, L.; Minzoni, M.; Anderson, J.E. Rotation in biphenyls with a single ortho-substituent. *J. Org. Chem.* **2006**, *71*, 5474–5481. [CrossRef] [PubMed]
37. Antonucci, J.M.; Regnault, W.F.; Skrtic, D. Polymerization shrinkage and stress development in amorphous calcium phosphate/urethane dimethacrylate polymeric composites. *J. Compos. Mater.* **2010**, *44*, 355. [CrossRef] [PubMed]
38. Da Silva, E.M.; Almeida, G.S.; Poskus, L.T.; Guimaraes, J.G. Relationship between the degree of conversion, solubility and salivary sorption of a hybrid and a nanofilled resin composite. *J. Appl. Oral Sci.* **2008**, *16*, 161–166. [CrossRef] [PubMed]
39. Fu, J.; Liu, W.; Hao, Z.; Wu, X.; Yin, J.; Panjiyar, A.; Liu, X.; Shen, J.; Wang, H. Characterization of a low shrinkage dental composite containing bismethylene spiroorthocarbonate expanding monomer. *Int. J. Mol. Sci.* **2014**, *15*, 2400–2412. [CrossRef] [PubMed]
40. Braga, R.R.; Ferracane, J.L. Contraction stress related to degree of conversion and reaction kinetics. *J. Dent. Res.* **2002**, *81*, 114–118. [CrossRef] [PubMed]
41. O'Donnell, J.N.; Langhorst, S.E.; Fow, M.D.; Antonucci, J.M.; Skrtic, D. Light-cured dimethacrylate-based resins and their composites: Comparative study of mechanical strength, water sorption and ion release. *J. Bioact. Compat. Polym.* **2008**, *23*, 207–226. [CrossRef] [PubMed]
42. Berridge, M.V.; Tan, A.S. Characterization of the cellular reduction of 3-(4,5-dimethylthiazol-2-yl)-2,5-diphenyltetrazolium bromide (MTT): Subcellular localization, substrate dependence, and involvement of mitochondrial electron transport in MTT reduction. *Arch. Biochem. Biophys.* **1993**, *303*, 474–482. [CrossRef] [PubMed]
43. Wang, Z.; Landis, F.A.; Giuseppetti, A.A.; Lin-Gibson, S.; Chiang, M.Y. Simultaneous measurement of polymerization stress and curing kinetics for photo-polymerized composites with high filler contents. *Dent. Mater.* **2014**, *30*, 1316–1324. [CrossRef] [PubMed]
44. Wang, Z.; Chiang, M.Y. Correlation between polymerization shrinkage stress and C-factor depends upon cavity compliance. *Dent. Mater.* **2016**, *32*, 343–352. [CrossRef] [PubMed]
45. Wang, Z.; Chiang, M.Y. System compliance dictates the effect of composite filler content on polymerization shrinkage stress. *Dent. Mater.* **2016**, *32*, 551–560. [CrossRef] [PubMed]

6

Electrospun Scaffolds Containing Silver-Doped Hydroxyapatite with Antimicrobial Properties for Applications in Orthopedic and Dental Bone Surgery

Thomas E. Paterson [1,†], Rui Shi [2,†], Jingjing Tian [3,4,†], Caroline J. Harrison [1], Mailys De Sousa Mendes [5], Paul V. Hatton [1,*], Zhou Li [3,*] and Ilida Ortega [1]

1. School of Clinical Dentistry, University of Sheffield, Shefield 0114, UK; t.paterson@sheffield.ac.uk (T.E.P.); c.j.harrison@sheffield.ac.uk (C.J.H.); i.ortega@sheffield.ac.uk (I.O.)
2. Beijing Laboratory of Biomedical Materials, Institute of Traumatology and Orthopaedics, Beijing Jishuitan Hospital, Beijing 100083, China; shirui@jst-hosp.com.cn
3. Beijing Key Laboratory of Micro-nano Energy and Sensor, Beijing institute of Nanoenergy and Nanosystems, Chinese Academy of Sciences, Beijing 100083, China; tianjingjing@pumch.cn
4. Central Laboratory, Peking Union Medical College Hospital, Peking Union Medical College and Chinese Academy of Medical Sciences, Beijing 100730, China
5. Certara, Simcyp division, Sheffield 0114, UK; mailys.mendes@certara.com

* Correspondence: paul.hatton@sheffield.ac.uk (P.V.H.); zli@binn.cas.cn (Z.L.)

† These authors have contributed equally to the work.

Abstract: Preventing the development of osteomyelitis while enhancing bone regeneration is challenging, with relatively little progress to date in translating promising technologies to the clinic. Nanoscale hydroxyapatite (nHA) has been employed as a bone graft substitute, and recent work has shown that it may be modified with silver to introduce antimicrobial activity against known pathogens. The aim of this study was to incorporate silver-doped nHA into electrospun scaffolds for applications in bone repair. Silver-doped nHA was produced using a modified, rapid mixing, wet precipitation method at 2, 5, 10 mol.% silver. The silver-doped nHA was added at 20 wt.% to a polycaprolactone solution for electrospinning. Bacteria studies demonstrated reduced bacterial presence, with *Escherichia coli* and *Staphylococcus aureus* undetectable after 96 h of exposure. Mesenchymal stem cells (MSCs) were used to study both toxicity and osteogenicity of the scaffolds using PrestoBlue® and alkaline phosphatase (ALP) assays. Innovative silver nHA scaffolds significantly reduced *E. coli* and *S. aureus* bacterial populations while maintaining cytocompatibility with mammalian cells and enhancing the differentiation of MSCs into osteoblasts. It was concluded that silver-doped nHA containing scaffolds have the potential to act as an antimicrobial device while supporting bone tissue healing for applications in orthopedic and dental bone surgery.

Keywords: electrospinning; antimicrobial; nano-hydroxyapatite; silver; toxicity; bone regeneration

---

1. Introduction

Preventing deep bone infections after surgery and enhancing bone regeneration reduces the time required for patient recovery and the costs associated with long hospital stays. Deep bone infections are very challenging to treat once established due to the difficulty of achieving a suitable antibiotic concentration in the affected area and ensuring all bacteria have been removed. Bacteria such as *Staphylococcus aureus* (*S. aureus*) and *Escherichia coli* (*E. coli*) are responsible for causing bone infections post-surgery [1,2], and the application of excessive antibiotics can lead to antimicrobial resistance. Antibacterial poly(methyl methacrylate) beads have been used routinely for treating infections in a reactive manner with additional disadvantages of requiring surgical removal after the treatment ends [3]. Silver has often been used to successfully treat bacterial and fungal infections [4,5] and can be delivered in a localized area. Metallic implants coated with silver have been investigated to prevent infections [6]. However, silver by itself does not enhance wound healing and can have a toxic effect on mammalian cells at higher concentrations [7,8].

To facilitate bone healing, surgeons currently employ hydroxyapatite in granular or paste form to stimulate bone regrowth. Hydroxyapatite is the mineral component of bone and can be manufactured synthetically and has been demonstrated to aid in bone regeneration [9]. Nanoscale hydroxyapatite (nHA) is an increasingly popular biomaterial due to its similarity to the hydroxyapatite in human bone and tooth enamel. Our group recently produced a bioinspired nHA material through a rapid mix preparation, which is slightly calcium deficient to better mimic biological apatite [10]. Using nHA-based medical devices to increase the regeneration rate of the bone after surgery could greatly decrease patient healing times. Unfortunately, despite its success in aiding bone regeneration, hydroxyapatite has no innate antimicrobial properties to prevent infection. Moreover, the implantation of medical devices provides an increased risk of bacterial colonization and eventual biofilm formation if left untreated [11]. Once a biofilm has been established it is very difficult to treat using antibiotics and even surgical intervention involves a high risk of reoccurrence [12].

There is growing interest in using a combination of silver and hydroxyapatite to produce a material with both antimicrobial/antifungal [13,14] and bone-regenerating properties [15–18]. Jiang et al. [19] produced foamed polyurethane scaffolds containing up to 40 wt.% silver phosphate particles (Ag_3PO_4) and nHA. These mold-formed scaffolds were porous and eluted silver for up to 22 days without toxic effects on the human osteosarcoma cell line MG63. Saravanan et al. [20] produced scaffolds using the freeze-drying technique incorporating nano-hydroxyapatite with nanoparticles of silver. Wilcock et al. [21] developed a novel, rapid mixing, wet precipitation method of producing bioinspired, nanoscale hydroxyapatite crystals doped with silver for antimicrobial action. A degradable scaffold could be placed against existing implants or used to hold packed bone substitutes (e.g., bone chips) into a bone defect.

The biomaterials' research community has been keenly interested in using electrospinning as a containment system for ceramic-derived materials including hydroxyapatite [22]. Electrospinning is a technique for producing fibrous scaffolds that roughly resemble the body's extracellular matrix. These can be made porous to allow cell thoroughfare or nanoscale to act as a barrier to cells, fulfilling a wide variety of applications. Ciraldo et al. [23] investigated three different manufacturing approaches using mesoporous glasses containing silver. These were glass coatings prepared using electrospraying, sol-gel methods, and directly spinning with polycaprolactone (PCL). For electrospinning, the authors were limited to 5% mesoporous glasses in PCL but did not investigate antimicrobial action. However, a recent paper by the same group demonstrated that the mesoporous glasses loaded with silver were antimicrobial [24]. Anjaneyulu et al. [25] manufactured doped hydroxyapatite through the sol-gel method and electrospun with poly(vinyl alcohol). Schneider et al. [26] electrospun tricalcium phosphate nanoparticles into poly(lactic-co-glycolic acid) (PLGA) scaffolds, looking at a single concentration of silver, but did not investigate mammalian toxicity of the scaffold. Furtos et al. [27] electrospun a PCL scaffold to contain both nHA and amoxicillin, which they tested against four bacterial strains and found that increasing the nHA content reduced the loading efficiency of the antibiotic.

A variety of polymers and calcium compounds have been used for producing these antimicrobial scaffolds. Different manufacturing technologies have also been employed to produce these as scaffolds. A relatively small number of the above publications have reported testing their material with primary mesenchymal stem cells (MSCs), which are key to understanding bone-healing mechanisms. Few of the published reports have investigated microbiological testing beyond agar diffusion assays with no time course elution antimicrobial testing.

Here we present the fabrication of novel, dual-function scaffolds that combine silver to impart antimicrobial properties and hydroxyapatite to enhance bone regeneration. Our laboratory previously developed a silver-doped nano-hydroxyapatite material formed by the wet precipitation method [21].

Here we show the incorporation of this innovative material into an electrospun scaffold alongside a thorough investigation of metal ion release, antimicrobial activity against clinically relevant bacterial strains, and in vitro biocompatibility using cultured mammalian MSCs. This research has provided an important proof-of-concept study that has the potential to underpin the development of a new generation of dual-action medical devices to address the growing challenges of deep bone infection and antimicrobial resistance.

2. Materials and Methods

2.1. Silver Nano-Hydroxyapatite ($Ca_{10}(PO_4)_6(OH)_2$) Manufacture via Wet Precipitation

This was based on our previously published methods [10,21]. In brief, calcium hydroxide (Sigma Aldrich, Dorset, UK) (50 mmol) was suspended in 500 mL deionized water (dH_2O) into which 0, 1, 2.5, or 5 mmol silver nitrate (Sigma Aldrich, UK) (corresponding to 0, 2, 5, or 10 mol%, respectively) was added and stirred at 400 rpm for 1 h on a hotplate (Fisher Scientific, Loughborough, UK) at 90 °C. Phosphoric acid (Sigma Aldrich, UK) (30 mmol) was dissolved in 250 mL dH_2O, poured into the calcium and silver preparation, and stirred for a further hour. The suspension was left to settle overnight, after which the supernatant was poured off and the silver-doped nHA suspension was washed with dH_2O (3 × 500 mL). The silver-doped nHA suspensions were dried at 60 °C and ground in an agate mortar and pestle.

2.2. Imaging the Silver Nano-Hydroxyapatite and Electrospun Fibers Using SEM

Dried nHA powder or a 5 × 5 mm section of electrospun scaffold was attached to a carbon tab and sputter gold coated and then imaged using a TESCAN VEGA3 SEM (Tescan, Brno, Czech Republic) with an accelerating voltage of 15 kV.

2.3. Imaging the Silver Nano-Hydroxyapatite Using Transmission Electron Microscopy (TEM) and Energy-Dispersive X-Ray Spectroscopy (EDX)

The nHA powder (0.1 g) was dispersed in ethanol in an ultrasonic bath (ThermoFisher, Shanghai, China) for 1 h and a drop was placed onto a copper mounting grid with carbon film and allowed to dry under ambient conditions. Samples were then imaged on a transmission electron microscope (Tecnai G2 F30, ThermoFisher, Shanghai, China) under standard imaging and EDX detecting elements Ca, P, Ag, and O. EDX settings used were 20 kV, takeoff 14.8, amp time 7 µs, and 126.5 eV resolution.

2.4. Analyzing Crystal Phases Present Using X-Ray Diffraction (XRD)

Phase analysis was performed on powdered samples using XRD (STOE IP, Darmstadt, Germany) with Cu Kα λ = 1.5418 Å radiation to determine the crystal structure of the materials. The diffractometer was operated at 40 kV and 35 mA, with a 2θ range of 20–50°. The following The International Centre for Diffraction Data Powder Diffraction (ICDD-PDF) cards were used for phase identification: 9-432 hydroxyapatite, 6-505 silver phosphate.

2.5. Electrospinning Polycaprolactone (PCL) and Incorporating the Ag–nHA

Polycaprolactone (average 80,000 Mn, Sigma, UK) was dissolved in a specific solvent and then propelled by an electric field onto a collector where polymer fibers formed as the solvent evaporated. Adding both the silver-doped and undoped nHA powder to the solution at 20 wt.% allowed it to be incorporated into the electrospun scaffold. PCL (1.5 g) was dissolved into a solvent mixture (90% Dichloromethane [DCM], 10% Dimethylformamide [DMF]) (Sigma Aldrich, UK) and stirred using a magnetic stirrer bar (5 mm bar, Sigma Aldrich, UK) for 2 h. The nHA powders were incorporated at 20 wt.% of the PCL component and added into the dissolved PCL solution. The polymer-ceramic-solvent mixtures were placed in an ultrasonic bath for 30 min, before stirring using a magnetic stirrer bar for 30 min to ensure even distribution of powder in the solution. A 1-mL Luer-Lok syringe (BD, EU) was loaded with 1 mL of the PCL/nHA solution and this was electrospun using a custom electrospinning rig described previously [28]. In total, 2 mL of solution at 1 mL/hr was used to fabricate each scaffold at 17 kV with a spinning gap between the needle and collector of 20 cm.

2.6. *Accelerated Degradation Study of Electrospun Scaffolds and Release Profile*

To investigate the rate at which nHA was released during scaffold degradation, an accelerated degradation study was performed over 30 days. Samples were weighed and added to a 5-mL solution of 0.1 M NaOH (Sigma Aldrich, UK) in dH_2O and placed in an oven at 37 °C. At each time point (days 0, 1, 7, 14, 21, and 28) material was also weighed and 0.5 mL of solution was removed, which was replaced with fresh solution. The solutions obtained were diluted to 5 mL using dH_2O.

2.7. *Inductively Coupled Plasma (ICP) Measurement of Material and Degradation Product*

To ascertain the presence and abundance of various elements within the sample, ICP was utilized. Solid samples (e.g., 0.25 g–0.5 g) were weighed into a glass tube and 9 mL of concentrated hydrochloric acid (Sigma Aldrich, UK) added and 3 mL of concentrated nitric acid (Sigma Aldrich, UK) added. The samples were then placed into the heating block and the temperature was gradually raised to 150 °C and maintained at this temperature for 30 min. After removal from the block and cooling, the samples were diluted to 50 mL with 1% nitric acid. Samples were diluted down to 1 in 100 for analysis. Samples were analyzed using an ICP-OES (Spectro-Ciros-Vision Optical Emission Spectrometer (Spectro, Kleve, Germany) using a procedure with a detection limit of at least 10 ppm.

2.8. *Scaffold Preparation for Cell Culture*

Disks of each electrospun scaffold were prepared and sterilized prior to culture with cells. Using a 13 mm cork borer, disks (13 mm) of each scaffold were punched out of the primary collector sheet. On the day of use, the culture scaffolds were disinfected with 70% ethanol (Sigma Aldrich, UK) in dH_2O for 30 min and then washed three times in dH_2O for 5 min.

2.9. *Contact Bacterial Toxicity Test*

Antimicrobial activity was investigated using a classical diffusion agar assay. Isolates of *E. coli* and *S. aureus* were purchased from the China Center of Industrial Culture Collection (CICC, Beijing, China): *E. coli*, CICC23657 and *S. aureus*, CICC10384. The bacterial suspensions at stationary phase were firstly obtained by culture in LB (Luria-Bertani) medium overnight at 37 °C in a 120-rpm shaker. Then 1 mL of the *E. coli* and *S. aureus* suspensions were pipetted from the overnight phase into another 100-mL flask containing 50 mL of fresh LB. The mixture was then cultured at 37 °C for another 6 h to obtain bacterial suspensions at exponential growth phase. After that, the bacterial suspension was centrifuged at 8000 rpm, washed, and resuspended in sterilized physiological saline to reach a concentration of 1×10^7 colony forming units (CFU)/mL. Then, 0.1 mL of the bacteria suspension with 1×10^7 CFU/mL was pipetted and plated on the agar plate uniformly. Three disks of the electrospun material (12 mm diameter) were placed on each Petri dish. These were incubated at 37 °C for 24 h. The zone of inhibition ring around the electrospun scaffolds was measured.

2.10. *Antimicrobial Diffusion Toxicity Test*

A disk of the electrospun scaffold (12 mm diameter) was immersed into the bacteria suspension (10 mL) containing 1 mL 10^7 CFU/mL and 9 mL sterile physiological saline in a 15-mL falcon tube. The falcon tubes were placed on a carousel (IKA, Staufen, Germany) and rotated 360° in the z axis at 30 rpm in an incubator at 37 °C. At the time points 3, 18, 24, 48, 72, and 96 h, 200 μL of phosphate buffered saline (PBS) was removed and serially diluted to 10^{-7} before 100 μL of diluted solutions were added to an agar plate and incubated for 24 h before imaging. The CFUs on plates were counted using the dilution, which was the highest with all bacterial colonies visible as single entities.

2.11. Rat Mesenchymal Stem Cell (MSC) Isolation and Passage

MSCs were isolated from four 4–5-week-old male Wistar rat femurs following the method previously described in literature [29,30]. Briefly, the femur was removed from the rats, opened at both ends, and flushed with media. This was then cultured to collect adherent cells, cells from all rats were intermixed, and cells were passaged twice before use. Cells were cultured in minimum essential medium (αMEM) supplemented with 10 U/mL penicillin (Sigma Aldrich, UK), 0.1 mg/mL streptomycin (Sigma Aldrich, UK), 20 mM alanyl-glutamine (Sigma Aldrich, UK), and 10% v/v fetal bovine serum (FBS; Biosera, Heathfield, UK). Cells were passaged 1:5 using trypsin-EDTA (ethylenediaminetetraacetic acid, Sigma Aldrich) and used below passage 10 for toxicity studies and below passage 5 for differentiation studies.

2.12. Noncontact Mammalian Cell Toxicity Study

Toxicity of elution from the electrospun scaffolds was measured by suspending the material over on cultured cells for 24 h. Both primary rat MSCs and the established fibroblast 3T3 cell line were used to test this material. Both cell lines were treated the same in the experiment apart from the rat MSCs were cultured in αMEM as described above and the 3T3 cells were cultured in high-glucose Dulbecco's Modified Eagle Medium (DMEM) with 10% FBS, both supplemented with 20 mM alanyl-glutamine (Sigma Aldrich, UK) and 0.1 mg/mL of streptomycin (Sigma Aldrich, UK). Cells were trypsinized and added to a 24-well plate (ThermoFisher, Loughborough, UK) at 30,000 cells per well in 1 mL of respective media. The cells were cultured for 24 h in an incubator at 37 °C and 5% CO_2. Media was replaced and a Transwell® insert (Millicell Hanging Cell Culture Insert, polyethylene terephthalate (PET) 0.4 μm, 24-well) was added to each well containing cells. In triplicate, the following were added to the Transwell® inserts: No scaffold (positive), 1 mL 70% industrial methylated spirit (IMS) (negative), 0% Ag nHA scaffold, 5% Ag nHA scaffold, and 10% Ag nHA scaffold. One mL of media was added to each Transwell® insert and plates were incubated for 48 h at 37 °C and 5% CO_2. After 48 h the cells within the wells were imaged and metabolic activity was assessed using PrestoBlue™ (ThermoFisher, UK). Media was removed and 700 μL of PrestoBlue™ (10% in complete media) was added to each well and the well plate was incubated for two hours. From the wells, 200 μL of PrestoBlue™ was added in triplicate to a 96-well plate. The fluorescence of the solutions was measured using a plate reader (FLx 800 Bio-Tek Instruments; Thermo Fisher Scientific, UK) with an excitation wavelength of 535 nm and an emission wavelength of 590 nm. The experiment was repeated four times (N = 4, n = 3).

2.13. Contact Biocompatibility Study on Rat MSCs

A direct-contact biocompatibility study was used to assess the toxicity of the scaffolds on cells over 21 days. Rat MSCs were used for this study. Disks of each scaffold were added in triplicate to a 24-well plate and 1 mL of media was added to each for 30 min (including a tissue culture plastic [TCP] control). Cells were trypsinized, suspended in media, and then 30,000 cells were added to each well. Well plates were agitated to aid even cell-seeding across the scaffold. Well plates were incubated for 24 h before cell metabolic activity was measured using PrestoBlue™. The scaffolds were transferred to a new well plate before PrestoBlue™ to avoid interference of cells growing on the tissue culture plastic surrounding the scaffold. PrestoBlue™ was measured at 4, 7, 14, and 21 days in culture. N = 2, n = 3.

2.14. Live and Dead Cell Staining

Cells were stained with two dyes to identify if the cell was alive or if the cell scaffold was disrupted (dead). Cells were stained using the LIVE/DEAD™ Viability/Cytotoxicity Kit (Thermofisher, UK) as per the instructions. In brief, cells were washed in PBS and then Calcien and Ethidium homodimer-1 (both at 5 μM concentration) were incubated with cells in media for 30 min. Samples were imaged using a fluorescent microscope (Axioplan 2, Zeiss, Jena, Germany) using the built-in filters for FITC (calcein) and TRITC (Ethidium homodimer-1).

2.15. Total Sample DNA and Alkaline Phosphatase Production Measurements

Alkaline phosphatase (ALP) is an early indicator of MSC differentiation to osteoblasts and can be measured using an ALP detection test. ALP was normalized to DNA to give a reading of alkaline phosphatase activity per cell regardless of cell number. Media was removed and samples washed three times with PBS. Cell digestion buffer was made up using deionized water and 1% triton X-100 (Sigma, UK). Samples were incubated at 4 °C for 1 h in the cell digestion buffer. The samples were then subjected to two freeze–thaw cycles (−20 °C to room temperature), which included solution agitation by pipetting when thawed to ensure thorough lysis of cells. After the second freeze–thaw cycle, an alkaline phosphatase diethanolamine detection kit was used to assess the alkaline phosphatase activity of the cultures. Then, 40 µL of cell culture lysate solution was placed in a 96-well plate in triplicate with 210 µL alkaline phosphatase reaction buffer. A standard curve of para-nitrophenyl (pNP) product was prepared with concentrations of 250, 100, 50, 10, and 0 nmole.ml^{-1} pNP in the alkaline phosphate reaction buffer. Then, 250 µL of the standard solutions were added in triplicate to the 96-well plate. The para-nitrophenylphosphate (pNPP) substrate solution was prepared by dissolving 6.6 mg pNPP per 1 mL of dH_2O. Then, 10 µL substrate was then added to each well using a multichannel pipette and the plate was incubated in the dark at 37 °C. The plate was monitored for color change and, at an appropriate time point, the absorbance at 405 nm was read, ensuring that the readings were within the range provided by the standard solutions. The amount of pNP in the sample wells was then calculated using the standard curve and used as a measure of ALP activity.

After a further freeze–thaw cycle, Quant-iT™ PicoGreen® dsDNA assay (ThermoFisher, UK) was used in accordance with the manufacturer's instructions to quantify the DNA content of the cultures. In detail, 50 µL of cell culture lysate was placed in a 96-well plate in triplicate along with 50 µL dH_2O. A standard curve of DNA was also prepared in triplicate with final concentrations of 1000, 500, 100, 50, 10, 5, and 0 ng.mL^{-1} when 100 µL of PicoGreen reagent was added to the 100 µL of standard solution in each well. Then, 100 µL of freshly made PicoGreen reagent was added to all the wells using a multichannel pipette. The plate was incubated in the dark for 4 min, after which the fluorescence was read using an excitation wavelength of 485 nm and an emission wavelength of 528 nm. The standard curve was plotted and used to convert the fluorescence units of the wells into the DNA content of the original cultures.

2.16. Statistical Methodology

Statistical analysis was conducted using ANOVA run with multiple comparisons using GraphPad Prism 8 (GraphPad Software, Inc., San Diego, CA, USA) with significance indicated with * when $p < 0.05$. No demarcation of lower p values was used as all were tested with $p = 0.05$.

3. Results

3.1. Analysis of Prepared Nanoscale Hydroxyapatite

Nano-hydroxyapatite was prepared via the rapid mixing technique previously published [10]. Using TEM, the nanoscale hydroxyapatite particles were visualized and contained crystalline and amorphous regions, typically less than 100 nm in size. Silver was found within the nanoscale hydroxyapatite particles, with the visible formation of nanoparticles of silver. Both materials showed the peaks associated with hydroxyapatite in XRD patterns. XRD showed the presence of silver phosphate peaks but only for the 10 mol.% silver-containing material (Figure 1a). Despite this, in both materials silver nanoparticles were visible under TEM; EDX confirmed that the darker regions found under the TEM contained silver. See Supplementary Figure S1 for EDX mapping of all elements found in sample Figure 1e. The size distribution of particles' diameter between nHA and nHA with 10 mol.% silver substituted in was found to be similar, with an average of 37 and 40 nm, respectively (Figure 1f).

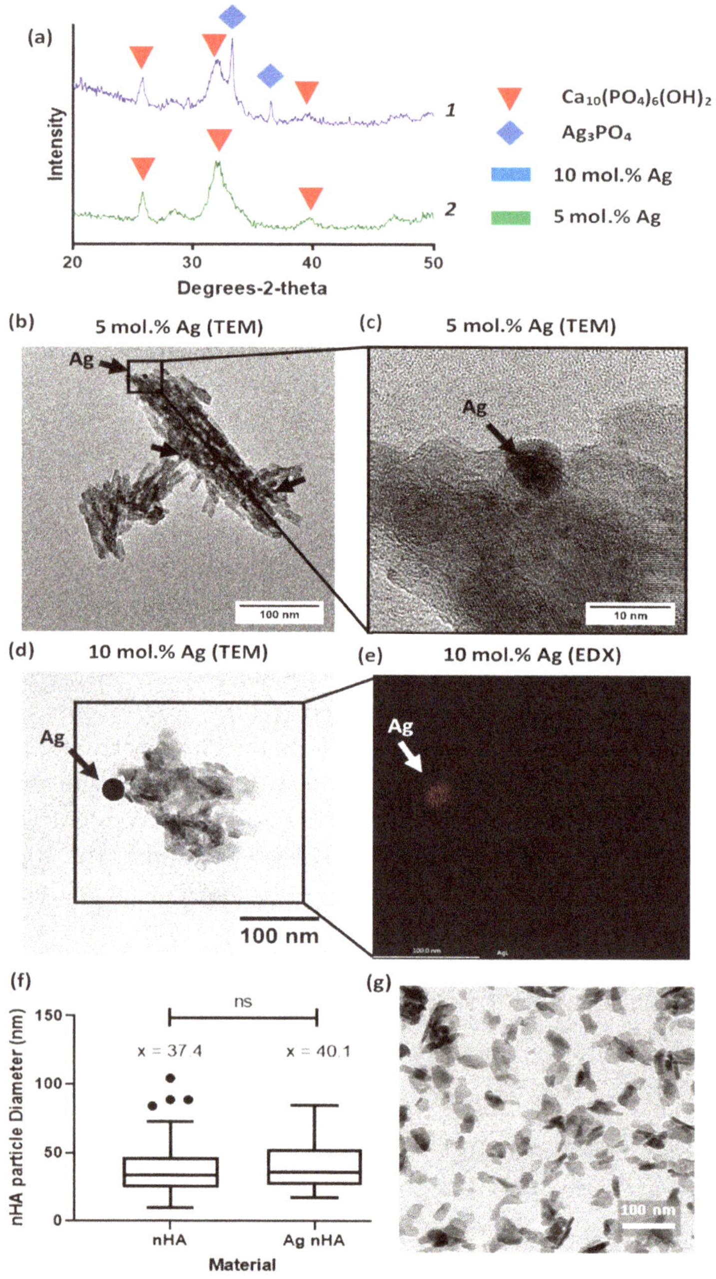

Figure 1. Evaluation of silver-containing nanoscale hydroxyapatite (**a**) XRD patterns of 5 and 10 mol.% silver doped nanoscale hydroxyapatite (Ag nHA), identifying peaks for hydroxyapatite $Ca_{10}(PO_4)_6(OH)_2$ and silver phosphate (Ag_3PO_4) phases within the sample. Silver phosphate was only identified in the 10 mol.% silver-containing material. Plot line 1 (blue) is 10 mol.% Ag nHA and plot line 2 (green) is 5 mol.% Ag nHA; (**b**) TEM image of nHA sample containing 5 mol.% silver. Silver deposits visible and highlighted by black arrows; (**c**) TEM at higher magnification on one of the silver deposit areas; (**d**) TEM image of nHA sample containing 10 mol.% silver. Larger silver deposit noted by black arrow; (**e**) Spatial EDX map of location of silver, mapped over the same location as that boxed in (**d**); (**f**) Particle diameter comparison between nHA and nHA with 10 mol.% silver shown as a Tukey box plot, ns = not significant; (**g**) TEM micrograph of nHA nanoscale particles.

3.2. Ensuring Encapsulation of nHA by Electrospun Fibers

Both silver and nondoped nHA were electrospun into polycaprolactone (PCL) scaffolds with a thickness of between 150 and 200 μm. SEM images showed incorporation of large particles in the fibers that were not observed in plain PCL scaffolds (Figure 2a). When digested, ICP analysis showed that plain PCL had very low levels of elements found within Ag-nHA (Figure 2b). The electrospun nHA showed the presence of calcium and phosphorus but not silver. Both electrospun scaffolds with silver-containing nHA showed the presence of silver alongside calcium and phosphorus (Figure 2b). This demonstrated that nHA was successfully incorporated into the electrospun fibers.

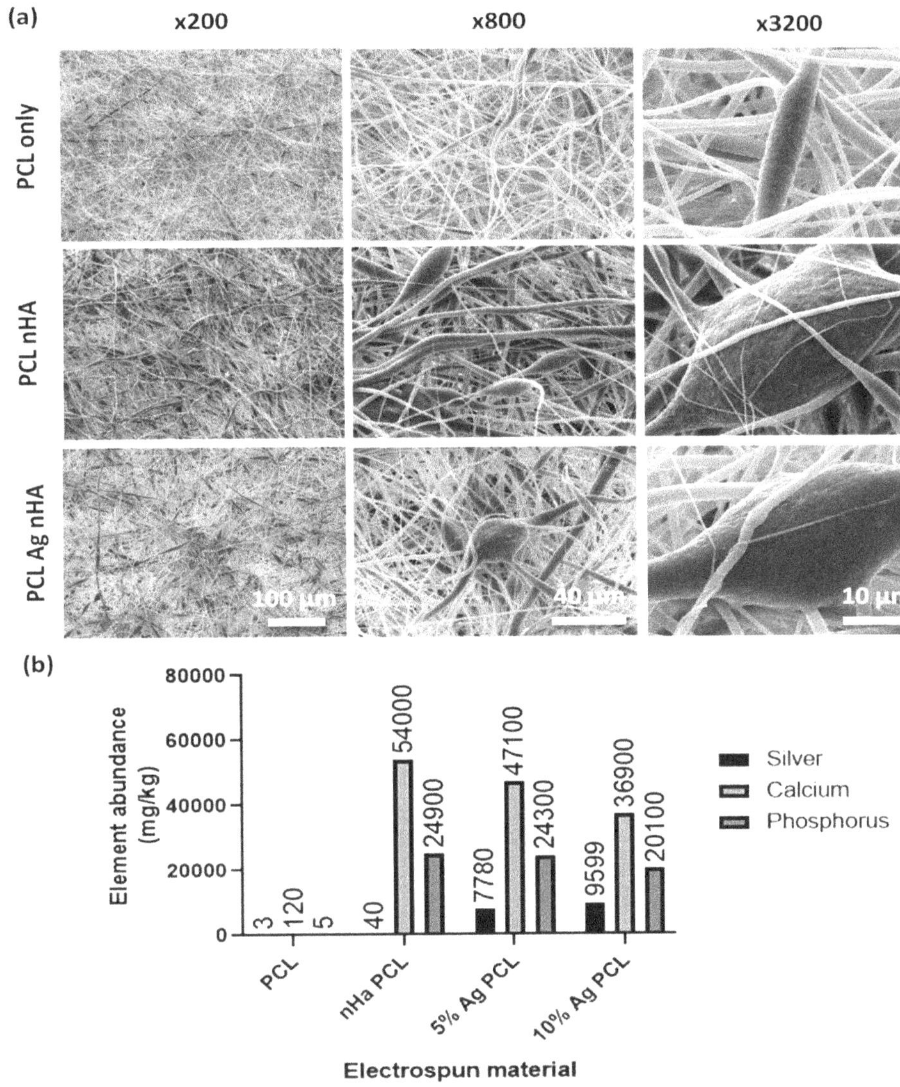

Figure 2. Scaffold fibers containing nHA (**a**) SEM micrographs of electrospun scaffold. Top: Polycaprolactone (PCL) scaffold. Middle: PCL scaffold containing nHA. Bottom: PCL scaffold containing 10 mol.% Ag nHA. Different magnifications were used to visualize encapsulation of nHA particles into the electrospun scaffold; (**b**) Inductively coupled plasma (ICP) analysis of dissolved electrospun scaffolds showing mg/kg of elements present. All % Ag materials are in mol.%.

3.3. Investigation of Silver Release and Scaffold Loss in Accelerated Degradation Study

An accelerated degradation assay was performed using sodium hydroxide at 37 °C to understand the degradation profile of the electrospun scaffolds and to observe release profiles (Figure 3). All scaffolds degraded at the same rate with the presence of nHA having no apparent effect on degradation profile (Figure 3a). Cumulative release of silver was observed for the full 30 days (Figure 3b). The plot of release rate (Figure 3c) indicated that in the early period of days 1 to 5 the release was from surface-bound origins, whereas from days 7 onwards the release was from silver within the polymer that was then released through degradation. Mass loss from degradation was nonexistent in the 1- to

7-day period and then rapidly degraded from there, which reinforced the conclusions drawn from the silver release rate.

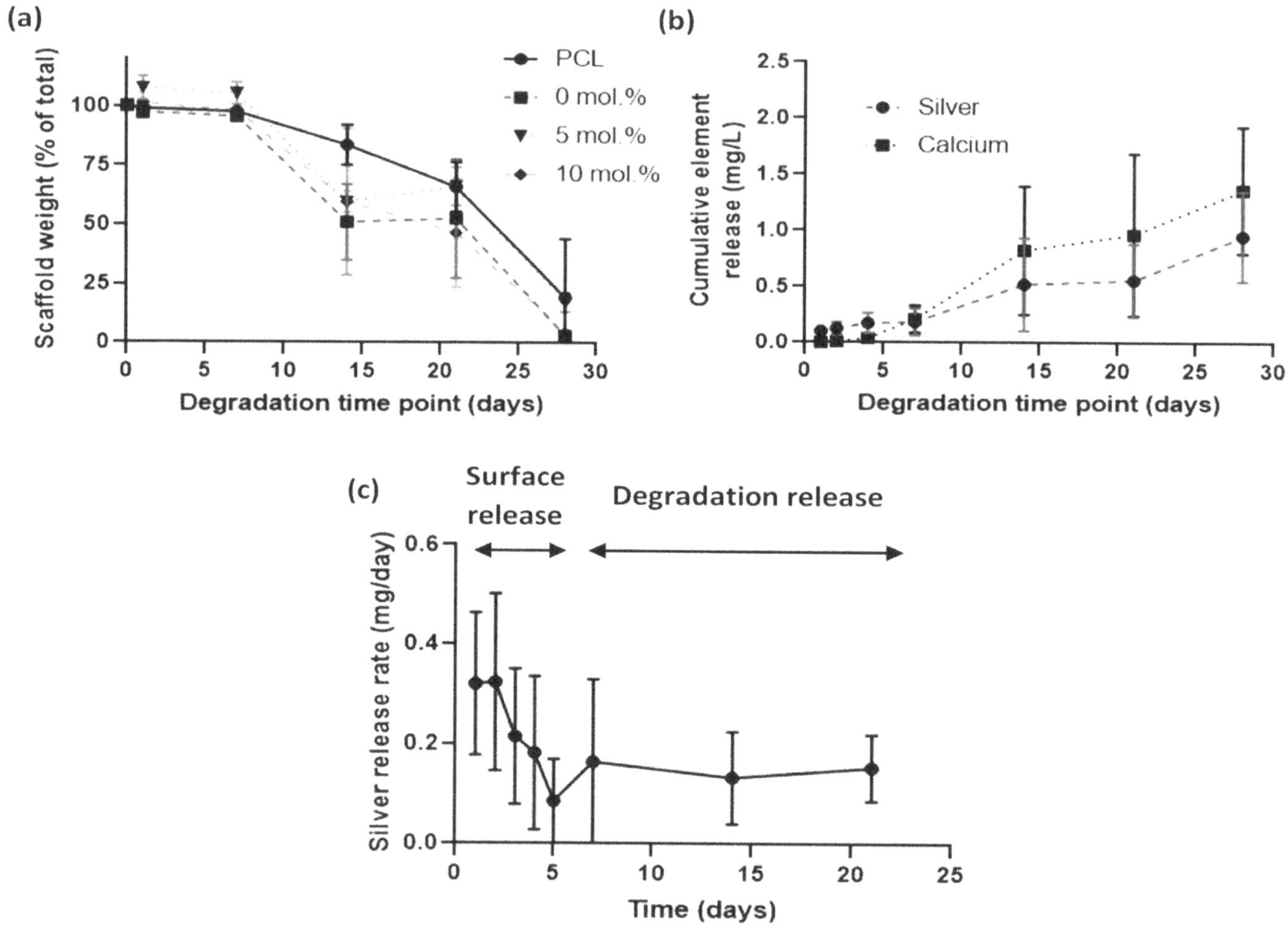

Figure 3. Accelerated degradation study of electrospun scaffolds containing nHA, over a 28-day period in 0.1 M sodium hydroxide. (**a**) Remaining weight over degradation time of different mol.% silver scaffolds; (**b**) Release profile of silver from an electrospun scaffold containing 10 mol.% Ag nHA over a 28-day period; (**c**) Plot of the silver release rate per day. All % Ag materials are in mol.%.

3.4. Antimicrobial Impact of Scaffolds

Both silver-containing scaffolds showed an antibacterial effect on both agar diffusion and on bacterial suspensions. PCL-only scaffolds and those with undoped nHA showed no innate antimicrobial action. Scaffolds containing silver of any concentration showed an antimicrobial response on agar diffusion (Figure 4a,b). Bacterial suspension cultures in PBS exposed to scaffolds for 24 h demonstrated the antimicrobial properties of the scaffolds containing silver. The 10 mol.% silver nHA was studied in a time course assay against bacteria and this showed a significant reduction in bacteria over time (Figure 4e,f). The scaffold reduced the viable bacteria count to undetectable levels by 48 h for *E. coli* and 96 h for *S. aureus*.

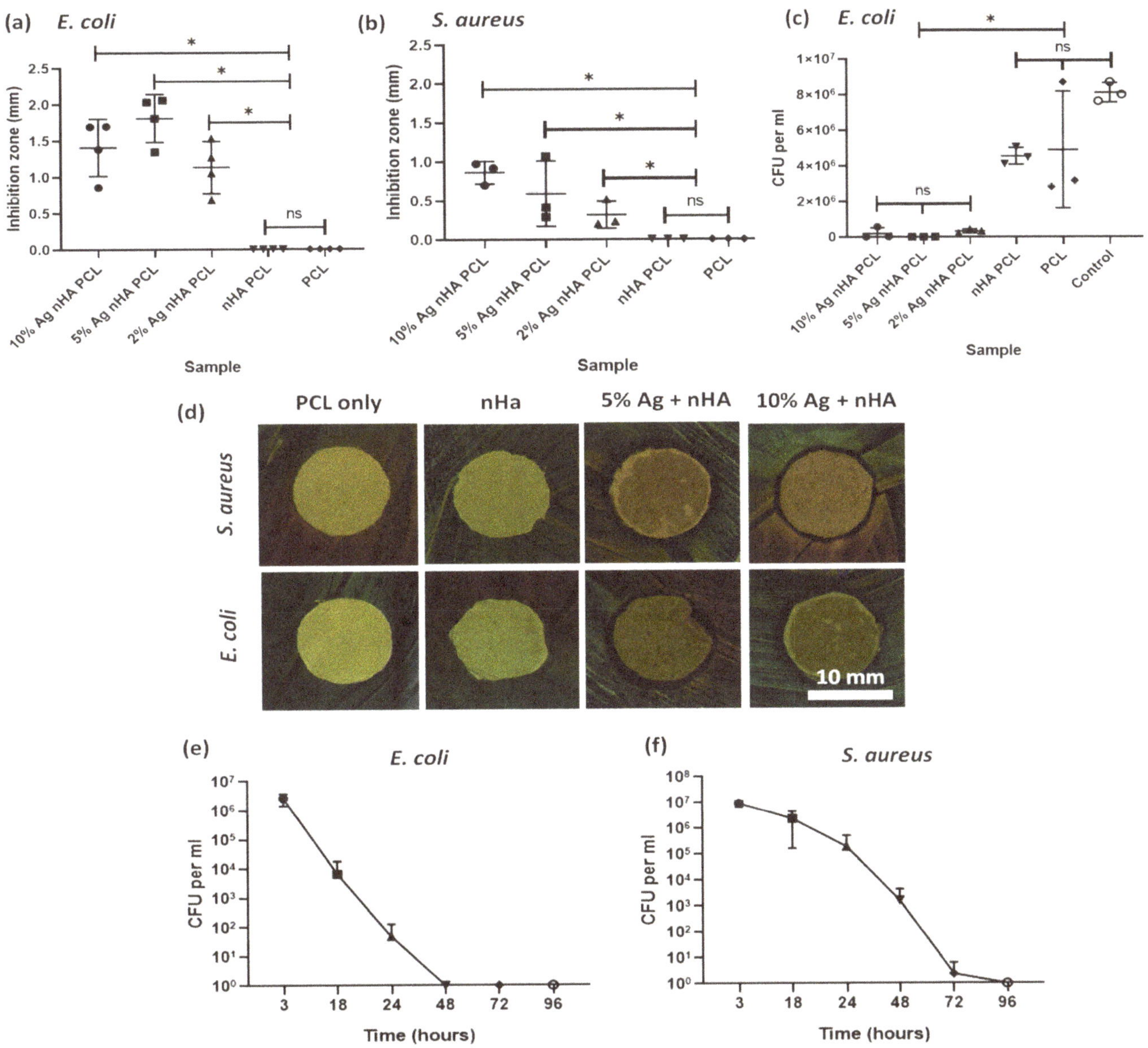

Figure 4. Antibacterial studies on *E. coli* and *S. aureus* bacteria using the electrospun scaffold. (**a**) Agar diffusion test using disks of the electrospun samples against *E. coli* bacteria. Graph displaying individual data plots with a line demarking the mean value; (**b**) Agar diffusion test using disks of the electrospun samples against *S. aureus*; (**c**) Disks of electrospun samples suspended in PBS containing bacteria, measuring viable colonies after 24 h; (**d**) Optical images of the area of inhibition ring surrounding a 12-mm disk of scaffold containing either 10 mol.% silver or plain PCL and tested against *S. aureus* and *E. coli*; (**e**) Bacteria count after *E. coli* are suspended in PBS and exposed to a disk of electrospun 10 mol.% silver nHA for 3, 18, 24, 48, 72, and 96 h; (**f**) Same as (**e**) but using *S. aureus* bacteria. All graphs show mean ± standard deviation. All % Ag materials are in mol.%.

3.5. Antimicrobial Impact of Scaffolds

Indirect toxicity assays found that higher silver concentrations were more toxic to both cell types while a longer, 21-day direct growth experiment showed a reduced toxic impact of these high silver samples on cells over time. When tested using fibroblast 3T3 cells, all scaffolds had a significantly higher viability than the negative (cytotoxic) control (Figure 5a). However, the scaffold containing 10 mol.% silver was also significantly different to the cell-only positive control, indicating some toxic impact. When the materials were tested on primary rat MSCs the toxic impact was more pronounced. The scaffold with 10 mol.% silver was significantly different to the cell-only positive control, but no statistical difference was found with the negative cell death control (Figure 5b). All the remaining materials were statistically different to the negative cell death controls. A longer, 21-day direct growth experiment found that cell metabolic activity for 5 mol.% silver-containing scaffolds were significantly increased compared to the PCL-only scaffolds (Figure 5c). The 10 mol.% silver-containing scaffolds reduced the metabolic activity when compared to 5 mol.% silver but did not show a toxic impact when compared to the PCL-only scaffold. Live cell morphology can be observed from live fluorescent images (Figure 5d) along with the proportion of live to dead cells. Cells appeared to have a more spread out morphology on the nHA silver-containing material than in the PCL-only control.

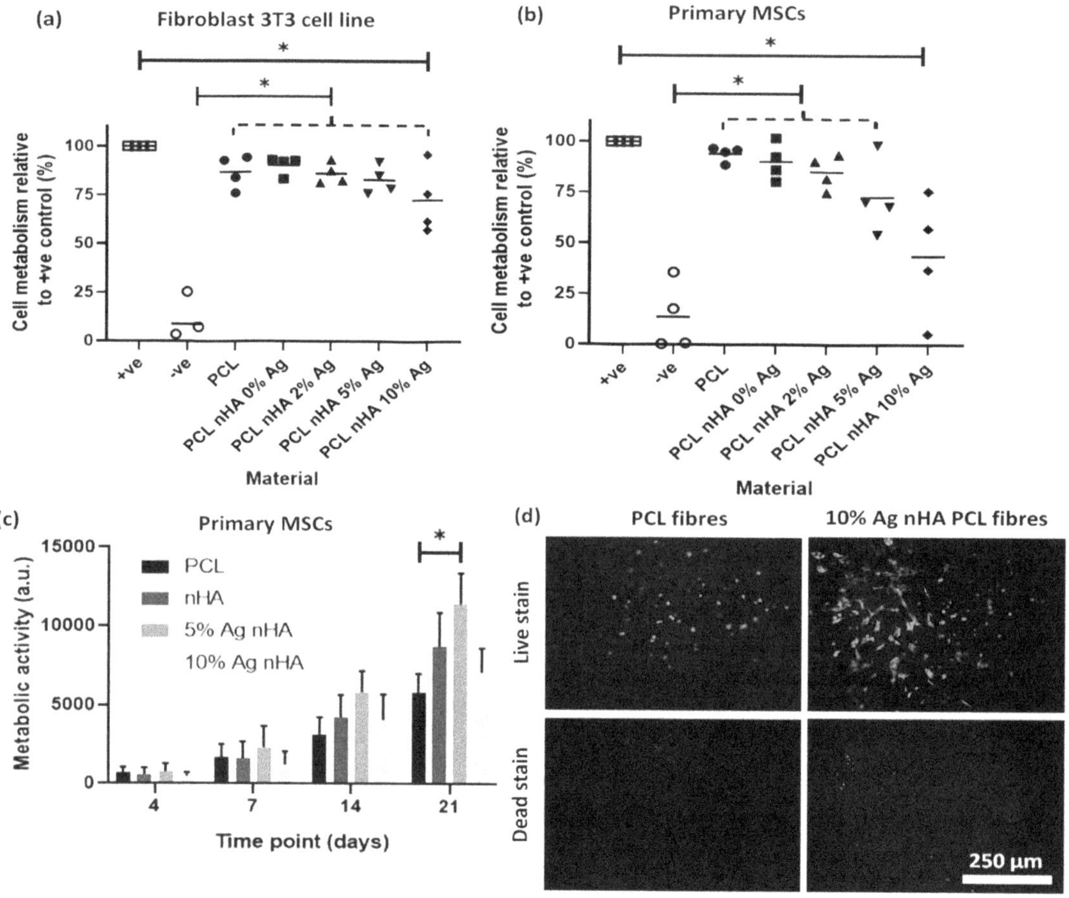

Figure 5. Cell toxicity from the electrospun scaffold with different concentrations of silver nHA assessed by cell metabolic activity via PrestoBlue™ assay. (**a**) A 48-h noncontact toxicity test with the scaffold in the media above a monolayer of 3T3 cells. Graph displaying individual data plots with a line demarking the mean value. Dotted line contains each scaffold under it to be compared to another condition; (**b**) A 48-h noncontact toxicity test with the scaffold in the media above a monolayer of primary rat MSCs. Graph displaying individual data plots with a line demarking the mean value. Dotted line without star contains each scaffold to be compare to another condition; (**c**) Cell metabolism after 21 days of direct culture with the cells seeded on top of the scaffold using metabolic activity at each time point. Statistics (ANOVA) conducted on the day 21 measurements; (**d**) Live/dead staining of MSCs cultured on electrospun scaffolds after 21 days.

3.6. MSC Osteogenic Differentiation Study by ALP Quantification

The impact of silver on the differentiation of primary MSCs down the osteoblast linage was measured after 21 days in culture by quantifying ALP content per unit of DNA (Figure 6). ANOVA showed a significant difference with 5 mol.% and the lower silver concentrations in regard to ALP production. Scaffolds with 10 mol.% silver are not significantly different to 5 mol.% silver scaffolds.

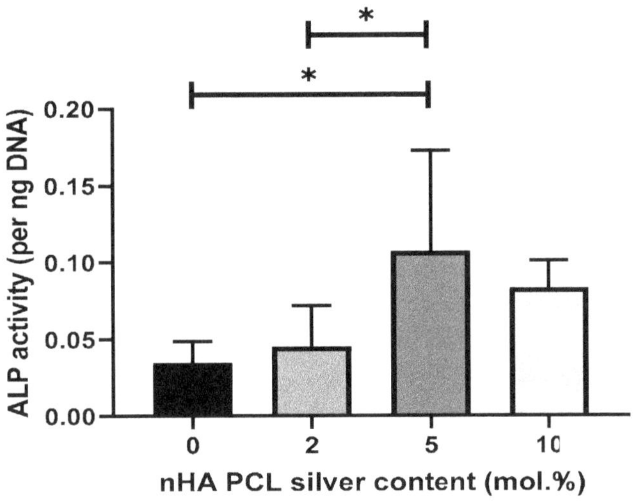

Figure 6. Cell differentiation potential of scaffolds containing different silver contents regarding ALP presence per unit of DNA after 21 days in culture with primary MSCs. Cells were cultured on top of the scaffolds. Graph displaying mean value ± standard deviation. N = 2, n = 3.

4. Discussion

Electrospun scaffolds with incorporated silver nano-hydroxyapatite are nontoxic to cells at a concentration that was antimicrobial, making them suitable for use as antimicrobial bone implants. In 2017, Anjaneyulu et al. [25] published a study looking into nanoscale electrospun fibers containing silver-doped hydroxyapatite and its hemocompatibility. Our study took a different direction, producing scaffolds with fibers to allow ingrowth of cells with larger pore sizes having positive impact on osteoblast cell growth [31]. Our study also included an in-depth microbiology study looking at both contact and noncontact tests. Investigating the impact of the scaffolds on bone regeneration via analyzing the toxicity on primary MSCs, for relevant cell toxicity, and 3T3 fibroblasts allowed toxicity comparison between labs.

The rapid manufacturing of nHA pioneered by Wilcock et al. [10] was replicated to produce silver-doped nHA powder. The characterization of nanoscale hydroxyapatite indicated it was comparable to that produced in previous studies. We were able to go one step further by confirming via TEM XRD that the denser (black) areas on the TEM contained silver. This had been hypothesized by the previous paper but not directly confirmed [21]. Under XRD we confirmed that the material was both hydroxyapatite and that it contained silver. TEM analysis showed that the nHA was in a nanoscale particulate form. The lack of an XRD-measurable silver phosphate phase in the 5 mol.% Ag nHA demonstrated that the silver had been incorporated into the nHA, either by substitution of silver into the HA crystal lattice for calcium or by doping of the silver ions onto the HA structure (i.e., not replacing the ions of the HA crystal). This result was expected for our method as our previous reports demonstrated a pure hydroxyapatite phase precipitated at 5 mol.% using this reaction [21].

The silver-doped nHA was successfully electrospun into PCL scaffolds. PCL is a popular material used in bone-related applications as its long-term degradation profile is suited to the slower healing rate of bone compared to soft tissues. Incorporating silver-containing tricalcium phosphate was reported by Schneider et al. [26], who found it effective against *E. coli* but did not test against the more common bone infection-related pathogen *S. aureus*. Jiang et al. [19] assessed antibacterial activity using both of these bacteria with a scaffold formed by in situ foaming, which allowed inclusion of silver/nHA up to 40% of total weight. This technique does not produce scaffolds, however, instead producing a monolithic block that would need to be carved to dimensions required during theater. Anjaneyulu et al. [25] investigated using both bacteria types and manufactured formed scaffolds but did not assess bone cell biocompatibility.

Our scaffolds degraded in an accelerated degradation study and showed a two-phase silver release system. Initially, a rapid burst of silver was released, decreasing in rate until day 7. During the same initial period of degradation, the polymer had not lost any mass. This rapid silver release is likely to arise from surface- (or near surface-) bound material. After the initial 7 days, the material lost mass and silver was released for the remainder of the experiment. Rothstein et al. described this in a model of an initial surface erosion system, which then transitions into bulk erosion [32]. The combination of the two allows for a rapid release when first implanted to clear immediate microorganisms and then a slower sustained release of the remainder of the implant life to prevent colonization from opportunistic bacteria, which may later attach to the device through a hematogenous route. Liu et al. [15] used electrochemical deposition of silver onto their electrospun fibers to provide an initial burst of silver over two days instead of a continual release. This would help prevent potential buildup of silver toxicity but would not prevent later infections from occurring. A continuous release of calcium and phosphorus was detected using ICP, which has been widely reported to stimulate bone regeneration [33]. An implanted material can act as a desirable location for bacteria to colonize with an infection requiring far fewer bacteria to start than in a normal tissue [34]. A continuous silver release would prevent opportunistic bacteria from infecting the implant at a later date. Due to the limited nature of our degradation method we cannot report on the exact amount of silver released per unit of time in vivo, as physiological conditions would impose a more complicated environment that may impact silver release. Despite not knowing the exact amount released, we showed that it is sufficient to prevent bacteria growth in non-accelerated studies.

Antimicrobial tests using both Gram-positive and Gram-negative bacteria showed that an antimicrobial response was found for 2, 5, and 10 mol.% incorporated silver-doped nHA. In a contact agar diffusion assay, both the silver-containing materials were found to produce an area of inhibition, whereas hydroxyapatite by itself does not [35]. Looking at the reduction of bacteria in solution, both bacteria were reduced beyond detection within 96 h. In our study we found silver was far more effective against *S. aureus* than against the *E. coli* bacteria. This was unexpected, as the thicker wall of the Gram-positive *S. aureus* is arguably better defended against the uptake of silver particles than thinner Gram-negative cell walls [36]. Resistance to silver can be acquired by bacteria [37], although it is a relatively broad spectrum medicant. This is significant, as *S. aureus* is among the most common pathogens found in bone infections [1,2]. Recent studies have shown that treating the motile *S. aureus* in an infected 3D tissue model is more challenging than treating a monolayer bacteria assay [38]. Therefore, this would be the logical progression for the testing of this material. One side effect of silver is that it can also be toxic to mammalian cells at elevated concentrations, which we investigated with our scaffolds.

The toxicity of the scaffolds was related to both the silver concentration and on the cell type being tested. Against the standard cell line of mouse fibroblast 3T3 cells there was a small indication of toxicity with scaffolds containing 10 mol.% silver. When using a primary rat MSCs there was clear toxicity detected with this highest concentration of silver. This shows the importance of not just using a single cell line to determine toxicity of a material but also of the correct choice of relevant cells. For a more in-depth review of the different modes of action of silver nanoparticles on various cell types, see Zhang et al. [39]. Using 3T3 cells is a useful method of comparing relative toxicities between different laboratories as they are well known and utilized in international standards for cytotoxicity (ISO 10993-5). The primary MSCs are more difficult to standardize between labs and are, therefore, harder to use to compare toxicity. They do give a more realistic insight on what levels of toxicity might be harmful in the environment the medical device is intended for. From the results presented, 5 mol.% silver-doped material at 20 wt. mol.% to PCL had an antimicrobial impact without being toxic to mammalian MSCs.

Using a longer study of 21 days, the 10 mol.% silver nHA scaffolds maintained a viable and growing cell population on par with the plain PCL material. Hydroxyapatite appeared to boost the metabolic activity of the MSCs by day 21 with the combination of 5 mol.% silver and hydroxyapatite, resulting in even higher levels of cell activity. Increasing the amount of silver to 10 mol.% did not increase the trend of increased proliferation. The initial high release rate from the material was potentially too toxic for the cells early on but, once the release level had fallen to a consistent 50 mol.%, surviving cells would then have been able to proliferate. After this period, the metabolic activity of cell on the 10 mol.% silver nHA scaffold increased at a similar growth rate to other materials. This is highly advantageous in a wound-healing application as it would allow an initially high burst to clear bacteria, which then lowers to allow the mammalian cells to begin the healing process.

Hydroxyapatite is widely reported to increase MSC differentiation into osteoblasts [40–42] so we focused on investigating the impact of silver on this process showing increased ALP production. Huge disparity can be found in the literature on whether silver has a significant impact on differentiation of MSCs. Some authors find that silver nanoparticles have no impact on MSC differentiation [43,44]. Other papers report on an impact of silver nanoparticles on MSC differentiation down the osteogenic lineage [45,46]. Conversely, some authors argue that silver particles can cause adipogenic differentiation [47] of MSCs, whereas others have found no impact at all on adipogenic differentiation [48]. One aspect that varies between these papers is the size of the silver nanoparticles, which might be a reason between the widely different reporting of the impact of silver on differentiation. Powers et al. found impact on neurodevelopment from silver on zebrafish PC12 cells, which was very dependent on both silver composition and silver nanoparticle size [49]. Another variation between papers is the wide range of different MSCs that are tested for differentiation, from both different tissue and animal origins. As even MSCs from different tissue origins vary in behavior, it is not surprising that different conclusions have been reported by multiple studies [50]. We found that 5 mol.% silver had the highest ALP production at day 21, although there was no significant difference to 10 mol.% silver. It is possible that either diminishing returns or an already reached optimum concentration of silver is the reason for no further increase at 10 mol.% silver. Another explanation is that the slightly more toxic impact of 10 mol.% silver offsets any additional osteogenic stimulation. Our study demonstrated that silver-doped nHA incorporated into PCL scaffolds may have a positive effect regarding MSC differentiation along an osteoblastic lineage due to increased levels of ALP production.

Limitations to the study include no mapping of elements within the electrospun membrane containing nHA. However, Figure 2b does show evidence that the material is present within the electrospun membranes but the precise location of the nHA is not known. Another limitation is that, while using bacteria typical of infections in bone, neither of the isolates was taken from a patient bone infection. Another limitation on the microbiology side is the simple nature of the tests used; it should be considered that (along with other disparities) osteomyelitis is associated with a hypoxic environment, which was not reflected by our experiments. Further work is needed to address these issues, including the use of a bone infection model to more accurately reproduce the conditions found in vivo. In a recent study we found that a material with antimicrobial impact on planktonic bacteria and simple biofilm models was then not effective on *P. aeruginosa* in tissue-engineered skin models, believed to be due to the bacteria motility [24]. This is something we intend to investigate in future work.

This research found that silver nHA containing scaffolds has the potential to act as an antimicrobial scaffold while stimulating bone tissue regeneration. The scaffolds degrade slowly and release a continuous amount of silver into the local environment over time. They are nontoxic to mammalian cells at a concentration that is toxic to both Gram-negative and Gram-positive bacterial strains. Investigating the impact of silver on MSC differentiation has suggested that higher values of silver promote MSC differentiation.

5. Conclusions

Silver-doped nanoscale hydroxyapatite may be incorporated into electrospun PCL scaffolds to fabricate a device that is both nontoxic to cultured mammalian cells and capable of inhibiting the growth of pathogenic microorganisms. The scaffold demonstrated antibacterial activity against both Gram-positive and Gram-negative bacterial strains commonly found in bone infections. The material was shown to release silver in an initial burst followed by a more sustained bulk degradation release. Silver appeared to enhance MSC differentiation down an osteogenic path when used in nontoxic concentrations. Silver-doped nHA containing scaffolds exhibited antimicrobial activity while stimulating bone tissue regeneration, which shows promise as a dual-action medical device to address unmet clinical needs in orthopedic and dental bone surgery.

Author Contributions: Conceptualization, T.E.P., R.S., P.V.H., and I.O.; Formal analysis, M.d.S.M.; Funding acquisition, T.E.P, R.S., and P.V.H.; Investigation, T.E.P. and J.T.; Methodology, T.E.P., J.T., and C.J.H.; Resources, P.V.H., Z.L., and I.O.; Supervision, R.S., Z.L., and I.O.; Validation, C.J.H.; Writing—original draft, T.EP. and J.T.; Writing—review & editing, R.S., C.J.H., P.V.H., Z.L., and I.O. All authors have read and agreed to the published version of the manuscript.

Acknowledgments: Mass spectrometry analyses were performed by the biOMICS/chemMS Facility of the Faculty of Science Mass Spectrometry Centre at the University of Sheffield.

References

1. Bouza, E.; Muñoz, P. Micro-organisms responsible for osteo-articular infections. *Best Pract. Res. Clin. Rheumatol.* **1999**, *13*, 21–35. [CrossRef] [PubMed]
2. Malone, M.; Bowling, F.L.; Gannass, A.; Jude, E.B.; Boulton, A. Deep wound cultures correlate well with bone biopsy culture in diabetic foot osteomyelitis. *Diabetes Metab Res. Rev.* **2013**, *29*, 546–550. [PubMed]
3. Stone, P.A.; Mousa, A.Y.; Hass, S.M.; Dearing, D.D.; Campbell, J.R., II; Parker, A.; Thompson, S.; AbuRahma, A.F. Antibiotic-loaded polymethylmethacrylate beads for the treatment of extracavitary vascular surgical site infections. *J. Surg.* **2012**, *55*, 1706–1711. [CrossRef] [PubMed]
4. Burdușel, A.-C.; Gherasim, O.; Grumezescu, A.; Mogoantă, L.; Ficai, A.; Andronescu, E. Biomedical applications of silver nanoparticles: An up-to-date overview. *Nanomaterials* **2018**, *8*, 681. [CrossRef]
5. Li, Z.; Tang, H.Y.; Yuan, W.W.; Song, W.; Niu, Y.S.; Yan, L.; Yu, M.; Dai, M.; Feng, S.Y.; Wang, M.H.; et al. Ag nanoparticle-ZnO nanowire hybrid nanostructures as enhanced and robust antimicrobial textiles via a green chemical approach. *Nanotechnology* **2014**, *25*. [CrossRef]
6. Chou, T.G.R.; Petti, C.A.; Szakacs, J.; Bloebaum, R.D. Evaluating antimicrobials and implant materials for infection prevention around transcutaneous osseointegrated implants in a rabbit model. *J. Biomed. Mater. Res. Part A* **2010**, *92*, 942–952. [CrossRef]
7. Ivask, A.; Kurvet, I.; Kasemets, K.; Blinova, I.; Aruoja, V.; Suppi, S.; Vija, H.; Käkinen, A.; Titma, T.; Heinlaan, M. Size-dependent toxicity of silver nanoparticles to bacteria, yeast, algae, crustaceans and mammalian cells in vitro. *PLoS ONE* **2014**, *9*, e102108. [CrossRef]
8. Milić, M.; Leitinger, G.; Pavičić, I.; Zebić Avdičević, M.; Dobrović, S.; Goessler, W.; Vinković Vrček, I. Cellular uptake and toxicity effects of silver nanoparticles in mammalian kidney cells. *J. Appl. Toxicol.* **2015**, *35*, 581–592. [CrossRef]
9. Thorwarth, M.; Schultze-Mosgau, S.; Kessler, P.; Wiltfang, J.; Schlegel, K.A. Bone regeneration in osseous defects using a resorbable nanoparticular hydroxyapatite. *J. Oral Maxillofac. Surg.* **2005**, *63*, 1626–1633. [CrossRef]
10. Wilcock, C.J.; Gentile, P.; Hatton, P.V.; Miller, C.A. Rapid Mix Preparation of Bioinspired Nanoscale Hydroxyapatite for Biomedical Applications. *J. Vis. Exp.* **2017**. [CrossRef]
11. Schierholz, J.; Beuth, J. Implant infections: A haven for opportunistic bacteria. *J. Hosp. Infect.* **2001**, *49*, 87–93. [CrossRef] [PubMed]
12. Zimmerli, W.; Sendi, P. Orthopaedic biofilm infections. *APMIS* **2017**, *125*, 353–364. [CrossRef] [PubMed]
13. Ciobanu, C.S.; Iconaru, S.L.; Le Coustumer, P.; Constantin, L.V.; Predoi, D. Antibacterial activity of silver-doped hydroxyapatite nanoparticles against gram-positive and gram-negative bacteria. *Nanoscale Res. Lett.* **2012**, *7*, 324. [CrossRef] [PubMed]
14. Predoi, D.; Iconaru, S.L.; Predoi, M.V. Bioceramic layers with antifungal properties. *Coatings* **2018**, *8*, 276. [CrossRef]

15. Liu, F.; Wang, X.; Chen, T.; Zhang, N.; Wei, Q.; Tian, J.; Wang, Y.; Ma, C.; Lu, Y. Hydroxyapatite/silver electrospun fibers for anti-infection and osteoinduction. *J. Adv. Res.* **2020**, *21*, 91–102. [CrossRef]
16. Singh, R.P.; Singh, M.; Verma, G.; Shukla, S.; Singh, S.; Singh, S. Structural Analysis of Silver Doped Hydroxyapatite Nanopowders by Rietveld Refinement. *Trans. Indian Inst. Met.* **2017**, *70*, 1973–1980. [CrossRef]
17. Ciobanu, C.S.; Iconaru, S.L.; Chifiriuc, M.C.; Costescu, A.; Le Coustumer, P.; Predoi, D. Synthesis and Antimicrobial Activity of Silver-Doped Hydroxyapatite Nanoparticles. *BioMed. Res. Int.* **2013**, *2013*, 916218. [CrossRef]
18. Jelínek, M.; Weiserová, M.; Kocourek, T.; Zezulová, M.; Strnad, J. Biomedical properties of laser prepared silver-doped hydroxyapatite. *Laser Phys.* **2011**, *21*, 1265–1269. [CrossRef]
19. Jiang, J.; Li, L.; Li, K.; Li, G.; You, F.; Zuo, Y.; Li, Y.; Li, J. Antibacterial nanohydroxyapatite/polyurethane composite scaffolds with silver phosphate particles for bone regeneration. *J. Biomater. Sci. Polym. Ed.* **2016**, *27*, 1584–1598. [CrossRef]
20. Saravanan, S.; Nethala, S.; Pattnaik, S.; Tripathi, A.; Moorthi, A.; Selvamurugan, N. Preparation, characterization and antimicrobial activity of a bio-composite scaffold containing chitosan/nano-hydroxyapatite/nano-silver for bone tissue engineering. *Int. J. Biol. Macromol.* **2011**, *49*, 188–193. [CrossRef]
21. Wilcock, C.; Stafford, G.; Miller, C.; Ryabenkova, Y.; Fatima, M.; Gentile, P.; Möbus, G.; Hatton, P. Preparation and antibacterial properties of silver-doped nanoscale hydroxyapatite pastes for bone repair and augmentation. *J. Biomed. Nanotechnol.* **2017**, *13*, 1168–1176. [CrossRef] [PubMed]
22. Zhang, S.; Jiang, G.; Prabhakaran, M.P.; Qin, X.; Ramakrishna, S. Evaluation of electrospun biomimetic substrate surface-decorated with nanohydroxyapatite precipitation for osteoblasts behavior. *Mater. Sci. Eng. C* **2017**, *79*, 687–696. [CrossRef] [PubMed]
23. Ciraldo, F.; Liverani, L.; Gritsch, L.; Goldmann, W.; Boccaccini, A. Synthesis and characterization of silver-doped mesoporous bioactive glass and its applications in conjunction with electrospinning. *Materials* **2018**, *11*, 692. [CrossRef] [PubMed]
24. Zheng, K.; Balasubramanian, P.; Paterson, T.E.; Stein, R.; MacNeil, S.; Fiorilli, S.; Vitale-Brovarone, C.; Shepherd, J.; Boccaccini, A.R. Ag modified mesoporous bioactive glass nanoparticles for enhanced antibacterial activity in 3D infected skin model. *Mater. Sci. Eng. C* **2019**, *103*, 109764. [CrossRef]
25. Anjaneyulu, U.; Priyadarshini, B.; Grace, A.N.; Vijayalakshmi, U. Fabrication and characterization of Ag doped hydroxyapatite-polyvinyl alcohol composite nanofibers and its in vitro biological evaluations for bone tissue engineering applications. *J. Sol Gel Sci. Technol.* **2017**, *81*, 750–761. [CrossRef]
26. Schneider, O.D.; Loher, S.; Brunner, T.J.; Schmidlin, P.; Stark, W.J. Flexible, silver containing nanocomposites for the repair of bone defects: Antimicrobial effect against E. coli infection and comparison to tetracycline containing scaffolds. *J. Mater. Chem.* **2008**, *18*, 2679–2684. [CrossRef]
27. Furtos, G.; Rivero, G.; Rapuntean, S.; Abraham, G.A. Amoxicillin-loaded electrospun nanocomposite membranes for dental applications. *J. Biomed. Mater. Res. Part B Appl. Biomater.* **2017**, *105*, 966–976. [CrossRef]
28. Paterson, T.E.; Beal, S.N.; Santocildes-Romero, M.E.; Sidambe, A.T.; Hatton, P.V.; Asencio, I.O. Selective laser melting–enabled electrospinning: Introducing complexity within electrospun membranes. *Proc. Inst. Mech. Eng. Part h J. Eng. Med.* **2017**, *231*, 565–574. [CrossRef]
29. Maniatopoulos, C.; Sodek, J.; Melcher, A.H. Bone formation in vitro by stromal cells obtained from bone marrow of young adult rats. *Cell Tissue Res.* **1988**, *254*, 317–330. [CrossRef]
30. Santocildes-Romero, M.E.; Crawford, A.; Hatton, P.V.; Goodchild, R.L.; Reaney, I.M.; Miller, C.A. The osteogenic response of mesenchymal stromal cells to strontium-substituted bioactive glasses. *J. Tissue Eng. Regen. Med.* **2015**, *9*, 619–631. [CrossRef]
31. Oh, S.H.; Park, I.K.; Kim, J.M.; Lee, J.H. In vitro and in vivo characteristics of PCL scaffolds with pore size gradient fabricated by a centrifugation method. *Biomaterials* **2007**, *28*, 1664–1671. [CrossRef] [PubMed]
32. Rothstein, S.N.; Federspiel, W.J.; Little, S.R. A unified mathematical model for the prediction of controlled release from surface and bulk eroding polymer matrices. *Biomaterials* **2009**, *30*, 1657–1664. [CrossRef] [PubMed]

33. LeGeros, R.Z. Calcium phosphate-based osteoinductive materials. *Chem. Rev.* **2008**, *108*, 4742–4753. [CrossRef] [PubMed]
34. Costerton, J.; Montanaro, L.; Arciola, C.R. Biofilm in implant infections: Its production and regulation. *Int. J. Artif. Organs* **2005**, *28*, 1062–1068. [CrossRef]
35. Kim, T.; Feng, Q.L.; Kim, J.; Wu, J.; Wang, H.; Chen, G.; Cui, F. Antimicrobial effects of metal ions (Ag+, Cu2+, Zn2+) in hydroxyapatite. *J. Mater. Sci. Mater. Med.* **1998**, *9*, 129–134. [CrossRef]
36. Feng, Q.L.; Wu, J.; Chen, G.; Cui, F.; Kim, T.; Kim, J. A mechanistic study of the antibacterial effect of silver ions on Escherichia coli and Staphylococcus aureus. *J. Biomed. Mater. Res.* **2000**, *52*, 662–668. [CrossRef]
37. Li, X.-Z.; Nikaido, H.; Williams, K.E. Silver-resistant mutants of Escherichia coli display active efflux of Ag+ and are deficient in porins. *J. Bacteriol.* **1997**, *179*, 6127–6132. [CrossRef]
38. Paterson, T.E.; Bari, A.; Bullock, A.J.; Turner, R.; Montalbano, G.; Fiorilli, S.; Vitale-Brovarone, C.; MacNeil, S.; Shepherd, J. Multifunctional Copper-Containing Mesoporous Glass Nanoparticles as Antibacterial and Proangiogenic Agents for Chronic Wounds. *Front. Bioeng. Biotechnol.* **2020**, *8*, 246. [CrossRef]
39. Zhang, X.-F.; Shen, W.; Gurunathan, S. Silver Nanoparticle-Mediated Cellular Responses in Various Cell Lines: An in Vitro Model. *Int. J. Mol Sci.* **2016**, *17*, 1603. [CrossRef]
40. Venugopal, J.; Rajeswari, R.; Shayanti, M.; Low, S.; Bongso, A.; Giri Dev, V.R.; Deepika, G.; Choon, A.T.; Ramakrishna, S. Electrosprayed hydroxyapatite on polymer nanofibers to differentiate mesenchymal stem cells to osteogenesis. *J. Biomater. Sci. Polym. Ed.* **2013**, *24*, 170–184. [CrossRef]
41. Guo, H.; Su, J.; Wei, J.; Kong, H.; Liu, C. Biocompatibility and osteogenicity of degradable Ca-deficient hydroxyapatite scaffolds from calcium phosphate cement for bone tissue engineering. *Acta Biomater.* **2009**, *5*, 268–278. [CrossRef] [PubMed]
42. Lin, L.; Chow, K.L.; Leng, Y. Study of hydroxyapatite osteoinductivity with an osteogenic differentiation of mesenchymal stem cells. *J. Biomed. Mater. Res. Part A* **2009**, *89*, 326–335. [CrossRef] [PubMed]
43. Liu, X.; He, W.; Fang, Z.; Kienzle, A.; Feng, Q. Influence of silver nanoparticles on osteogenic differentiation of human mesenchymal stem cells. *J. Biomed. Nanotechnol.* **2014**, *10*, 1277–1285. [CrossRef] [PubMed]
44. Samberg, M.E.; Loboa, E.G.; Oldenburg, S.J.; Monteiro-Riviere, N.A. Silver nanoparticles do not influence stem cell differentiation but cause minimal toxicity. *Nanomedicine* **2012**, *7*, 1197–1209. [CrossRef]
45. Qin, H.; Zhu, C.; An, Z.; Jiang, Y.; Zhao, Y.; Wang, J.; Liu, X.; Hui, B.; Zhang, X.; Wang, Y. Silver nanoparticles promote osteogenic differentiation of human urine-derived stem cells at noncytotoxic concentrations. *Int. J. Nanomed.* **2014**, *9*, 2469. [CrossRef]
46. Zhang, R.; Lee, P.; Lui, V.C.; Chen, Y.; Liu, X.; Lok, C.N.; To, M.; Yeung, K.W.; Wong, K.K. Silver nanoparticles promote osteogenesis of mesenchymal stem cells and improve bone fracture healing in osteogenesis mechanism mouse model. *Nanomed. Nanotechnol. Biol. Med.* **2015**, *11*, 1949–1959. [CrossRef]
47. Sengstock, C.; Diendorf, J.; Epple, M.; Schildhauer, T.A.; Köller, M. Effect of silver nanoparticles on human mesenchymal stem cell differentiation. *Beilstein J. Nanotechnol.* **2014**, *5*, 2058–2069. [CrossRef]
48. He, W.; Kienzle, A.; Liu, X.; Müller, W.E.; Elkhooly, T.A.; Feng, Q. In vitro effect of 30 nm silver nanoparticles on adipogenic differentiation of human mesenchymal stem cells. *J. Biomed. Nanotechnol.* **2016**, *12*, 525–535. [CrossRef]
49. Powers, C.M.; Badireddy, A.R.; Ryde, I.T.; Seidler, F.J.; Slotkin, T.A. Silver nanoparticles compromise neurodevelopment in PC12 cells: Critical contributions of silver ion, particle size, coating, and composition. *Environ. Health Perspect.* **2010**, *119*, 37–44. [CrossRef]
50. Ribeiro, A.; Laranjeira, P.; Mendes, S.; Velada, I.; Leite, C.; Andrade, P.; Santos, F.; Henriques, A.; Grãos, M.; Cardoso, C.M.P.; et al. Mesenchymal stem cells from umbilical cord matrix, adipose tissue and bone marrow exhibit different capability to suppress peripheral blood B, natural killer and T cells. *Stem Cell Res. Ther.* **2013**, *4*, 125. [CrossRef]

7

Early Polylysine Release from Dental Composites and its Effects on Planktonic *Streptococcus mutans* Growth

Nikos N. Lygidakis [1], Elaine Allan [2], Wendy Xia [3], Paul F. Ashley [1] and Anne M. Young [3,*]

1 Unit of Paediatric Dentistry, Department of Craniofacial Growth and Development, UCL Eastman Dental Institute, London WC1X 8LD, UK; nikos.lygidakis@gmail.com (N.N.L.); p.ashley@ucl.ac.uk (P.F.A.)
2 Division of Microbial Diseases, UCL Eastman Dental Institute, London WC1X 8LD, UK; e.allan@ucl.ac.uk
3 Department of Biomaterials and Tissue Engineering, UCL Eastman Dental Institute, London WC1X 8LD, UK; wendy.xia2011@yahoo.co.uk
* Correspondence: anne.young@ucl.ac.uk

Abstract: The study aim was to assess the effect of incorporating polylysine (PLS) filler at different mass fractions (0.5, 1 and 2 wt%) on PLS release and *Streptococcus mutans* planktonic growth. Composite containing PLS mass and volume change and PLS release upon water immersion were assessed gravimetrically and via high-performance liquid chromatography (HPLC), respectively. Disc effects on bacterial counts in broth initially containing 8×10^5 versus 8×10^6 CFU/mL *Streptococcus mutans* UA159 were determined after 24 h. Survival of sedimented bacteria after 72 h was determined following LIVE/DEAD staining of composite surfaces using confocal microscopy. Water sorption-induced mass change at two months increased from 0.7 to 1.7% with increasing PLS concentration. Average volume increases were 2.3% at two months whilst polylysine release levelled at 4% at 3 weeks irrespective of composite PLS level. Early percentage PLS release, however, was faster with higher composite content. With 0.5, 1 and 2% polylysine initially in the composite filler phase, 24-h PLS release into 1 mL of water yielded 8, 25 and 93 ppm respectively. With initial bacterial counts of 8×10^5 CFU/mL, this PLS release reduced 24-h bacterial counts from 10^9 down to 10^8, 10^7 and 10^2 CFU/mL respectively. With a high initial inoculum, 24-h bacterial counts were 10^9 with 0, 0.5 or 1% PLS and 10^7 with 2% PLS. As the PLS composite content was raised, the ratio of dead to live sedimented bacteria increased. The antibacterial action of the experimental composites could reduce residual bacteria remaining following minimally invasive tooth restorations.

Keywords: polylysine; antibacterial; dental composites

---

1. Introduction

Dental caries is one of the most common diseases affecting humans. Traditionally, treatment involved the removal of all the affected tooth structure followed by replacement with amalgam. Silver mercury amalgam is a highly effective restorative material due to both its good mechanical and antibacterial properties. Following the Minamata agreement in 2013 on global mercury reduction signed by 140 counties, amalgam is being phased out. In Europe, amalgam use in primary teeth was banned in 2018 [1].

Modern dentistry advocates for the removal of highly infected surface dentine but not underlying demineralized and less infected dentine that may be close to the pulp [2]. Effective cavity sealing with Glass Ionomer Cement (GIC) restorations can reduce any underlying residual bacterial contamination. It can also encourage remineralization but have insufficient strength for larger cavities.

Conversely, dental composites have greater strength, but their placement is complex and their technique sensitive. Multiple adhesion-promoting steps are required, in addition to material placement and light curing in several increments to reduce polymerization shrinkage consequences [3]. Composite failure is usually due to secondary caries at the restoration margins. This is attributed to a combination of residual bacteria, shrinkage and enzyme-activated degradation of demineralized dentine, which may compromise the bonding interface, enabling further bacterial penetration and growth [4]. A composite material that could provide surface release of antibacterial and remineralizing agents upon damage of the tooth/restoration interface might therefore be beneficial.

Antibacterial components such as chlorhexidine, fluoride, quaternary ammonium methacrylate, silver and triclosan have previously been added to dental composites [5–9]. Polylysine (PLS) is an alternative antibacterial agent that has been included in composites more recently. Polylysine-greater eukaryotic cell-compatibility may address the limited biocompatibility of some other antibacterial agents [10,11]. Studies suggest electrostatic adsorption of polylysine on bacterial surfaces, and its abnormal distribution within their cytoplasm, leads to their cell damage [12,13]. Polylysine, however, is generally recognized as safe (GRAS). It is a natural polypeptide that is biodegradable, water-soluble, nontoxic and edible. Additionally, polylysine is extensively used in eukaryotic cell culture to promote cell attachment and as a food preservative [12,14]. In the human body, polylysine degrades harmlessly to give the essential amino acid, lysine [12,14]. Furthermore, polylysine addition into calcium phosphate-containing composites can enhance apatite precipitation on their surfaces from simulated body fluid. Polylysine may therefore also enhance composite remineralizing potential [10].

Whilst many properties of polylysine-containing dental composites have now been investigated [10,11], publications on their actions against bacteria are limited. In this study, therefore, the ability of composites with increasing levels of polylysine to affect bacterial growth was investigated. Effects on planktonic bacteria are assessed to model the feasibility of surface polylysine release reducing bacterial microleakage in gaps at the tooth restoration interface. Polylysine release kinetics are provided to help explain the varying levels of antibacterial action. Potential polylysine addition and release effects on set material stability are monitored through mass and volume changes in water.

2. Materials and Methods

2.1. Components

The resin matrix was prepared using Urethane Dimethacrylate (UDMA) (DMG, Hamburg, Germany) as a base monomer and PolyPropylene Glycol Dimethacrylate (PPGDMA) (Polysciences, Inc., Warrington, FL, USA) as a diluent monomer. 4-methacryloxyethyl trimellitate anhydride (4-META) (Polysciences, Inc., Warrington, FL, USA) and Camphorquinone (CQ) (DMG, Hamburg, Germany) were added at low level. The filler consisted of two different sizes of aluminosilicate glass of 7 μm and 0.7 μm (DMG, Hamburg, Germany), fumed silica (Aerosil OX 50, Evonik, Essen, Germany), monocalcium phosphate monohydrate (MCPM) (Himed, Old Bethpage, NY, USA) and polylysine (PLS) (Handary, Brussels, Belgium).

UDMA is a common base monomer, that has been used as an alternative to bisphenol A-glycidyl methacrylate (Bis-GMA) [15]. In previous studies, PPGDMA, a diluent monomer that can be used instead of triethylene glycol dimethacrylate (TEGDMA), enhanced paste stability, increased light activated polymerization and reduced associated shrinkage [11]. 4-META is an adhesion-promoting monomer [16]. Monocalcium phosphate monohydrate (MCPM) particles added to composites can promote water sorption and react to produce brushite crystals of greater volume thereby giving expansion to compensate polymerisation shrinkage. Furthermore, release of its phosphate ions can promote apatite precipitation from simulated dentinal fluid to remineralize dentine [17].

2.2. Paste Preparation

Four formulations with 1 variable (PLS) were prepared. The resin (liquid) phase consisted of UDMA (72 wt%), PPGDMA (24 wt%), 4-META (3 wt%), and CQ (1 wt%) [11]. This was prepared by mixing the components and stirring for 24 h at room temperature on a magnetic stirrer hot plate (Jeo Tech) until a clear liquid was achieved. The filler phase contained glass of 7 μm, 0.7 μm and fumed silica in the ratio 6:3:1. 10 wt% MCPM was added to the filler as in F2 in previous work [11] but the tricalcium phosphate was removed. Additionally, the filler PLS level was varied (0, 0.5, 1 or 2 wt%) instead of being fixed at 2 wt%. Filler: resin were mixed in the weight ratio 5:1 for 45 s at 3500 rpm using a centrifugal mixer (Speedmixer, Hauschild Engineering, Hamm, Germany). This high ratio produced pastes with a consistency comparable with the commercial packable composite Filtek Z250 (3M, Bracknell, UK) used as an additional control in antibacterial studies.

2.3. Composite Discs Preparation

Disc-shaped specimens were formed by applying the composite pastes within metal circlips with internal diameter 10 mm and thickness of 1 mm and pressing them between two sheets of acetate (Figure 1). The specimens were then photopolymerized using a blue light-emitting diode curing unit with a wavelength of 450–470 nm and power of 1100–1300 mW/cm^2 (Demi Plus, Kerr Dental, Bioggio, Switzerland) with the tip in contact with the acetate sheet. The curing duration was 40 s on each side of each disc. This method gives 72% monomer conversion for the formulations [11]. The discs were then removed from the circlip, any excesses were trimmed with a no.11 blade, and stored at room temperature in the dark until required.

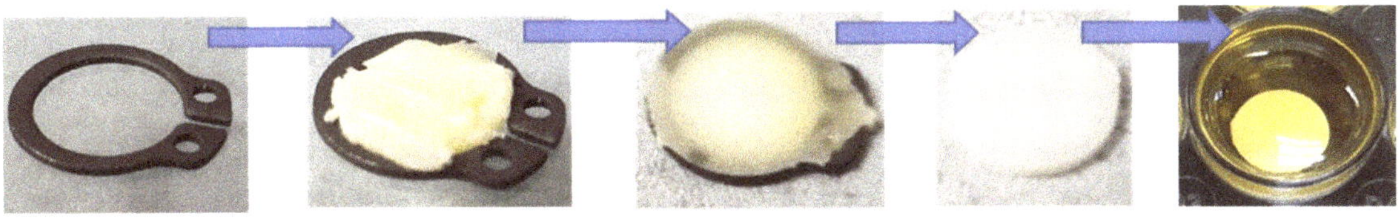

Figure 1. Preparation of composite disc and disc placed in well.

2.4. Mass and Volume Change

The mass and volume change of set discs versus time in deionised water (DW) were determined using a density kit and four-figure digital balance (AG204, Mettler, Toledo, OH, USA) according to the ISO 17304:2013. 1% sodium dodecyl sulphate (Sigma-Aldrich, Gillingham, UK) in DW was used as the buoyancy medium.

Discs (n = 3), prepared as above, were immersed in 1 mL of DW in individual sterilin tubes at 23 °C. At 1, 3, 6 h, 1, 2, 5, 7 days, 2, 4 and 8 weeks, the discs were removed from the solution, their surfaces blot dried using absorbent paper, weighed in air and in the buoyancy medium and then placed into new tubes with fresh 1 mL of DW. Initial mass and volume were calculated by extrapolation of early data versus square root of time to zero. Mass and volume change were then calculated as percentages of original mass as shown in detail in previous publications [10,11].

2.5. Polylysine Release

High-performance liquid chromatography (HPLC) (Shimadzu corporation, Kyoto, Japan) was used to measure polylysine release from composite discs. The composite discs (n = 3) were prepared as above, weighed and then immersed in 1 mL deionized water (DW) in individual sterilin tubes. The discs were removed from the DW and placed in a new tube with 1 mL of fresh DW at 1, 3, 6 h, 1, 2, 5, 7 days and 3 weeks. The storage solutions were stored at 23 °C prior to analysis.

A normal phase column in hydrophilic interaction liquid chromatography (HILIC) mode was used. The mobile phase was 50 vol% acetonitrile in DW with 0.1 vol% of phosphoric acid (97%) added. Flow rate, run time, temperature, and UV detection wavelength were 1.0 mL/min, 43 min, 30 °C and 210 nm respectively. PLS solutions of 10 to 100 ppm were used to generate a calibration curve which was then employed to determine PLS concentrations in each storage solution. Cumulative PLS versus time, as a percentage of that calculated to be in the original specimen, was then determined [10].

2.6. Bacterial Growth Inhibition

A single colony of *S. mutans* UA159 was inoculated into brain heart infusion broth (BHI, Oxoid, Basingstoke, UK) and incubated statically at 37 °C for 16 h in air enriched with 5% CO_2. The culture was diluted in BHI broth to generate an inoculum of 8×10^5 and 8×10^6 CFU/mL which was confirmed by viable counting.

On the day of each experiment the discs ($n = 3$) were placed in a custom made ultraviolet light box and irradiated for 30 min on each side to ensure sterility. Decontamination was verified by plating on agar. The discs were then placed into a 24 well plate as seen in Figure 1. 1 mL of the *S. mutans* inoculum was added to each well and the plates placed in the incubator on a shaking tray at 200 rpm at 37 °C in air. At 24 h, the cultures were 10-fold serially diluted and plated out on BHI agar (Oxoid, Basingstoke, UK). Bacterial colonies were counted after 3 days of incubation at 37 °C in 5% CO_2.

2.7. Surface Bacteria Observations

To assess viability of attached bacteria on material surfaces, composite discs ($n = 2$) were immersed in an *S. mutans* suspension with concentration of 5×10^6 CFU/mL and incubated statically for 72 h in air at 37 °C. The discs were removed and gently immersed in fresh BHI broth to remove unattached bacteria before placing in a clean well plate for staining using LIVE/DEAD Viability kit (Thermofisher Scientific, Loughborough, UK). Confocal laser scanning microscopy (Radiance 2100, Biorad, Hercules, CA, USA) with an objective lens of 10×–20× magnification was used to visualize bacteria. Images were saved and processed using Lasersharp 2000 (Biorad, Hercules, CA, USA) and ImageJ (ImageJ Developers).

2.8. Statistical Analysis

Data analysis was undertaken for volumetric analysis, polylysine release and bacterial viable counts using Analysis of Variance (ANOVA) and SPSS (IBM, Armonk, NY, USA) with $p < 0.05$ considered significant. To perform multiple comparisons of multiple formulations, the Bonferroni adjustment was used.

3. Results

3.1. Mass and Volume

Mass and volume change both increased proportional to the square root of time. Final mass change at 2 months increased linearly with polylysine content from 0.7 to 1.7 wt% (RSQ = 0.96). Final volume change, however, was not significantly affected by PLS level ($p > 0.05$) and was between 2.2 and 2.5 vol% (Figure 2).

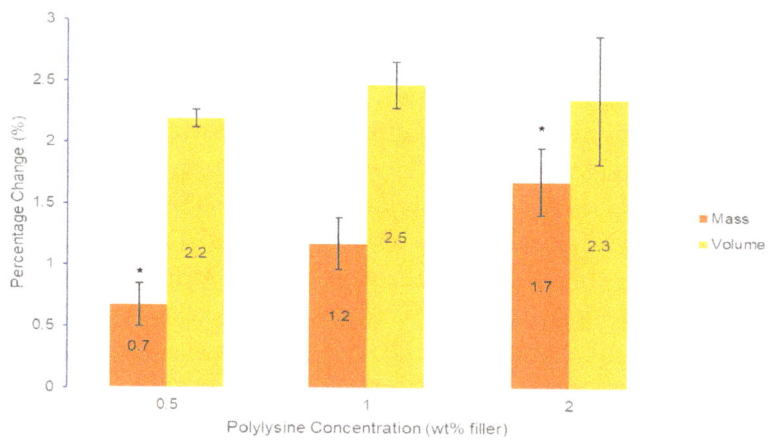

Figure 2. Graph of percentage change in mass and volume of the three formulations containing polylysine after 2 months. Error bars = st. dev. ($n = 3$). * indicates significance between results ($p < 0.05$).

3.2. Polylysine Release

Cumulative polylysine release was initially proportional to the square root of time but then levelled between 2 and 3 weeks (Figure 3). Cumulative percentage release was higher with 2% PLS at 1 and 2 days at 2.4 and 2.7% but within experimental error independent of concentration and 4% by 3 weeks. In Figure 4, the percentage release is converted to provide a calculated total concentration per disc that would have been released into 1 mL of storage solution by 6 h, 24 h and three weeks. At 3 weeks, the PLS release in grams was proportional to the level in the filler. At earlier time points, however, doubling the filler PLS content more than doubled the release in grams (see Figure 4).

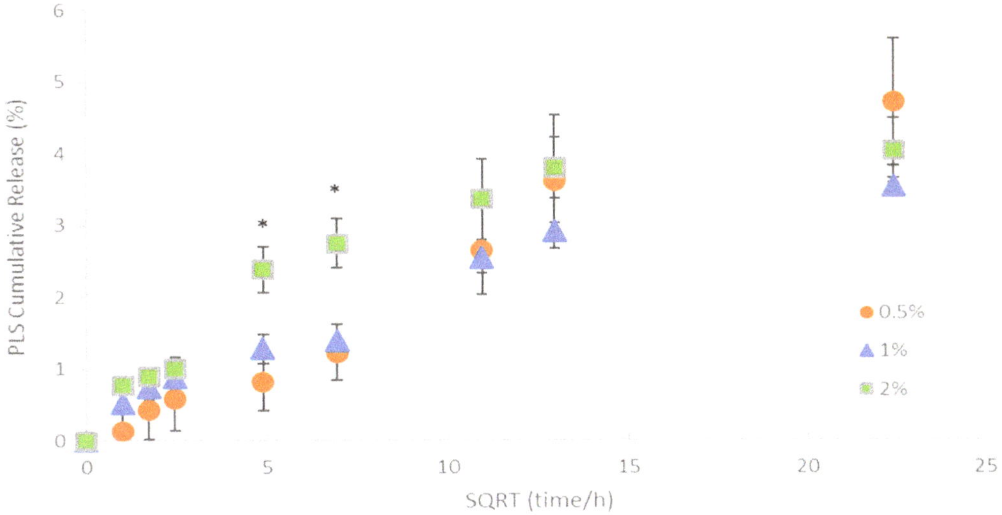

Figure 3. Cumulative percentage release of polylysine (PLS) versus the square root (SQRT) of time. Error bars = st. dev ($n = 3$). * indicates that formulation with 2% PLS has significantly higher percentage release at 24 and 48 h but not at early or later times.

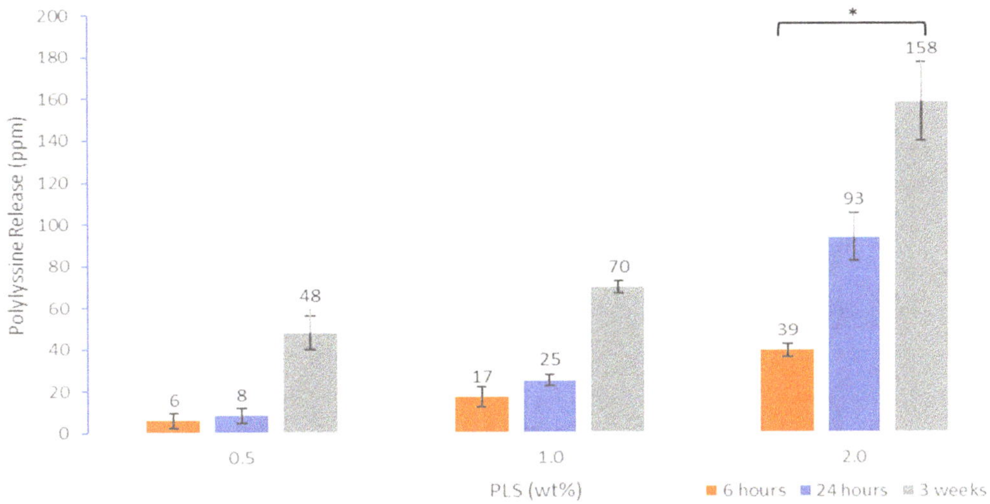

Figure 4. Cumulative polylysine release after 6 h, 24 h and 3 weeks at 23 °C for formulations with 0.5, 1 or 2% PLS. Error bars = st. dev ($n = 3$). * indicates 2% PLS containing formulation has significantly higher release at all time points compared with the other 2 formulations.

3.3. Determination of Antibacterial Activity

Colony forming units are shown in Figure 5, after 24 h incubation in air with different composite formulations for two different initial inoculum bacterial levels. Irrespective of initial inoculum level, CFU increased to 10^9 for all controls with no PLS. This was also observed with 0.5% and 1% PLS with the higher initial inoculum. Conversely, 0.5 and 1% PLS in the composite filler caused a 90 and

99% reduction in CFU with the lower initial inoculum concentration. With 2% PLS, the 24 h CFU count was down to 10^7 and 10^2 with high versus low initial inoculum levels, respectively. The 2% PLS formulations had statistically significantly less bacteria at 24 h when compared to all other composites at both inoculum concentrations.

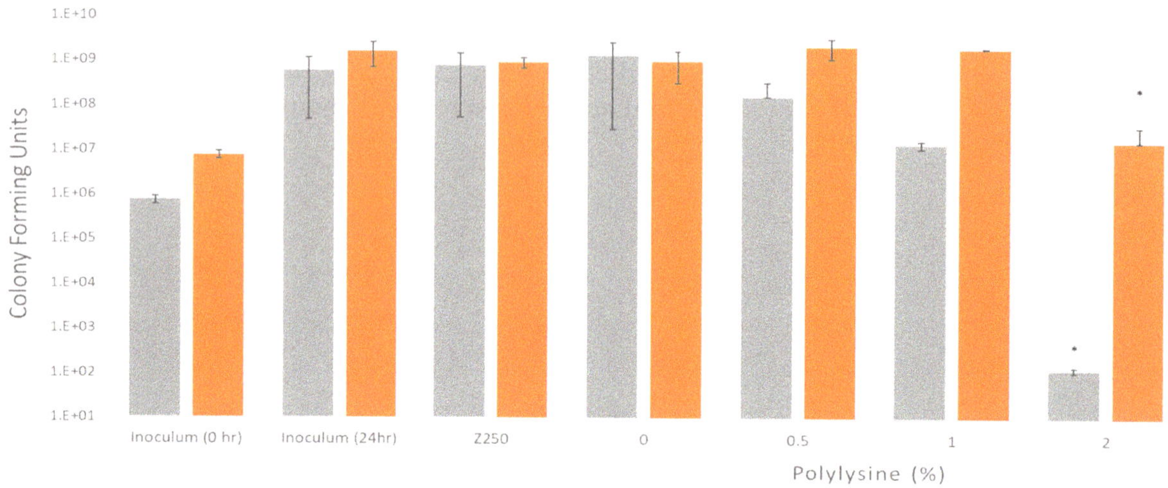

Figure 5. Bacterial growth after 24 h with two different inoculum concentrations of *S. mutans*, 8×10^5 and 8×10^6 CFU/mL. Four different formulations and a commercial composite were tested. Plates with discs and inoculum were incubated in air for 24 h at 37 °C while being shaken. Error bars = st. dev (n = 3), * indicates 2% is significantly different when compared to other formulations.

3.4. Confocal Laser Scanning Microscopy

Figure 6 shows confocal images of composite surfaces stained with live/dead stain. The bacteria do not form a biofilm due to the lack of sucrose but are seen as individual bacteria on the material surface. As the concentration of polylysine in the composite disc increases, an increase in the proportion of dead bacteria is seen.

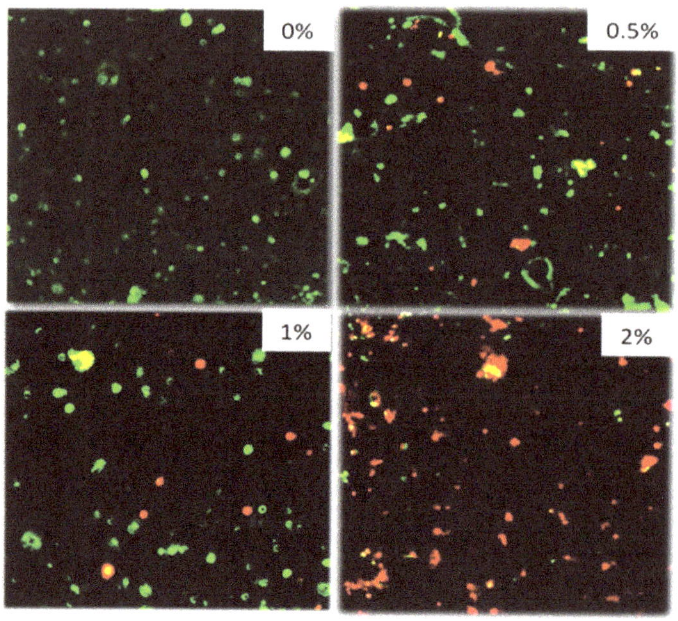

Figure 6. From top left to bottom right 0, 0.5, 1, 2% formulations. Inoculum: *S. mutans* 5×10^6 CFU/mL. Plates with discs and inoculum were incubated for 72 h in air at 37 °C before staining. Stained with Live/Dead staining. (n = 2).

4. Discussion

4.1. Mass and Volume Change

Dental restorations are exposed to fluids from the oral cavity continuously. Any dental composite will have micro voids after the setting reaction has taken place. When immersed in solution (i.e., deionized water), over time, the water will be absorbed by the voids in the composite as well as the composite matrix phase and the mass and volume will increase. Excessive expansion can result in a reduction in mechanical properties [18].

Mass and volume changes were undertaken for 2 months, as previous work has shown they tend to level off after this time [19]. With low PLS, the volume change, approximately double the mass change, suggests water is mostly expanding the matrix phase [19]. This is a consequence of the composite density being double that of water. With higher PLS, the mass increase, more comparable with the volume change, suggests there are more pores being filled by water which would cause mass increase but no expansion. The porosity may be caused by poor wetting and dispersion of the hydrophilic PLS particles by the monomer phase. The lack of change in the volume with increasing PLS level suggests it has minimal effect on the surrounding matrix expansion. The final levels of mass and volume change with 2% PLS (1.7 wt% and 2.3 vol%) are approximately two thirds of those seen with an earlier similar formulation (F2) (2.5 wt% and 3.5 vol%) that had an additional 10 wt% tricalcium phosphate [11]. This suggests the mass and volume changes are related to the total calcium phosphate levels in these composites. A previous study has shown that the commercial composite Z250 shows an increase in mass and volume after 7 weeks of 1.1 and 1.6% respectively [11]. The mass and volume changes of the experimental composites were comparable or above those observed for Z250.

4.2. Antibacterial Activity and Polylysine Release

Polylysine has been added to dental composites in previous research [10,11], but reports on the optimum concentration have not been carried out. This study attempts to replicate the conditions at the interface between the composite and the sealed affected dentine in which sucrose will be excluded. In this situation, the formation of biofilm on the discs was not observed. One recent study demonstrated that polylysine had satisfactory antibacterial efficacy against *S. mutans* in a liquid culture medium and as an application on biofilm–dentin surfaces. The study demonstrated that the susceptibility of microorganisms to polylysine was dependent on polylysine concentrations [20]. Additionally, it showed that polylysine can kill and inhibit the growth of the periodontal pathogen *Porphyromonas gingivalis* [20].

Increased polylysine release from the composite can have a negative effect on the mechanical properties of the material [11], so the minimum amount to cause bacterial kill would need to be used. This is a common issue for formulations with a released soluble antibacterial agent [5,6]. Other antibacterial agents, such as quaternary ammonium methacrylate, are non-released and their effect on physical properties is less evident [8,21]. Additionally, their surface antibacterial properties could be more stable over time. Surface antibacterial benefits, however, may be neutralized by a biofilm or adhesive covering. Conversely, the benefit of high early polylysine release is a greater chance of an effective reduction in residual bacteria deep within minimally excavated cavities. The above studies suggest, however, that higher levels of polylysine release may be required for highly infected cavities.

Previous experiments have shown greater early burst release and a higher release over time from a 2.5% PLS formulation with approximately 5.5% after 24 h and 9% at 3 weeks of being observed. As this was not previously affected by monocalcium and tricalcium phosphate addition, the differences may instead be due to the use of the more standard TEGDMA monomer. This can cause lower conversions [10] than seen with PPGDMA [11]. In this new study, the composite formulation with 2% PLS released 2.4% of polylysine in the first 24 h and after 3 weeks this had increased to just 4%. Initial polylysine release, proportional to the square root of time with no early burst release, is more in agreement with a recent report using the same monomer system as this study [22]. The work showed that increasing the polylysine concentration from 4 to 6 and then 8 wt% of the filler caused final release percentages to level at values of 13, 28 and 42% after 1, 2 and 3 months respectively [22]. This was attributed to surface release from layers of 65, 140 and 210 micron thick. The PLS release levelling between 1 and 3 weeks in this study fits with this trend. Given that the sample thickness is 100 microns, a final release of 4% suggests the PLS release may be from surface layers of just 20 microns thick.

Due to the initially higher concentration of PLS, the release in grams is higher as the concentration of polylysine in the formulations increased from 0.5 to 2%. The Minimum Inhibitory Concentration of polylysine on *S. mutans* in air with inoculum density of 5×10^5 CFU/mL is 20 µg/mL [23]. After 24 h, the 0.5%, 1% and 2% formulations had an average ($n = 3$) of 8, 25 and 93 µg/mL of polylysine released. This could explain why the 1% and 2% formulations inhibit growth in air conditions as they release more than 20 µg/mL of polylysine. Conversely, the 0.5% formulations which released less than 20 µg/mL did not inhibit growth. It is therefore expected that higher PLS concentrations will be required to inhibit growth of higher inoculum concentrations. This was also demonstrated in a recent study [20].

The aim of using Confocal was to visualize the live/dead state of bacteria sedimented on the composite disc surfaces. In many other studies, additional sucrose is added to promote biofilm formation [8,9]. The method chosen in this study with no additional sucrose, however, better replicates the environment beneath the restoration after effective sealing. With these conditions, largely only well-spaced individual bacteria were seen on the material surfaces and not biofilms. With the 0.5% and 1% PLS discs, some dead bacteria were present on disc surfaces at 72 h, whereas on the 2% PLS discs, the majority were dead. At the high level of initial inoculum chosen for the confocal study, the 2% PLS disc prevents any change in bacterial numbers in suspension at 24 h indicating bacterial increase is exactly balanced by killing. It is possible, therefore, that dead bacteria on the composite surfaces were killed when they made contact with remaining PLS on the composite surfaces or through more prolonged and increasing contact with PLS in the suspension.

5. Conclusions

Increasing polylysine concentration from 0.5% to 2% in composite discs leads to an increase in mass but not volume change over three weeks. Whilst the PLS-release percentage was faster in the first 24 h with 2% in the filler, the final percentage release was not affected by increasing composite PLS level. With 2% PLS, the amount released into 1 mL of broth in 24 h was sufficient to display significantly reduced bacterial levels when the initial inoculum level was at 8×10^5, but their growth in number was only inhibited when the initial bacterial counts were raised 10-fold. With an initial inoculum of 5×10^6 bacteria, those detected on the composite surfaces after 72 h were mostly live with 1% or less PLS in the composite but dead with 2% PLS. Higher PLS may enable the greater killing of residual bacteria when composites are used for minimally invasive tooth restorations. Considering the limitations of this study and taking into account work completed in previous studies [24–26], future research should include sucrose in the experiments to allow for biofilm growth on the discs to determine the effectiveness of PLS against biofilms, test multispecies biofilms and assess long term polylysine release and how this may affect the integrity of the restoration.

6. Patents

The work is covered by the following licensed patent families: Formulations and composites with reactive fillers (US8252851 B2, EP2066703B1, US20100069469, WO2008037991A1), and Formulations and materials with cationic polymers (PCT/GB2014/052349, WO2015015212 A1, EP3027164A1, US20160184190).

Author Contributions: Conceptualization, N.N.L., E.A., W.X., P.F.A., A.M.Y.; Methodology, N.N.L., E.A., W.X., P.F.A., A.M.Y.; Validation, N.N.L., E.A., P.F.A., A.M.Y.; Formal Analysis, N.N.L.; Investigation, N.N.L.; Resources, N.N.L., E.A., P.F.A., A.M.Y.; Writing—original Draft Preparation, N.N.L.; Writing—review & Editing, N.N.L., E.A.,

P.F.A., A.M.Y.; Supervision, E.A., W.X., P.F.A., A.M.Y.; Project Administration, A.M.Y.; Funding Acquisition, A.M.Y. All authors have read and agreed to the published version of the manuscript.

References

1. Bourguignon, D. Briefing EU Legislation in Progress Mercury Aligning EU Legislation with Minamata. 2017. Available online: http://www.europarl.europa.eu/RegData/etudes/BRIE/2017/595887/EPRS_BRI(2017)595887_EN.pdf (accessed on 16 February 2020).
2. Ricketts, D.; Lamont, T.; Innes, N.; Kidd, E.; Clarkson, J.E. Operative caries management in adults and children. *Cochrane Database Syst. Rev.* **2013**, *28*. [CrossRef] [PubMed]
3. Ferracane, J.L. Resin composite—State of the art. *Dent. Mater.* **2011**, *27*, 29–38. [CrossRef]
4. Chisini, L.A.; Collares, K.; Cademartori, M.G.; de Oliveira, L.J.C.; Conde, M.C.M.; Demarco, F.F.; Corrêa, M.B. Restorations in primary teeth: A systematic review on survival and reasons for failures. *Int. J. Paediatr. Dent.* **2018**, *28*, 123–139. [CrossRef] [PubMed]
5. Leung, D.; Spratt, D.; Pratten, J.; Gulabivala, K.; Mordan, N.; Young, A.M. Chlorhexidine-releasing methacrylate dental composite materials. *Biomaterials* **2005**, *26*, 7145–7153. [CrossRef] [PubMed]
6. Zhang, J.F.; Wu, R.; Fan, Y.; Liao, S.; Wang, Y.; Wen, Z.T.; Xu, X. Antibacterial Dental Composites with Chlorhexidine and Mesoporous Silica. *J. Dent. Res.* **2014**, *93*, 1283–1289. [CrossRef] [PubMed]
7. Nedeljkovic, I.; Teughels, W.; De Munck, J.; Van Meerbeek, B.; Van Landuyt, K.L. Is secondary caries with composites a material-based problem? *Dent. Mater.* **2015**, *31*, e247–e277. [CrossRef] [PubMed]
8. Wang, H.; Wang, S.; Cheng, L.; Jiang, Y.; Melo, M.A.; Weir, M.; Oates, T.; Zhou, X.; Xu, H.K. Novel dental composite with capability to suppress cariogenic species and promote non-cariogenic species in oral biofilms. *Mater. Sci. Eng. C* **2019**, *94*, 587–596. [CrossRef]
9. Balhaddad, A.A.; Ibrahim, M.S.; Weir, M.D.; Xu, H.H.K.; Melo, M.A.S. Concentration dependence of quaternary ammonium monomer on the design of high-performance bioactive composite for root caries restorations. *Dent. Mater.* **2020**, *36*, e266–e278. [CrossRef]
10. Panpisut, P.; Liaqat, S.; Zacharaki, E.; Xia, W.; Petridis, H.; Young, A.M. Dental Composites with Calcium/Strontium Phosphates and Polylysine. *PLoS ONE* **2016**, *11*, e0164653. [CrossRef]
11. Kangwankai, K.; Sani, S.; Panpisut, P.; Xia, W.; Ashley, P.; Petridis, H.; Young, A.M. Monomer conversion, dimensional stability, strength, modulus, surface apatite precipitation and wear of novel, reactive calcium phosphate and polylysine-containing dental composites. *PLoS ONE* **2017**, *12*, e0187757. [CrossRef]
12. Ye, R.; Xu, H.; Wan, C.; Peng, S.; Wang, L.; Xu, H.; Aguilar, Z.; Xiong, Y.; Zeng, Z.; Wei, H. Antibacterial activity and mechanism of action of poly-l-lysine. *Biochem. Biophys. Res. Commun.* **2013**, *439*, 148–153. [CrossRef]
13. Bo, T.; Han, P.; Su, Q.; Fu, P.; Guo, F.; Zheng, Z.; Tan, Z.; Zhong, C.; Jia, S. Antimicrobial ε-poly-l-lysine induced changes in cell membrane compositions and properties of Saccharomyces cerevisiae. *Food Control* **2016**, *61*, 123–134. [CrossRef]
14. Sayed, S.; Jardine, M. Antimicrobial biopolymers. In *Advanced Functional Materials*; John Wiley & Sons Inc.: Hoboken, NJ, USA, 2015; pp. 493–533.
15. Walters, N.; Xia, W.; Salih, V.; Ashley, P.; Young, A.M. Poly(propylene glycol) and urethane dimethacrylates improve conversion of dental composites and reveal complexity of cytocompatibility testing. *Dent. Mater.* **2016**, *32*, 264–277. [CrossRef]
16. Van Landuyt, K.; Snauwaert, J.; De Munck, J.; Peumans, M.; Yoshida, Y.; Poitevin, A.; Coutinho, E.; Suzuki, K.; Lambrechts, P.; Van Meerbeek, B. Systematic review of the chemical composition of contemporary dental adhesives. *Biomaterials* **2007**, *28*, 3757–3785. [CrossRef] [PubMed]
17. Aljabo, A.; Abou Neel, E.A.; Knowles, J.C.; Young, A.M. Development of dental composites with reactive fillers that promote precipitation of antibacterial-hydroxyapatite layers. *Mater. Sci. Eng. C Mater. Biol. Appl.* **2016**, *60*, 285–292. [CrossRef] [PubMed]
18. Sideridou, I.D.; Karabela, M.M.; Bikiaris, D.N. Aging studies of light cured dimethacrylate-based dental resins and a resin composite in water or ethanol/water. *Dent. Mater.* **2007**, *23*, 1142–1149. [CrossRef] [PubMed]

19. Aljabo, A.; Xia, W.; Liaqat, S.; Khan, M.A.; Knowles, J.C.; Ashley, P.; Young, A.M. Conversion, shrinkage, water sorption, flexural strength and modulus of re-mineralizing dental composites. *Dent. Mater.* **2015**, *31*, 1279–1289. [CrossRef]
20. Dima, S.; Lee, Y.-Y.; Watanabe, I.; Chang, W.-J.; Pan, Y.-H.; Teng, N.-C. Antibacterial Effect of the Natural Polymer ε-Polylysine Against Oral Pathogens Associated with Periodontitis and Caries. *Polymers* **2020**, *12*, 1218. [CrossRef]
21. Chen, L.; Suh, B.I.; Yang, J. Antibacterial dental restorative materials: A review. *Am. J. Dent.* **2018**, *31*, 6B–12B.
22. Yaghmoor, R.B.; Xia, W.; Ashley, P.; Allan, E.; Young, A.M. Effect of Novel Antibacterial Composites on Bacterial Biofilms. *J. Funct. Biomater.* **2020**, *11*, accepted.
23. Badaoui Najjar, M.; Kashtanov, D.; Chikindas, M.L. Natural Antimicrobials ε-Poly-l-lysine and Nisin A for Control of Oral Microflora. *Probiotics Antimicrob. Proteins* **2009**, *1*, 143–147. [CrossRef] [PubMed]
24. Balhaddad, A.A.; Kansara, A.A.; Hidan, D.; Weir, M.D.; Xu, H.; Melo, M. Toward dental caries: Exploring nanoparticle-based platforms and calcium phosphate compounds for dental restorative materials. *Bioact. Mater.* **2018**, *4*, 43–55. [CrossRef] [PubMed]
25. Dahl, J.E.; Stenhagen, I. Optimizing quality and safety of dental materials. *Eur. J. Oral Sci.* **2018**, *126* (Suppl. S1), 102–105. [CrossRef] [PubMed]
26. Ibrahim, M.S.; Garcia, I.M.; Kensara, A.; Balhaddad, A.A.; Collares, F.M.; Williams, M.A.; Ibrahim, A.S.; Lin, N.J.; Weir, M.D.; Xu, H.H.K.; et al. How we are assessing the developing antibacterial resin-based dental materials? A scoping review. *J. Dent.* **2020**, e103369. [CrossRef] [PubMed]

8

Myristyltrimethylammonium Bromide (MYTAB) as a Cationic Surface Agent to Inhibit *Streptococcus mutans* Grown over Dental Resins: An In Vitro Study

Paola Andrea Mena Silva [1,2,3], Isadora Martini Garcia [1], Julia Nunes [4], Fernanda Visioli [4], Vicente Castelo Branco Leitune [1], Mary Anne Melo [5,6,*] and Fabrício Mezzomo Collares [1,*]

1 Dental Materials Laboratory, School of Dentistry, Federal University of Rio Grande do Sul, 90035-003 Porto Alegre-RS, Brazil; pao_mena100@hotmail.com (P.A.M.S.); isadora.garcia@ufrgs.br (I.M.G.); vicente.leitune@ufrgs.br (V.C.B.L.)
2 Universidad Central del Ecuador, 170129 Quito, Ecuador
3 Postgraduate Department, Universidad Regional Autónoma de Los Andes, 170129 Quito, Ecuador
4 Oral Pathology Department, School of Dentistry, Federal University of Rio Grande do Sul, 90035-003 Porto Alegre-RS, Brazil; jusnunes@icloud.com (J.N.); fernanda.visioli@ufrgs.br (F.V.)
5 Operative Dentistry Division, General Dentistry Department, University of Maryland School of Dentistry, Baltimore, MD 21201, USA
6 Ph.D. Program in Biomedical Sciences, University of Maryland School of Dentistry, Baltimore, MD 21201, USA
* Correspondence: mmelo@umaryland.edu (M.A.M.); fabricio.collares@ufrgs.br (F.M.C.)

Abstract: This in vitro study evaluated the effect of myristyltrimethylammonium bromide (MYTAB) on the physical, chemical, and biological properties of an experimental dental resin. The resin was formulated with dental dimetacrylate monomers and a photoinitiator/co-initiator system. MYTAB was added at 0.5 ($G_{0.5\%}$), 1 ($G_{1\%}$), and 2 ($G_{2\%}$) wt %, and one group remained without MYTAB and was used as the control (G_{Ctrl}). The resins were analyzed for the polymerization kinetics, degree of conversion, ultimate tensile strength (UTS), antibacterial activity against *Streptococcus mutans*, and cytotoxicity against human keratinocytes. Changes in the polymerization kinetics profiling were observed, and the degree of conversion ranged from 57.36% (±2.50%) for $G_{2\%}$ to 61.88% (±1.91%) for $G_{0.5\%}$, without a statistically significant difference among groups ($p > 0.05$). The UTS values ranged from 32.85 (±6.08) MPa for $G_{0.5\%}$ to 35.12 (±5.74) MPa for G_{Ctrl} ($p > 0.05$). MYTAB groups showed antibacterial activity against biofilm formation from 0.5 wt % ($p < 0.05$) and against planktonic bacteria from 1 wt % ($p < 0.05$). The higher the MYTAB concentration, the higher the cytotoxic effect, without differences between G_{Ctrl} e $G_{0.5\%}$ ($p > 0.05$). In conclusion, the addition of 0.5 wt % of MYTAB did not alter the physical and chemical properties of the dental resin and provided antibacterial activity without cytotoxic effect.

Keywords: dental materials; dentistry; anti-bacterial agents; dental caries; biocompatible materials; biofilms; quaternary ammonium compounds

1. Introduction

Dental caries-linked bacteria growing in biofilms play a pivotal role in the initial formation and development of carious lesions. The demand for the development of antibacterial surfaces has gained prominence in order to reduce patients' susceptibility to new or repeated diseases [1–5]. In dentistry, dental materials have been developed with antibacterial agents to provide new preventive and treatment dynamics for patients [6–9]. The antibacterial approach for dental materials relies on biological interactions of the bacteria grown over the materials, and the contact with antibacterial agents presents in the surface or is released by the materials [10–13]. In this context, the achievement of surfaces able to reduce caries-linked biofilm formation over dental tissues or restorative structures has gained the attention of dental biomaterial researchers.

The current understanding of the dental caries disease process and the new advances in dental materials promote the preservation of dental structure and the application of minimally invasive techniques [14]. Under this framework, dental resins are the first option for the replacement of dental hard tissues that were lost due to carious lesions [15,16]. Dental resins are materials cured by chemical or physicochemical (via photo-activation) processes, and they present inorganic fillers depending on their purpose. In areas where it is necessary to increase strength (occlusal/chewing surfaces of teeth), a high amount of inorganic fillers is incorporated [17]. Dental resins with low viscosity can also be successfully used to seal the biting surfaces of teeth, decreasing the incidence of caries lesions [18].

The oral environment provides many challenges to the physical and chemical stability of dental resins, such as high humidity, temperature, and pH variations [19,20]. Likewise, acids leached by high acidogenic caries-linked bacteria such as *Streptococcus mutans*, conjointly with a degradative attack of enzymes, inherently present in the saliva, can jeopardize the materials' properties over time [21]. More expressively, acidic attack from high acidogenic caries-linked bacteria is a crucial step in tooth demineralization around the restorations [22]. On this basis, the search for long-lasting strategies challenging biofilm accumulation on dental resins, as well as the consequent caries lesion development around restorations, must be addressed.

Antibacterial surfaces with a bacteria-killing function have shown great promise in biological and biomedical applications, in particular for dental resin-based materials. This approach employs the incorporation of quaternary ammonium compounds (QACs) in the monomeric blend of the resin-based material formulation [9,11,23]. QACs have facile synthesis, antibacterial property, and a lack of a detrimental effect on the mechanical and physical properties when incorporated in concentrations. Typically, QAS exhibits a positive charge, which confers the surface with the ability to attach and kill bacteria efficiently. The killing effect is attributed to their electronically interaction and linking to bacteria membrane and wall, along with their possible diffusion into the cytoplasmic membrane, an increase of osmotic pressure, and the release of some cytoplasmic constituents [24,25].

Myristyltrimethylammonium bromide (MYTAB) is a QAC with an alkyl-chain length of 14 carbons presenting a chemical structure of $C_{17}H_{38}NBr$, a molecular weight of 336.39, and a cationic polar head group. Trimethyl alkylammonium compounds such as the MYTAB series can also strongly affect bacterial membrane properties of a wide range of microorganisms, including changes in electrokinetic potential as well as net surface charge [26]. A recent study has shown promising application for the sealing of dental roots during endodontic treatment with expressive bacterial reduction of the endodontic pathogen [27]. Additionally, the long-chain MYTAB presents the potential to act as a useful endocytosis inhibitor for cell biology, inhibiting different forms of endocytosis in multiple cell systems [26].

The present study aimed to evaluate the potential ability of MYTAB to impair bacterial reduction when incorporated into dental resin at increasing concentrations. Its antibacterial effects against *S. mutans*, a pivotal cariogenic pathogen presented in planktonic and biofilm stages, were assessed. The cytotoxicity effect on human keratinocytes was investigated. The chemical and physical effects of its incorporation on the materials were also explored.

2. Results

Figure 1 shows the results of polymerization kinetics (Figure 1a–c), degree of conversion (Figure 1d), and ultimate tensile strength (UTS) (Figure 1e). The experimental dental resins had different polymerization behavior throughout the 40 s of photoactivation. The degree of conversion per time is shown in Figure 1a. The results (Figure 2d) ranged from 57.36% (±2.50%) for $G_{2\%}$ to 61.88% (±1.91%) for $G_{0.5\%}$, without statistical difference among groups ($p > 0.05$). Figure 1b indicates the results of the polymerization rate per time, showing that the higher the concentration of MYTAB, the higher the delay in achieving the maximum polymerization rate. Moreover, the higher the concentration of MYTAB, the lower the maximum polymerization rate. Figure 1c displays these differences, showing that at the same degree of conversion among groups, the polymerization rate of G_{Ctrl} was higher than $G_{1\%}$ and $G_{2\%}$ and lower than $G_{0.5\%}$. In Figure 1d, the degree of conversion revealed similar behavior for the tested groups ($p > 0.05$). The mechanical property of the dental resins was evaluated under UTS and expressed in MPa, as shown in Figure 1e. The UTS ranged from 32.85 (±6.08) MPa for $G_{0.5\%}$ to 35.12 (±5.74) MPa for G_{Ctrl}. There was no statistical difference among groups ($p > 0.05$).

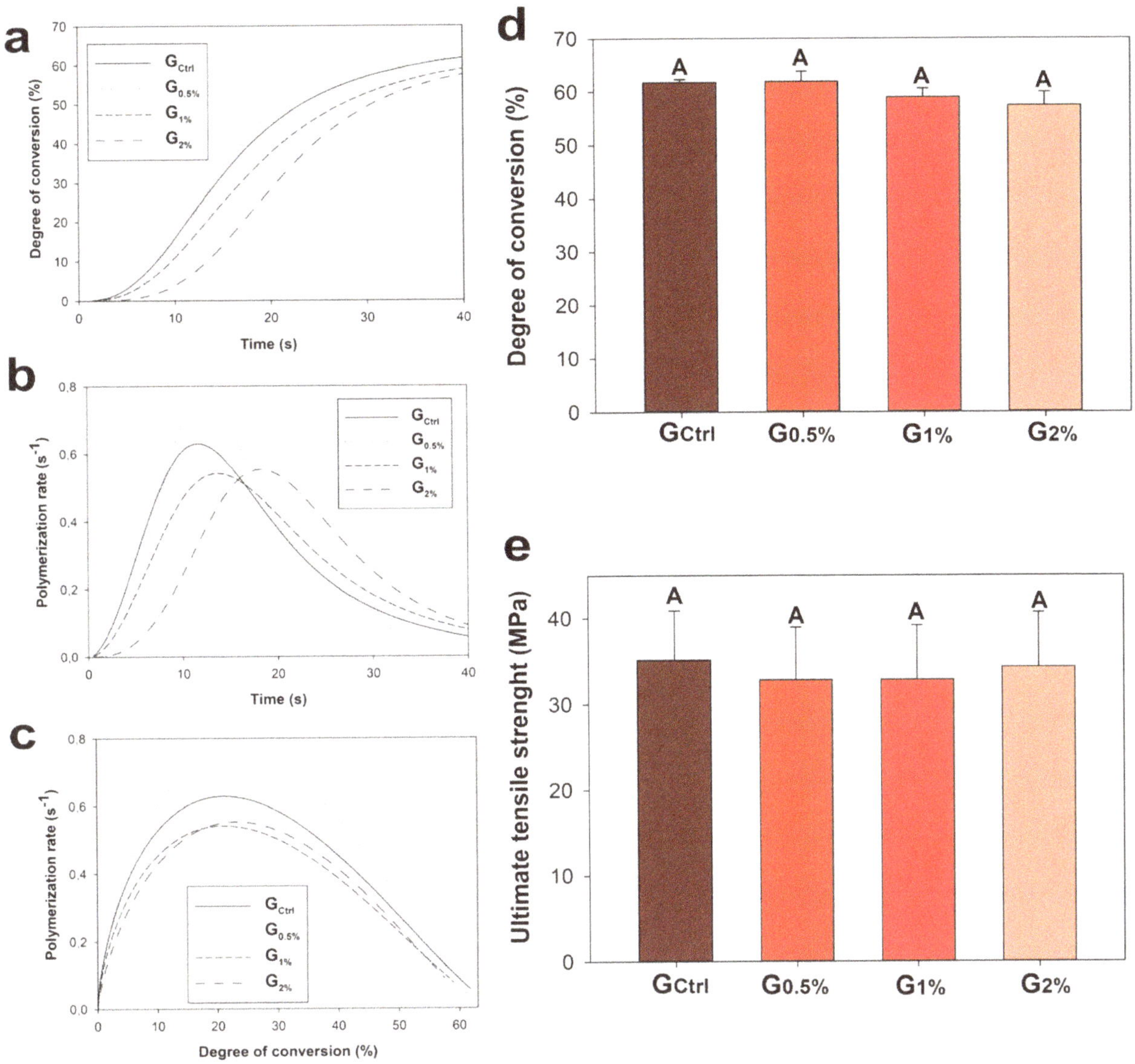

Figure 1. Comprehensive results of polymerization kinetics (**a**–**c**), degree of conversion after 40 s of photoactivation (**d**), and ultimate tensile strength (UTS) (**e**). Same capital letters indicate no statistical difference among groups ($p > 0.05$). The groups had different polymerization kinetics without statistical difference for the degree of conversion and UTS.

Figure 2 shows the results of the antibacterial activity of the experimental dental resins against biofilm formation of *S. mutans* and planktonic *S. mutans*, expressed by the log reduction in colony-forming unit per milliliter. In the microbiological assessment against biofilm formation (Figure 2a), the values ranged from 4.58 (±0.08) log CFU/mL for $G_{2\%}$ to 7.21 (±0.08) log CFU/mL for G_{Ctrl} ($p < 0.05$). A greater bacterial reduction ($p < 0.05$) was observed at the higher concentration of MYTAB incorporated into the dental resin. In the test against planktonic bacteria (Figure 2b), the values ranged from 6.68 (±0.58) log CFU/mL for $G_{2\%}$ to 8.28 (±0.05) log CFU/mL for G_{Ctrl} ($p < 0.05$). The group presenting MYTAB concentration at 2% expressed the highest *S. mutans* bacterial reduction ($p < 0.05$).

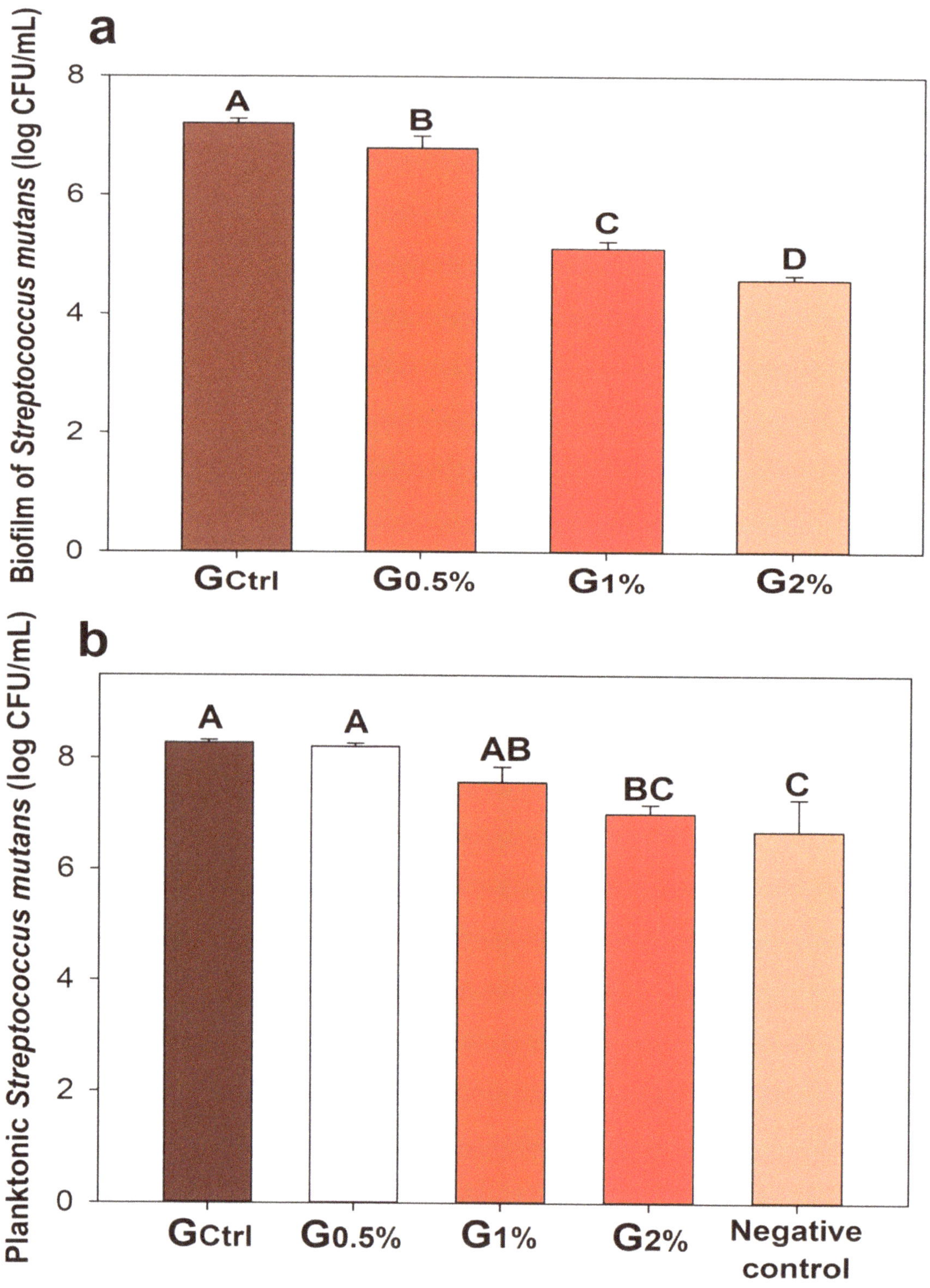

Figure 2. Bacterial colony forming unit counting: (**a**) *Streptococcus mutans* biofilms and (**b**) planktonic *S. mutans* that were in contact with the polymerized samples. Values indicated by different letters indicate statistical differences among the groups ($p < 0.05$).

Figure 3 presents the effects of MYTAB incorporated into a dental resin on normal human keratinocytes (HaCaT) for cytotoxicity assessed by sulforhodamine B (SRB) assay. The percentage of viability of the cells ranged from 45.26% (±14.11%) for $G_{2\%}$ to 110.16% (±14.64%) for G_{Ctrl} ($p < 0.05$). $G_{0.5\%}$ (91.82% ± 12.17%) presented no statistical difference in comparison to G_{Ctrl} ($p > 0.05$) for cytotoxicity against human keratinocytes.

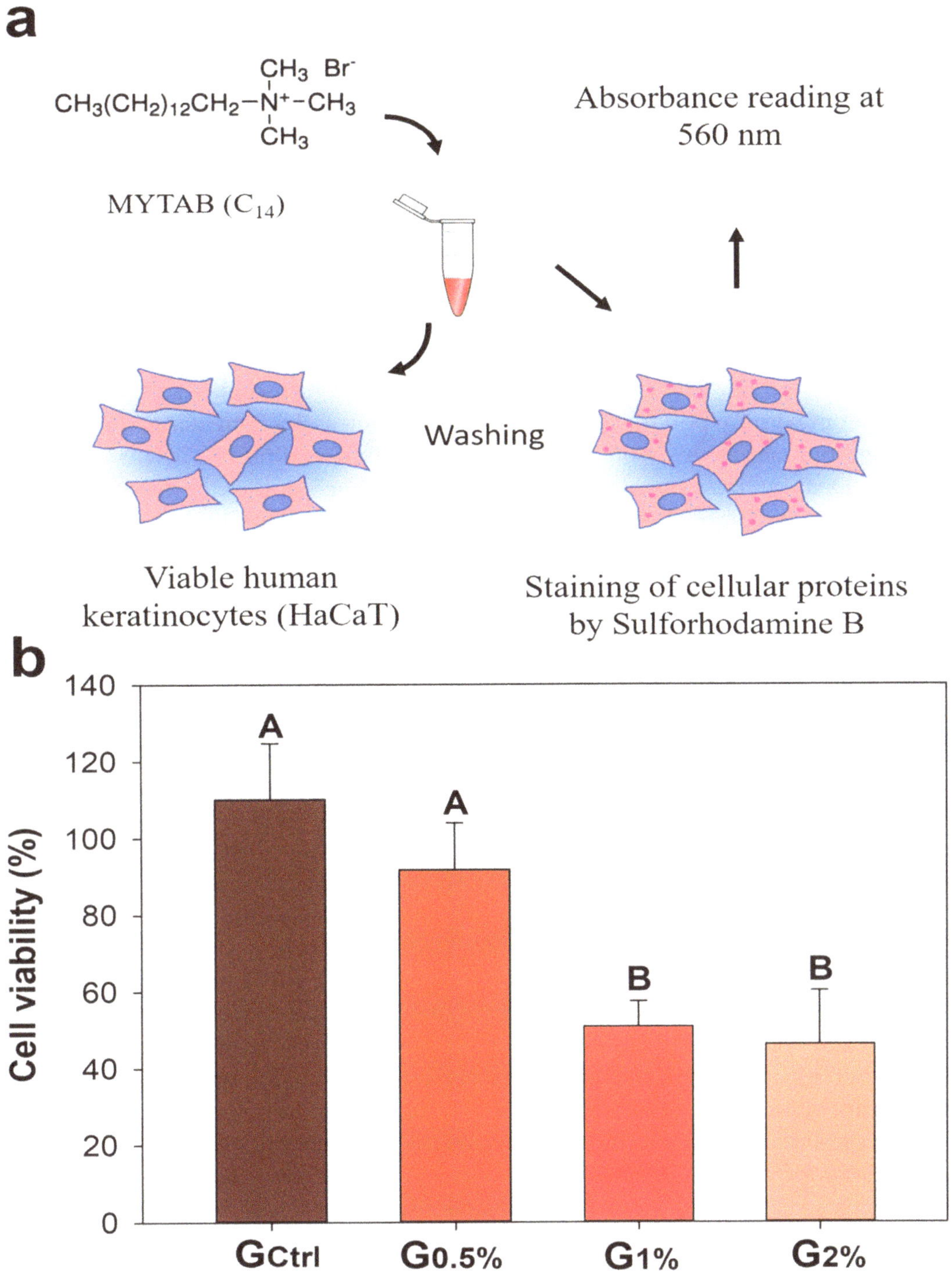

Figure 3. Cytotoxicity evaluation of the experimental dental resins expressed by percentage of cell viability: (**a**) structure of myristyltrimethylammonium bromide (MYTAB) and schematic drawing of sulforhodamine B (SRB) assay; and (**b**) MYTAB cytotoxicity assessed in normal human keratinocytes (HaCaT) line. Different capital letters indicate statistical differences among groups ($p < 0.05$).

3. Discussion

Dental resins are reliable materials to restore teeth, and, when used as pit and fissure sealants, could prevent new caries lesions [18,28,29]. Nevertheless, the formation of caries lesions around dental resins is still a major concern due to biofilm accumulation [22,30]. In order to prevent this issue, we investigated the effect of a cationic organic compound, MYTAB, in the properties of an experimental dental resin. The formulated resin is a suitable material for dental restorative purposes.

The longevity of dental restorative materials is strongly related to material rates of polymerization. High monomer conversion is essential for polymers to achieve reliable properties and stability [31]. The study of their polymerization behavior of modified formulations assists in understanding the effects of the incorporation of the compound on the functional aspect of the restorative material. Here, the formulated experimental dental resins showed different polymerization kinetics depending on the concentration of MYTAB. The effects were more evident with the addition of 1 wt % of MYTAB in the resin (Figure 2 A–C). From this concentration, the polymerization process was delayed, and the groups reached the maximum polymerization rate later compared to G_{Ctrl} and $G_{0.5\%}$.

On the other hand, $G_{0.5\%}$ showed a higher maximum polymerization rate compared to all groups (Figure 2 B). The rationale for this may be attributed to different viscosities among groups [32]. It was previously suggested that cationic surfactants could increase monomer chain mobility and modify polymerization behavior [33]. The lower viscosity and the higher monomer chain mobility for $G_{0.5\%}$ may lead to a higher maximum polymerization rate. Nevertheless, by increasing MYTAB incorporation, the spaces among monomer chains would be increased further, leading to a lower polymerization rate for $G_{1\%}$ and $G_{2\%}$. Despite these events, there was no difference in the degree of conversion among groups, and they achieved high values of conversion, similar to commercial dental resins [34].

Even though all groups presented a reliable degree of conversion, the delay during the polymerization kinetics observed for $G_{1\%}$ and $G_{2\%}$ could induce the formation of a more linear polymer, with lower crosslinking density [35]. Therefore, the mechanical evaluation of the formulated materials was essential in better understanding their performance. The specimens of dental resins were submitted to tensile strength until fracture in a universal testing machine with no statistical difference among groups. The UTS was a promising outcome because the incorporation of antibacterial agents could lead to lower mechanical properties [36]. The dental resins formulated in this study may be used in occlusal surfaces, where repetitive chewing stress is applied. The maintenance of resins' mechanical properties besides the antibacterial activity presented is essential in keeping the material in function.

In chewing sites, the experimental material proposed could be used not only for the prevention of caries lesions [18] but also to treat teeth already affected by the disease [29]. Pits and fissures are sites of difficult hygiene, favoring biofilm accumulation. Dental sealants successfully inhibit dental caries due to their ability to seal the demineralized tissue and form a mechanical barrier, inhibiting bacterial growth, hampering lesion progression, or preventing the demineralization of the sealed area [18,37]. The use of dental sealants in children and adolescents decreases the susceptibility to caries development in occlusal surfaces of permanent molars in comparison to people with no sealed teeth. Even among the people with sealed teeth, there are around 18% who present new lesions over time [18]. The composition of the sealants available in the market does not present antibacterial agents in their composition, which could be a strategy to reduce this percentage.

The parental composite resin formulated had its viscosity manually accessed for friendly use in clinical settings as a sealant. In the previous study with similar QAC, a high antibacterial effect of myristyltrimethylammonium bromide against *Enterococcus faecalis* was observed [27]. In both cases, these QACs have a long alkyl chain, which increases the QAC's hydrophobicity [38]. Consequently, when leached, these agents are more prone to penetrate bacterial walls and membranes [39]. With MYTAB, the higher its concentration in the dental resin, the lower the viability of *S. mutans* in biofilm and in planktonic stages.

For the assessment of antibacterial property, discs of the polymerized dental resins entered into contact with an enriched broth containing *S. mutans* as previously performed [13,33,40–42].

This bacterium is Gram-positive, and it is present in intraoral multispecies biofilms [43]. *S. mutans* group is the main bacteria associated with caries lesion development [44], and they can attach to dental and material surfaces [1,21]. The samples were exposed to planktonic as well as biofilm stages. During the contact with a dental resin containing MYTAB, planktonic bacteria reduction is suggested because of the leaching of some MYTAB molecules for the broth. The lack of assessment of the long-term antibacterial effect of the dental resins is a limitation of this study. Besides this, the quantities of MYTAB released over time from the polymerized resin is not known. The knowledge about this event could be valuable in order to understand the long-term behavior of the material and to assist in predicting the in vivo outcomes. However, the main goal of this study was to investigate the potential adverse effects of the addition of this compound into the composite to impart an antibacterial effect.

The cytotoxicity test was performed against human keratinocytes via the SRB method. Through this method, proteins of viable cells are stained, indicating increased viability when higher optical density is achieved [45]. The higher the incorporation of MYTAB, the higher the cytotoxic effect observed. This result corroborates with previous studies, which showed that cationic compounds with long-alkyl chains lead to high cytotoxic effects [46]. The International Organization for Standardization (ISO) recommends that biomaterials must promote up to 70% of cells' viability in order to not be considered cytotoxic [47]. It is worth mentioning that, despite the lower values of viability found for 1 and 2 wt % of MYTAB, all groups were directly treated with the eluates from the samples. In other words, we did not dilute the agent as other studies do [46], but we did somewhat increase the challenge by using the eluates on human cells during 72 h of contact.

A similar compound to MYTAB, a quaternary ammounium compound called ATAB, has been found to show antibacterial activity against *Enterococcus faecalis*, a relevant bacterium to endodontic infections [48]. The main difference between MYTAB and ATAB is the presence of mixing of QACs with different aliphatic chain lengths for ATAB, which does not occur in the case of MYTAB. In the previous study, ATAB was associated with halloysite nanotubes (HNT) that were incorporated in the sealer without the evaluation of ATAB alone [27], which might have repercussions for physical, chemical, or biological properties. In the same study, there were no cytotoxic effects for pulp cells with the incorporation of 10 wt % of ATAB/ halloysite nanotubes in the sealer, even when the proportion of ATAB/ halloysite nanotubes was 2:1 [27]. Here, MYTAB was not carried out by another system because we aimed to evaluate the QAC itself as a free drug, which may have increased the biological effects. $G_{0.5\%}$ showed no cytotoxicity in comparison to G_{Ctrl}, and both promoted viability higher than 70%. Therefore, the addition of 0.5 wt % of MYTAB may be a promising method for providing antibacterial activity for a dental resin without compromising its physical, chemical, and biological properties. The material here formulated is an exciting approach to be further translated for clinical trials.

4. Materials and Methods

4.1. Study Design and Formulation of Dental Resins

The study design is described in the flowchart presented in Figure 4. All reagents of the analytical grade for in vitro experiments were purchased from Sigma-Aldrich (Sigma-Aldrich Chemical Company, St. Louis, MO, USA) if not otherwise specified. First, a parental resin was formulated with two dimethacrylate monomers: bisphenol A glycol dimethacrylates (BisGMA) and triethylene glycol dimethacrylate (TEGDMA), at the proportion of 1:1. As a photoinitiator/co-initiator system, camphorquinone and ethyl 4-dimethylaminobenzoate were added to the resin at 1 mol % each. Butylated hydroxytoluene was added at 0.01 wt % as a polymerization inhibitor. Calcium tungstate ($CaWO_4$) was added as inorganic filler at 30 wt %. Colloidal silicon dioxide (SiO_2; Aerosil 200, Evonik, Essen, Germany) was incorporated at 0.7 wt % to adjust the resin's viscosity. After being hand-mixed for 5 min, they were sonicated for 180 s and hand-mixed for 5 min.

MYTAB with a purity of > 99% was added to the parental dental resin formulation at an increased double concentration of 0.5, 1, and 2% wt% mass fractions.

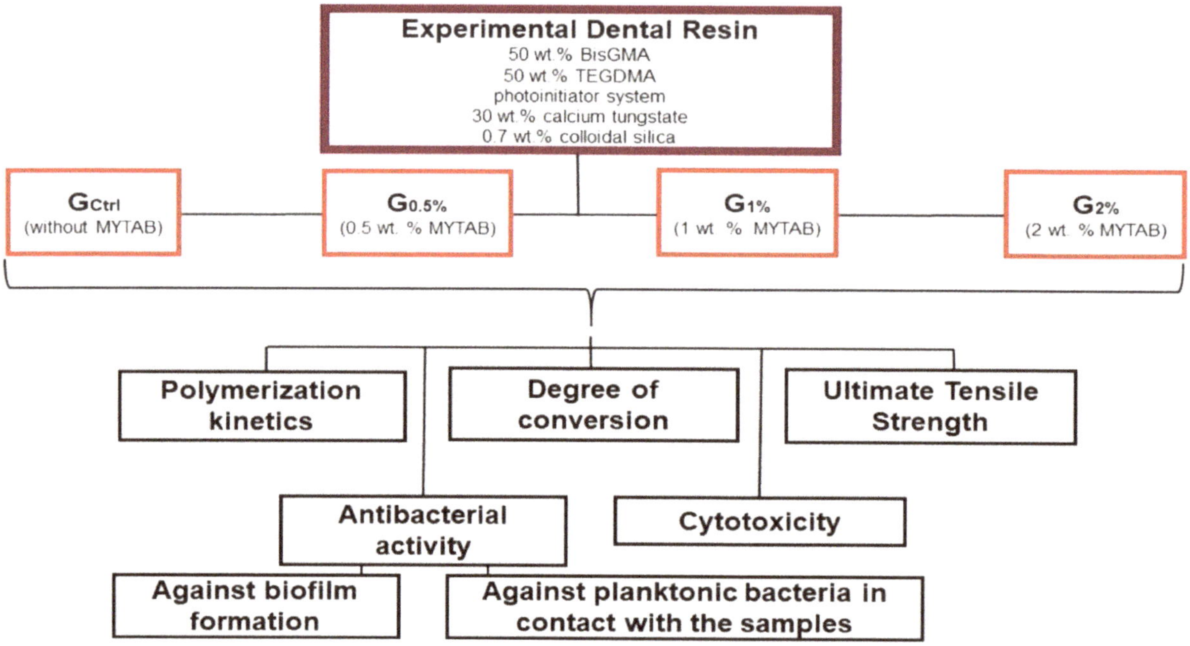

Figure 4. Flowchart of the study design. Experimental dental resins were formulated with different concentrations of a quaternary ammonium compound (MYTAB). Bisphenol A glycol dimethacrylates (BisGMA) and triethylene glycol dimethacrylate (TEGDMA) were used for the monomeric blend. The four experimental groups were evaluated for chemical, physical, and antibacterial properties, alongside their effect against human keratinocytes.

4.2. Polymerization Kinetics and Degree of Conversion

Fourier transform infrared spectroscopy (FTIR, Vertex 70, Bruker Optics, Ettinger, Germany) was used to evaluate the polymerization kinetics and the degree of conversion of the experimental dental resin. For this test, three samples per group were analyzed by dispensing them on the attenuated total reflectance (ATR) device in the polyvinylsiloxane matrix measuring 1 mm thickness and 4 mm in diameter. To perform the photoactivation of each sample, the light-cured unit (Radii Cal, SDI, Australia; 1200 mW/cm^2) was fixed using support to maintain 1 mm between the tip of the light-cured unit and the top of each sample. During the 40 s of photoactivation, two spectra were obtained per second in absorbance mode (10 kHz velocity, 4 cm^{-1} resolution; Opus 6.5 software, Bruker Optics, Ettlingen, Germany) in the range of 4000 to 400 cm^{-1}. The first spectrum obtained was used as "uncured resin dental resin", and the last spectrum as "cured resin dental resin" in the calculation of the degree of conversion. The peak at 1610 cm^{-1} from aromatic carbon–carbon double bond was used as an internal standard, and the peak at 1640 cm^{-1} was used as an aliphatic carbon–carbon double bond to calculate the conversion in percentage (Equation (1)) [31]. The polymerization rate was calculated using the degree of conversion at time *t* subtracted from the degree of conversion at time *t-1*.

Equation (1):

$$\mathbf{DC}\ (\%) = 100 \times \left(\frac{\text{peak height of cured aliphatic C=C/peak height of cured aromatic C=C}}{\text{peak height of uncured aliphatic C=C/peak height of uncured aromatic C=C}} \right) \quad (1)$$

4.3. Ultimate Tensile Strength (UTS)

Ten samples per group with hourglass shape were prepared in a metallic matrix that was 8.0 mm long, 2.0 mm wide, and of 1.0 mm thickness, with a cross-sectional area of ±1 mm^2. Each uncured sample was placed in the mold and photoactivated for 20 s on each side (bottom and top). The prepared samples were stored in distilled water at 37 °C for 24 h. The samples were fixed in jigs with cyanoacrylate resin, and they were submitted under tensile strength in a universal testing machine (EZ-SX Series,

Shimadzu, Kyoto, Japan) at 1 mm/min until fracture. The maximum force value (Newtons, N) achieved was divided by the constriction area of each sample, which was measured with a digital caliper (Mitutoyo, Kawasaki, Kanagawa, Japan) to calculate the maximum value of tensile strength (Equation (2)). The results were expressed in megapascals (MPa).

Equation (2):

$$\mathbf{UTS\ (MPa)} = \left(\frac{Force\ (N)}{Constriction\ area\ (mm^2)}\right) \tag{2}$$

4.4. Antibacterial Activity

Two in vitro assessments were performed to evaluate the antibacterial activity of the experimental dental resin: (1) planktonic bacteria and (2) against biofilm formation on the polymerized samples. The bacteria used in both tests were *S. mutans* (NCTC 10449). Three samples per group were prepared for the biofilm test, and the other three samples per group were used in the test against planktonic bacteria. *S. mutans* were prepared according to a previous study [13], and the initial inoculum used for the tests was assessed by serial dilution method and colony counting, which indicated an inoculum at 7.8×10^7 CFU/mL.

To evaluate the antibacterial activity against biofilm formation, the polymerized samples (1 mm thickness and 4 mm diameter) were fixed on Teflon specimens that were fixed on the cover of a 48-well plate, and this assembly was sterilized with hydrogen peroxide plasma (58%, 48 min, 56 °C) [13,49]. From the initial inoculum, 100 μL was added in each well of a 48-well plate with 900 μL of brain–heart infusion (BHI) broth with 1 wt % of sucrose. All reagents used in the antibacterial activity analysis were purchased from Aldrich Chemical Company (St. Louis, MO, USA). The sterile set of cover and samples was joined with this 48-well plate and kept for 24 h under 37 °C for biofilm formation on the samples. After this period, each sample was detached from the cover and vortexed for 1 min in 1 mL of sterile saline solution. The solution was serial diluted up to 10^{-6} mL and plated on Petri dishes containing BHI agar to count the colonies and to calculate (Equation 3) the colony-forming units per milliliter (CFU/mL).

Equation (3):

$$\mathbf{CFU/mL} = \left(\frac{\text{Avarage number of colonies x Dilution factor}}{\text{Volume of culture plate}}\right) \tag{3}$$

To evaluate the antibacterial activity against planktonic bacteria, the BHI broth that was in contact with the polymerized samples along the 24 h mentioned above was used. From each well of the 48-well plate, 100 μL was collected after the 24 h of bacteria–sample contact and was inserted into Eppendorf tubes with 900 μL of saline solution to be vortexed, diluted until 10^{-6}, and plated on BHI agar Petri dishes. For this test, an additional group was added as a negative control. The negative control was composed of BHI broth and *S. mutans* at the same proportion (10% of initial inoculum of bacteria in each well) without samples' contact. Colonies were visually counted, and the results were also expressed in CFU/mL.

4.5. Cytotoxicity

To evaluate the possible cytotoxic effect of the experimental dental resin, human keratinocytes (HaCaT, CLS Cell Lines Service GmbH, Eppelheim, Germany) were used in this test [40]. All reagents used to evaluate the possible cytotoxicity of the dental resins were purchased from Aldrich Chemical Company (St. Louis, MO, USA). The keratinocytes were kept in contact (5×10^3 cells/per well) with 100 μL of Dulbecco's modified Eagle's medium (DMEM) in 96-well plates for 24 h at 37 °C. On the same day, five samples per group (1 mm thickness and 4 mm diameter) were placed separately in Eppendorf tubes containing 1 mL of DMEM and kept for 24 h at 37 °C. Thus, eluates from possible leaching from the samples were formed. These eluates (100 μL) were kept in contact with the keratinocytes in the

96-well plates for 72 h at 37 °C. There was one group that was maintained without eluates with 100 μL of pure DMEM that was used as a control for the test. In addition to using five samples per group, the eluates were applied in five replications, totalizing 100 wells containing eluates from the samples. After 72 h, 50 μL of trichloroacetic acid/distilled water solution (50:50) was added in each well and kept at 4 °C for 1 hour to fix the cells on the bottom. Running water (30 s) was used to wash the 96-well plates six times. The 96-well plates were kept at room temperature until drying.

Sulforhodamine B at 0.4% (50 μL) was added in each well, and the 96-well plates were kept at room temperature for 30 min. The 96-well plates were washed four times with acetic acid at 1% and kept at room temperature until drying. Trizma solution at 10 mM (100 μL) was added in each well, and the 96-well plates were incubated for 1 hour at room temperature. The absorbance of plates' wells was analyzed at 560 nm, and the cell viability of the wells that contained eluates was compared to the wells without eluates. The viability of the keratinocytes used was normalized against the viability of cells without contact with eluates (negative control). The results were expressed in percentage using the viability of negative control as 100%.

4.6. Statistical Analysis

Data normality was evaluated by the Shapiro–Wilk test. One-way ANOVA and Tukey's post-hoc test was used to compare groups for all tests at a level of 0.05 of significance.

5. Conclusions

The present study incorporated a not yet investigated quaternary ammonium MYTAB into a dental resin, which achieved potent antibacterial effects against dental plaque microcosm biofilms for the first time. The results showed that (1) MYTAB at 2% greatly decreased *S. mutans* in planktonic and biofilm stages compared to G_{Ctrl}, (2) higher MYTAB mass fraction rendered the adhesive more strongly antibacterial, (3) MYTAB at 1% mass fraction greatly reduced the cell viability, and (4) the incorporation of MYTAB at a maximum concentration of 2% had no detrimental effect on the degree of conversion and ultimate tensile strength. MYTAB-containing dental resin is a promising strategy for dental applications.

Author Contributions: P.A.M.S. contributed to design, data acquisition, and analysis, and drafted the manuscript; I.M.G. contributed to design, data acquisition, and analysis, and drafted the manuscript; J.N. contributed to data acquisition and analysis; F.V. contributed to data acquisition and analysis; V.C.B.L. contributed to design, data analysis, and data interpretation; M.A.M. contributed to data analysis and data interpretation, and drafted the manuscript; F.M.C. contributed to conception, design, data acquisition, analysis, and interpretation, and drafted and critically revised the manuscript. All authors have read and agreed to the published version of the manuscript.

Acknowledgments: This study was financed in part by the Coordenação de Aperfeiçoamento de Pessoal de Nível Superior—Brasil (CAPES)—Finance Code 001.

References

1. Lin, N.J. Biofilm over teeth and restorations: What do we need to know? *Dent. Mater.* **2017**, *33*, 667–680. [CrossRef] [PubMed]
2. Pandey, V.K.; Srivastava, K.R.; Ajmal, G.; Thakur, V.K.; Gupta, V.K.; Upadhyay, S.N.; Mishra, P.K. Differential Susceptibility of Catheter Biomaterials to Biofilm-Associated Infections and Their Remedy by Drug-Encapsulated Eudragit RL100 Nanoparticles. *Int. J. Mol. Sci.* **2019**, *20*, 5110. [CrossRef] [PubMed]
3. Alves, D.; Vaz, A.T.; Grainha, T.; Rodrigues, C.F.; Pereira, M.O. Design of an Antifungal Surface Embedding Liposomal Amphotericin B Through a Mussel Adhesive-Inspired Coating Strategy. *Front. Chem.* **2019**, *7*, 431. [CrossRef] [PubMed]
4. Donlan, R.M. Biofilms and device-associated infections. *Emerg. Infect. Dis.* **2001**, *7*, 277–281. [CrossRef]

5. He, Y.; Wan, X.; Xiao, K.; Lin, W.; Li, J.; Li, Z.; Luo, F.; Tan, H.; Li, J.; Fu, Q. Anti-biofilm surfaces from mixed dopamine-modified polymer brushes: Synergistic role of cationic and zwitterionic chains to resist staphyloccocus aureus. *Biomater. Sci.* **2019**, *7*, 5369–5382. [CrossRef]
6. Jung, J.; Li, L.; Yeh, C.K.; Ren, X.; Sun, Y. Amphiphilic quaternary ammonium chitosan/sodium alginate multilayer coatings kill fungal cells and inhibit fungal biofilm on dental biomaterials. *Mater. Sci. Eng. C* **2019**, *104*, 109961. [CrossRef]
7. Melo, M.A.; Orrego, S.; Weir, M.D.; Xu, H.H.; Arola, D.D. Designing Multiagent Dental Materials for Enhanced Resistance to Biofilm Damage at the Bonded Interface. *ACS Appl. Mater. Interfaces* **2016**, *8*, 11779–11787. [CrossRef]
8. Degrazia, F.W.; Genari, B.; Leitune, V.C.B.; Arthur, R.A.; Luxan, S.A.; Samuel, S.M.W.; Collares, F.M.; Sauro, S. Polymerisation, antibacterial and bioactivity properties of experimental orthodontic adhesives containing triclosan-loaded halloysite nanotubes. *J. Dent.* **2018**, *69*, 77–82. [CrossRef]
9. Makvandi, P.; Jamaledin, R.; Jabbari, M.; Nikfarjam, N.; Borzacchiello, A. Antibacterial quaternary ammonium compounds in dental materials: A systematic review. *Dent. Mater.* **2018**, *34*, 851–867. [CrossRef]
10. Braga, R.R.; Fronza, B.M. The use of bioactive particles and biomimetic analogues for increasing the longevity of resin-dentin interfaces: A literature review. *Dent. Mater. J.* **2019**. [CrossRef]
11. Andre, C.B.; Chan, D.C.; Giannini, M. Antibacterial-containing dental adhesives' effects on oral pathogens and on Streptococcus mutans biofilm: Current perspectives. *Am. J. Dent.* **2018**, *31*, 37B–41B. [PubMed]
12. Chi, M.; Qi, M.; A, L.; Wang, P.; Weir, M.D.; Melo, M.A.; Sun, X.; Dong, B.; Li, C.; Wu, J.; et al. Novel Bioactive and Therapeutic Dental Polymeric Materials to Inhibit Periodontal Pathogens and Biofilms. *Int. J. Mol. Sci.* **2019**, *20*, 278. [CrossRef] [PubMed]
13. Garcia, I.M.; Souza, V.S.; Hellriegel, C.; Scholten, J.D.; Collares, F.M. Ionic Liquid-Stabilized Titania Quantum Dots Applied in Adhesive Resin. *J. Dent. Res.* **2019**, *98*, 682–688. [CrossRef] [PubMed]
14. Schwendicke, F.; Frencken, J.E.; Bjorndal, L.; Maltz, M.; Manton, D.J.; Ricketts, D.; Van Landuyt, K.; Banerjee, A.; Campus, G.; Domejean, S.; et al. Managing Carious Lesions: Consensus Recommendations on Carious Tissue Removal. *Adv. Dent. Res.* **2016**, *28*, 58–67. [CrossRef] [PubMed]
15. Lynch, C.D.; Opdam, N.J.; Hickel, R.; Brunton, P.A.; Gurgan, S.; Kakaboura, A.; Shearer, A.C.; Vanherle, G.; Wilson, N.H. Guidance on posterior resin composites: Academy of Operative Dentistry—European Section. *J. Dent.* **2014**, *42*, 377–383. [CrossRef]
16. Tyas, M.J.; Anusavice, K.J.; Frencken, J.E.; Mount, G.J. Minimal intervention dentistry—A review. FDI Commission Project 1–97. *Int. Dent. J.* **2000**, *50*, 1–12. [CrossRef]
17. Ferracane, J.L. Resin composite—State of the art. *Dent. Mater.* **2011**, *27*, 29–38. [CrossRef]
18. Ahovuo-Saloranta, A.; Forss, H.; Walsh, T.; Nordblad, A.; Makela, M.; Worthington, H.V. Pit and fissure sealants for preventing dental decay in permanent teeth. *Cochrane Database Syst. Rev.* **2017**, *7*, CD001830. [CrossRef]
19. De Munck, J.; Van Meerbeek, B.; Yoshida, Y.; Inoue, S.; Vargas, M.; Suzuki, K.; Lambrechts, P.; Vanherle, G. Four-year water degradation of total-etch adhesives bonded to dentin. *J. Dent. Res.* **2003**, *82*, 136–140. [CrossRef]
20. Frassetto, A.; Breschi, L.; Turco, G.; Marchesi, G.; Di Lenarda, R.; Tay, F.R.; Pashley, D.H.; Cadenaro, M. Mechanisms of degradation of the hybrid layer in adhesive dentistry and therapeutic agents to improve bond durability—A literature review. *Dent. Mater.* **2016**, *32*, e41–e53. [CrossRef]
21. Kusuma Yulianto, H.D.; Rinastiti, M.; Cune, M.S.; de Haan-Visser, W.; Atema-Smit, J.; Busscher, H.J.; van der Mei, H.C. Biofilm composition and composite degradation during intra-oral wear. *Dent. Mater.* **2019**, *35*, 740–750. [CrossRef] [PubMed]
22. Opdam, N.J.; van de Sande, F.H.; Bronkhorst, E.; Cenci, M.S.; Bottenberg, P.; Pallesen, U.; Gaengler, P.; Lindberg, A.; Huysmans, M.C.; van Dijken, J.W. Longevity of posterior composite restorations: A systematic review and meta-analysis. *J. Dent. Res.* **2014**, *93*, 943–949. [CrossRef] [PubMed]
23. Imazato, S.; Ma, S.; Chen, J.H.; Xu, H.H. Therapeutic polymers for dental adhesives: Loading resins with bio-active components. *Dent. Mater.* **2014**, *30*, 97–104. [CrossRef] [PubMed]
24. Kenawy, E.-R.; Abdel-Hay, F.I.; El-Shanshoury, A.E.-R.R.; El-Newehy, M.H. Biologically active polymers. V. Synthesis and antimicrobial activity of modified poly(glycidyl methacrylate-co-2-hydroxyethyl methacrylate) derivatives with quaternary ammonium and phosphonium salts. *J. Polym. Sci.* **2002**, *40*, 2384–2393. [CrossRef]

25. Lu, G.; Wu, D.; Fu, R. Studies on the synthesis and antibacterial activities of polymeric quaternary ammonium salts from dimethylaminoethyl methacrylate. *React. Funct. Polymer* **2007**, *67*, 355–366. [CrossRef]
26. Quan, A.; McGeachie, A.B.; Keating, D.J.; van Dam, E.M.; Rusak, J.; Chau, N.; Malladi, C.S.; Chen, C.; McCluskey, A.; Cousin, M.A.; et al. Myristyl trimethyl ammonium bromide and octadecyl trimethyl ammonium bromide are surface-active small molecule dynamin inhibitors that block endocytosis mediated by dynamin I or dynamin II. *Mol. Pharmacol.* **2007**, *72*, 1425–1439. [CrossRef]
27. Monteiro, J.C.; Garcia, I.M.; Leitune, V.C.B.; Visioli, F.; de Souza Balbinot, G.; Samuel, S.M.W.; Makeeva, I.; Collares, F.M.; Sauro, S. Halloysite nanotubes loaded with alkyl trimethyl ammonium bromide as antibacterial agent for root canal sealers. *Dent. Mater.* **2019**, *35*, 789–796. [CrossRef]
28. Pallesen, U.; van Dijken, J.W. A randomized controlled 27 years follow up of three resin composites in Class II restorations. *J. Dent.* **2015**, *43*, 1547–1558. [CrossRef]
29. Munoz-Sandoval, C.; Gambetta-Tessini, K.; Giacaman, R.A. Microcavitated (ICDAS 3) carious lesion arrest with resin or glass ionomer sealants in first permanent molars: A randomized controlled trial. *J. Dent.* **2019**, *88*, 103163. [CrossRef]
30. Chisini, L.A.; Collares, K.; Cademartori, M.G.; de Oliveira, L.J.C.; Conde, M.C.M.; Demarco, F.F. Restorations in primary teeth: A systematic review on survival and reasons for failures. *Int. J. Paediatr. Dent.* **2018**, *28*, 123–139. [CrossRef]
31. Collares, F.M.; Ogliari, F.A.; Zanchi, C.H.; Petzhold, C.L.; Piva, E.; Samuel, S.M. Influence of 2-hydroxyethyl methacrylate concentration on polymer network of adhesive resin. *J. Adhes. Dent.* **2011**, *13*, 125–129. [PubMed]
32. Barszczewska-Rybarek, I.M. Characterization of urethane-dimethacrylate derivatives as alternative monomers for the restorative composite matrix. *Dent. Mater.* **2014**, *30*, 1336–1344. [CrossRef] [PubMed]
33. Martini Garcia, I.; Jung Ferreira, C.; de Souza, V.S.; Castelo Branco Leitune, V.; Samuel, S.M.W.; de Souza Balbinot, G.; de Souza da Motta, A.; Visioli, F.; Damiani Scholten, J.; Mezzomo Collares, F. Ionic liquid as antibacterial agent for an experimental orthodontic adhesive. *Dent. Mater.* **2019**, *35*, 1155–1165. [CrossRef] [PubMed]
34. Borges, B.C.; Bezerra, G.V.; Mesquita Jde, A.; Pereira, M.R.; Aguiar, F.H.; Santos, A.J.; Pinheiro, I.V. Effect of irradiation times on the polymerization depth of contemporary fissure sealants with different opacities. *Braz. Oral Res.* **2011**, *25*, 135–142. [CrossRef] [PubMed]
35. Rodrigues, S.B.; Collares, F.M.; Leitune, V.C.; Schneider, L.F.; Ogliari, F.A.; Petzhold, C.L.; Samuel, S.M. Influence of hydroxyethyl acrylamide addition to dental adhesive resin. *Dent. Mater.* **2015**, *31*, 1579–1586. [CrossRef]
36. Vidal, M.L.; Rego, G.F.; Viana, G.M.; Cabral, L.M.; Souza, J.P.B.; Silikas, N.; Schneider, L.F.; Cavalcante, L.M. Physical and chemical properties of model composites containing quaternary ammonium methacrylates. *Dent. Mater.* **2018**, *34*, 143–151. [CrossRef]
37. Liang, Y.; Deng, Z.; Dai, X.; Tian, J.; Zhao, W. Micro-invasive interventions for managing non-cavitated proximal caries of different depths: A systematic review and meta-analysis. *Clin. Oral Investig.* **2018**, *22*, 2675–2684. [CrossRef]
38. Yoshimura, T.; Chiba, N.; Matsuoka, K. Supra-long chain surfactants with double or triple quaternary ammonium headgroups. *J. Colloid Interface Sci.* **2012**, *374*, 157–163. [CrossRef]
39. Wang, Y.; Costin, S.; Zhang, J.F.; Liao, S.; Wen, Z.T.; Lallier, T.; Yu, Q.; Xu, X. Synthesis, antibacterial activity, and biocompatibility of new antibacterial dental monomers. *Am. J. Dent.* **2018**, *31*, 17b–23b.
40. Garcia, I.M.; Rodrigues, S.B.; de Souza Balbinot, G.; Visioli, F.; Leitune, V.C.B.; Collares, F.M. Quaternary ammonium compound as antimicrobial agent in resin-based sealants. *Clin. Oral Investig.* **2019**. [CrossRef]
41. Garcia, I.M.; Rodrigues, S.B.; Leitune, V.C.B.; Collares, F.M. Antibacterial, chemical and physical properties of sealants with polyhexamethylene guanidine hydrochloride. *Braz. Oral Res.* **2019**, *33*, e019. [CrossRef] [PubMed]
42. Machado, A.H.S.; Garcia, I.M.; Motta, A.S.D.; Leitune, V.C.B.; Collares, F.M. Triclosan-loaded chitosan as antibacterial agent for adhesive resin. *J. Dent.* **2019**, *83*, 33–39. [CrossRef] [PubMed]
43. Metwalli, K.H.; Khan, S.A.; Krom, B.P.; Jabra-Rizk, M.A. Streptococcus mutans, Candida albicans, and the human mouth: A sticky situation. *PLoS Pathog.* **2013**, *9*, e1003616. [CrossRef] [PubMed]

44. Kirstila, V.; Hakkinen, P.; Jentsch, H.; Vilja, P.; Tenovuo, J. Longitudinal analysis of the association of human salivary antimicrobial agents with caries increment and cariogenic micro-organisms: A two-year cohort study. *J. Dent. Res.* **1998**, *77*, 73–80. [CrossRef]
45. van Tonder, A.; Joubert, A.M.; Cromarty, A.D. Limitations of the 3-(4,5-dimethylthiazol-2-yl)-2,5-diphenyl-2H-tetrazolium bromide (MTT) assay when compared to three commonly used cell enumeration assays. *BMC Res. Notes* **2015**, *8*, 47. [CrossRef]
46. Gindri, I.M.; Siddiqui, D.A.; Bhardwaj, P.; Rodriguez, L.C.; Palmer, K.L.; Frizzo, C.P.; Martins, M.A.P.; Rodrigues, D.C. Dicationic imidazolium-based ionic liquids: A new strategy for non-toxic and antimicrobial materials. *RSC Adv.* **2014**, *4*, 62594–62602. [CrossRef]
47. International Organization for Standardization (ISO). *Biological Evaluation of Medical Devices—Part 5: Tests for in vitro Cytotoxicity*; ISO 10993-5:2009(E); ISO: Vernier, Geneva, Switzerland, 2009; Volume 1, p. 34.
48. Stuart, C.H.; Schwartz, S.A.; Beeson, T.J.; Owatz, C.B. Enterococcus faecalis: Its role in root canal treatment failure and current concepts in retreatment. *J. Endod.* **2006**, *32*, 93–98. [CrossRef]
49. Genari, B.; Leitune, V.C.B.; Jornada, D.S.; Camassola, M.; Arthur, R.A.; Pohlmann, A.R.; Guterres, S.S.; Collares, F.M.; Samuel, S.M.W. Antimicrobial effect and physicochemical properties of an adhesive system containing nanocapsules. *Dent. Mater.* **2017**, *33*, 735–742. [CrossRef]

9

Effect of Novel Antibacterial Composites on Bacterial Biofilms

Rayan B. Yaghmoor [1,2], Wendy Xia [3], Paul Ashley [4], Elaine Allan [5] and Anne M. Young [3,*]

1 Department of Biomaterials and Tissue Engineering/Department of Microbial Diseases, UCL Eastman Dental Institute, London, NW3 2QG, UK; rayan.yaghmoor.18@ucl.ac.uk
2 Department of Restorative Dentistry, Umm Al-Qura University, College of Dental Medicine, Makkah 24381, Saudi Arabia
3 Department of Biomaterials and Tissue Engineering, UCL Eastman Dental Institute, London NW3 2QG, UK; wendy.xia2011@yahoo.co.uk
4 Unit of Paediatric Dentistry, UCL Eastman Dental Institute, London WC1E 6DE, UK; p.ashley@ucl.ac.uk
5 Department of Microbial Diseases, UCL Eastman Dental Institute, London NW3 2QG, UK; e.allan@ucl.ac.uk
* Correspondence: anne.young@ucl.ac.uk

Abstract: Continuing cariogenic bacterial growth demineralizing dentine beneath a composite filling is the most common cause of tooth restoration failure. Novel composites with antibacterial polylysine (PLS) (0, 4, 6, or 8 wt%) in its filler phase were therefore produced. Remineralising monocalcium phosphate was also included at double the PLS weight. Antibacterial studies involved set composite disc placement in 1% sucrose-supplemented broth containing *Streptococcus mutans* (UA159). Relative surface bacterial biofilm mass ($n = 4$) after 24 h was determined by crystal violet-binding. Live/dead bacteria and biofilm thickness ($n = 3$) were assessed using confocal laser scanning microscopy (CLSM). To understand results and model possible in vivo benefits, cumulative PLS release from discs into water ($n = 3$) was determined by a ninhydrin assay. Results showed biofilm mass and thickness decreased linearly by 28% and 33%, respectively, upon increasing PLS from 0% to 8%. With 4, 6, and 8 wt% PLS, respectively, biofilm dead bacterial percentages and PLS release at 24 h were 20%, 60%, and 80% and 85, 163, and 241 μg/disc. Furthermore, initial PLS release was proportional to the square root of time and levelled after 1, 2, and 3 months at 13%, 28%, and 42%. This suggested diffusion controlled release from water-exposed composite surface layers of 65, 140, and 210 μm thickness, respectively. In conclusion, increasing PLS release initially in any gaps under the restoration to kill residual bacteria or longer-term following composite/tooth interface damage might help prevent recurrent caries.

Keywords: dental composite; antibacterial; antibiofilm; polylysine

1. Introduction

Dental caries is a main public health issue worldwide [1]. In Europe, it affects almost 100% of adults and 20–90% of 6-year-old children [2]. Mercury silver amalgam was for nearly 200 years the most commonly used permanent direct dental filling material in the EU. European legislation, however, in July 2018, aligned with the Minamata convention on mercury reduction to ban the use of dental amalgam for children under 15 years old and pregnant or breastfeeding women. Complete dental amalgam phase out is planned for 2030 [3]. Mercury concerns in combination with growing demand for more conservative and aesthetic restorations have made the resin composite the new main direct long-term restorative of choice [4,5]. Composites, however, have higher failure rate with the most common cause being recurrent (secondary) caries [5–8]. This is largely due to the tendency of resin composite to accumulate bacterial biofilms more than amalgam, which is not only responsible for recurrent caries but also periodontal problems [9].

Dental plaque biofilms consist of microorganisms in an exopolymer matrix (EPM) [10]. These biofilms are three dimensional, spatially-organized microbial communities that show properties as a unit [11]. Metagenomics studies revealed that up to 19,000 bacterial species could be found in a mature dental plaque biofilm [12,13]. Shift in composition of the dental biofilm towards more acidogenic and aciduric bacteria leads to caries. Dentinal caries lesions contain primarily acid-producing and Gram-positive species, with *Streptococcus mutans* being particularly high [14,15]. Their lowering of pH enhances solubility and dissolution of apatite in enamel [16]. Subsequent demineralization of dentine activates enzymes that, over time, slowly hydrolyze remaining collagen [16].

Previously, tooth restoration involved removal of the soft, highly-infected as well as the underlying harder, acid-affected dentine through drilling. Tooth restoration became a major problem during the global SARS-Cov-2 pandemic in 2020, as drilling increases aerosol production that could spread the viral infection [17,18]. Additionally, acid-affected dentine is remineralizable [19]. Furthermore, current recommendations for management of cavitated caries advocate controlling the lesion [19]. This could be better achieved through minimally invasive treatment and bacterial inactivation instead of total demineralized dentine removal [19]. This would reduce the need for drilling, which both dentists and patients consider a major benefit [20].

Bacterial inactivation by composite restorations can be achieved by cavity sealing reducing nutrient ingress [19]. Composite shrinkage during placement or long-term cyclical loading, however, can damage this seal. Residual bacteria or bacterial leakage from surface plaque with sugars from food would then enable biofilm formation in gaps at the composite/tooth interface. Immediate release of antibacterial agents in response to interface damage could potentially reduce this risk. In combination with remineralising agents to seal any gaps, this could provide the time required for the tooth to self-heal.

(Poly-ε-lysine) (ε-PL) (PLS) is a naturally created antibacterial homopolypeptide of 25–30 L-lysine residues that is stable in basic and acidic environments as well as at high temperatures [21,22]. Moreover, it is biodegradable, water-soluble, edible, non-toxic, and has broad-spectrum antibacterial properties [21,23]. Polylysine has therefore recently been incorporated into resin composites with remineralising agents [22,24]. Chemical setting kinetics, volumetric stability, polylysine release kinetics, remineralising features, mechanical properties, and wear have already been investigated [22,24]. One recent study has also studied material effects on bacteria [25]. This previous investigation, however, was restricted to formulations with low PLS concentrations and planktonic *S. mutans* with none of the sucrose required for biofilm maturation [25]. Biofilms, in general, have been shown to be more resistant to antimicrobial agents compared to the same bacterium growing in planktonic culture [26].

The aim of this new study was to evaluate if higher levels of PLS and remineralising agents within composites have the potential to prevent residual bacteria in cavities depositing and forming biofilms early on the composite surface. This is achieved through investigation of new composites incubated with *S. mutans* and sucrose. PLS release kinetics are also provided to help explain the observations.

2. Materials and Methods

2.1. Composite Components

Resin-composite formulations were prepared as in previous studies [25] but with higher antibacterial and remineralising agents by combining two phases: liquid and powder. Liquid components included urethane dimethacrylate (UDMA) as the main base monomer and the initiator camphorquinone (CQ). Both were from DMG (Hamburg, Germany). Poly (propylene glycol) dimethacrylate (PPGDMA) was added to improve fluidity and polymerization kinetics. This and the adhesion promoting monomer, 4-methacryloyloxyethyl trimellitic anhydride (4-META), were from Polysciences (PA, Warrington, UK) [25].

The filler consisted primarily of silane-treated radiopaque strontium aluminosilicate glass filler of 7 and 0.7 μm from DMG. These were combined with silica nano-glass particles (Azelis, Hertford, UK). Monocalcium phosphate monohydrate (MCPM) (Himed, Old Bethpage, NY, USA) and polylysine (PLS) (Handary, Brussels, Belgium) were added as remineralising and antibacterial agents, respectively. Particle SEM images are provided in a previous work [24].

2.2. *Paste and Solid Sample Disc Composition and Preparation*

Four semi-fluid paste formulations were prepared using a powder to liquid weight ratio of 3:1. The clear liquid phase consisted of UDMA (72 wt%), PPGDMA, (24 wt%), 4-META (3 wt%), and CQ (1 wt%). This monomer system polymerizes effectively upon light activation without need of an amine activator [24]. Then, 7 μm glass, 0.7 μm glass, and silica were combined in the weight ratio 6:3:1 [24]. This maximized particle packing and provided flow and material handling characteristics approved by clinical focus groups. MCPM (0, 8, 12, and 16 wt%) and PLS (0, 4, 6, and 8 wt%) were added to this powder with the MCPM:PLS weight ratio fixed at 2:1.

Clear liquids were prepared by completely dissolving solid 4-META and CQ in PPGDMA followed by UDMA addition. The powder components were mixed first at 3500 rpm for 10 s using a Speedmixer (DAC600.2 CM51, Synergy Devices Ltd., High Wycombe, UK). Monomers and powders were then mixed at 3500 rpm for 40 s.

To prepare solid disc specimens (1 mm thick, 9.4 mm diameter, and mass 0.13 g), pastes were pressed within metal circlips sandwiched between two acetate sheets then light cured. Each surface was cured using a light-emitting diode (LED) with a wavelength of 450–470 nm and power of 1100–1300 mW/cm^2 (Demi Plus, Kerr Dental, Bioggio, Switzerland) in contact with the acetate sheet with 4 overlapping irradiation cycles according to ISO:4049 [27]. Then, 40 s per cycle was used to ensure maximum room temperature monomer conversion of 72% [24]. After curing, composite discs were removed from the moulds, and excess composite was trimmed.

2.3. *Biofilm Formation on Composite Discs*

S. mutans (UA159) was cultured on brain heart infusion (BHI) Agar (CM1136 by OXOID, Thermo Fisher Scientific, Loughborough, UK) at 37 °C in an atmosphere of air enriched with 5% CO_2 for 72 h. A single colony was inoculated into 10 mL BHI broth (CM1135 by OXOID) and allowed to grow for 18 h at 37 °C in air enriched with 5% CO_2. This was diluted to obtain a bacterial density of 8×10^7 CFU/mL, which was confirmed by colony forming unit (CFU) counting and calibrated optical density (caused by absorbance and light scatter) at 595 nm (OD_{595}). The OD_{595} was measured using a spectrophotometer (Biochrom WPA CO8000, Cambridge, UK).

Specimen discs were placed randomly in 24 well plates (Greiner bio-one, Cellstar, Kremsmunster, Austria) and sterilized through top and bottom surface exposure to UV light for 40 min. Biofilms were grown on each composite disc by adding 25 μL of 8×10^7 CFU/mL inoculum (containing 2×10^6 CFU) with 1 mL BHI broth (OXOID) containing 1% (*w*/*v*) sucrose. The well plate was incubated at 37 °C statically in air enriched with 5% CO_2. After 24 h, the medium was carefully removed. The resultant biofilms were washed twice with 1 mL of sterile phosphate buffered saline (PBS) and fixed by exposure to 1 mL methanol during 15 min.

2.4. *Crystal Violet (CV) Biofilm Assay*

A crystal violet (CV) assay was used to evaluate relative biofilm mass on composite surfaces [28]. Biofilms were produced on 4 separate days; 3 composite discs per formula were tested each day requiring 12 discs per formula in total.

The procedure involved addition of 1 mL of aqueous 0.1% CV (Pro-Lab Diagnostics, Bromborough, UK) to each disc for 5 min then washing with 1 mL of PBS twice. After drying, bound CV was solubilized in 1 mL of 30% aqueous acetic acid. Once fully dissolved, the resultant CV solutions were diluted to enable absorbance (OD_{595}) determination, and the OD_{595} of the undiluted solutions were calculated and reported.

2.5. Live/Dead and Biofilm Thickness Assessment

Live/dead assay and biofilm thickness were assessed using confocal laser scanning microscopy (CLSM, Lasersharp 2000) (Radiance 2100, Biorad, Hercules, CA, USA) with a 40× magnification wet lens. Biofilms were prepared and examined on different days in 3 independent assays with one disc per formulation each day.

Then, 20 μL of LIVE/DEAD stain (Viability Kit, Thermofisher Scientific, Loughborough, UK) and 10 mL of PBS were added to the biofilms on discs within wells. Green and red images of live versus dead bacteria were obtained from near the biofilm centre (260 × 260 μm^2). In the following, red and green images are shown overlapped. For analysis, the individual red or green images were converted to black (background) and white (stained bacteria), and the percentage area that was white was determined using ImageJ software. The ratio of live/dead bacteria was obtained by dividing the percentage of white areas from the green versus red images; this was then converted to percentages. Additionally, movement of the microscope stage in the z direction enabled determination of biofilm thickness. Average results at three random points within the image area were obtained. Normalised thickness was obtained by dividing biofilm thickness by that for the control with no PLS on each given day.

2.6. Polylysine Release

To quantify kinetics of PLS release, 6 composite discs of each formulation of known total mass were stored in plastic pots containing 5 mL of deionized water at room temperature (RT). A total of 2 discs per pot enabled sufficient release for ease of detection and a sample repetition number of $n = 3$. The discs were transferred to new plastic containers with fresh 5 mL of deionized water at the following time points: 6 h, 24 h, 3 days, and at 1, 2, 3, 4, 5, 6, 7, 8, 9, 10, 12, 14, and 18 weeks.

The concentration of PLS that had leached into the deionized water was determined using a ninhydrin assay that was modified from previously published work [29]. It involved adding 1 mL of 0.5% ethanolic Ninhydrin (Sigma-Aldrich, Gillingham, UK) solution to boiling tubes containing 4 mL of sample storage solution or aqueous polylysine solutions of known concentration. After vortex-mixing for 10 s, 1.5 g (± 0.1) of marble chips (BDH, Poole, England, UK) were added to each tube. All tubes were covered with aluminium foil and placed in a boiling water bath to accelerate a ninhydrin/PLS reaction. After 15 min, reactions were quenched by rapid cooling to RT.

Following sedimentation, supernatant liquids were analysed using a spectrophotometer (Thermo Spectronic Unicam UV 500 Spectrophotometer, Loughborough, England with Vision pro^{TM} software). The absorbance was recorded between 400–700 nm to ensure curves were consistent and free of background scattering (for example due to residual non sedimented marble chips). Absorbances at 570 nm (A_{570}) for known polylysine concentrations of 0, 4, 10, 16, 20, 40, 60, 80, and 100 ppm were used to establish a calibration graph (A_{570} = 0.023/ppm, Pearson correlation coefficient, RSQ = 0.96). This was then used to determine polylysine concentration in each storage solution and cumulative release in μg/disc versus time. Cumulative PLS (%) was also calculated using:

$$\%\ \text{PLS release} = \frac{100[\sum_0^t R_t]}{w_c} \quad (1)$$

where R_t is the amount of released PLS (g) at time t, w_c is the amount of *PLS* (g) in the composite disc.

2.7. Statistical Analysis

The 95% confidence intervals (95%CI) (equal to 2 SD/SQRT(n) where SD and SQRT are standard deviation and square root) are provided as error bars in Figures. Average percentage standard deviations (%SD) were 7%, 9%, and 15% and sample numbers n = 4, 3, and 3 for crystal violet (CV) absorbance, normalised biofilm thickness, and PLS release studies, respectively. Significance ($p < 0.05$) was determined using one-way Analysis of Variance (ANOVA) followed by pairwise comparisons (Kruskal–Wallis test). Excel was used for curve fitting and to calculate the Pearson correlation coefficient (RSQ).

3. Results

3.1. Biofilm Mass

CV adsorption and subsequent absorbance indicated an inverse relationship between the amount of biofilm mass and the concentration of PLS in composite formulations (Figure 1). All PLS-containing formulations (4, 6, and 8 wt%) had biofilms with significantly less CV adsorption than the control formula with no PLS. In addition, the formula containing 8% PLS had significantly less CV adsorption compared to the material containing 4% PLS.

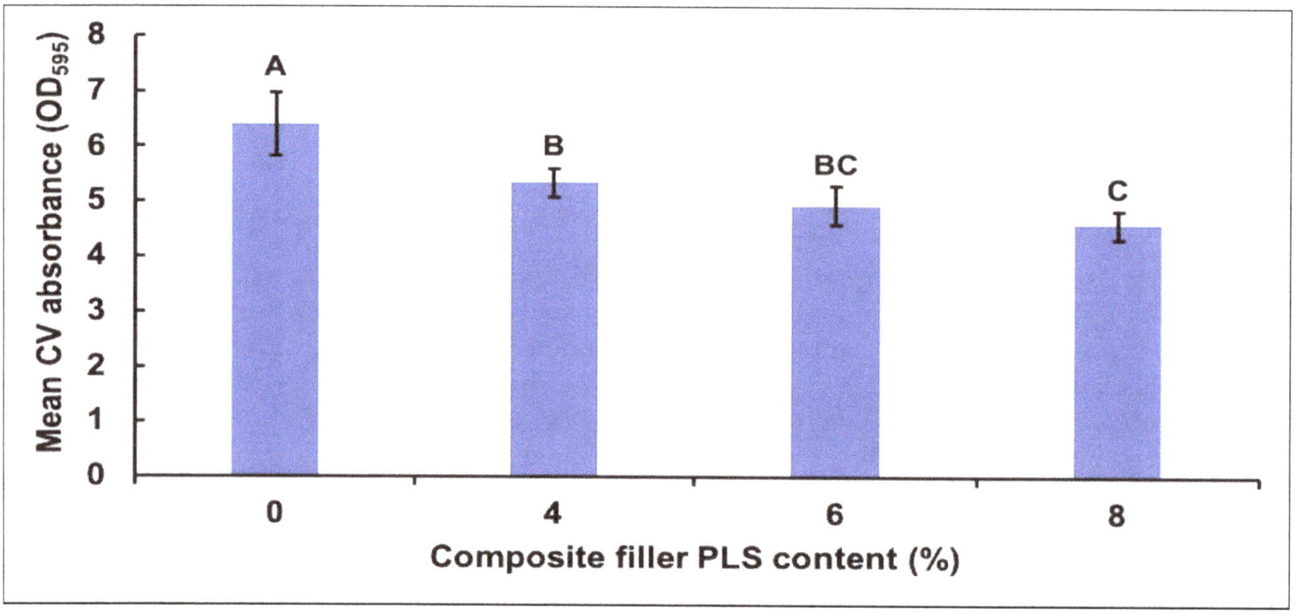

Figure 1. Mean ± (95%CI, n = 4) absorbance (OD_{595}) due to crystal violet (CV) adsorbed by biofilms on the four composite formulations with 0, 4, 6, or 8 wt% polylysine (PLS) in filler phase (error bars are for 4 repetitions on different days with an average result of 3 specimens per formulation each day). The absorbance values were 10 times those measured in the spectrometer to account for dilution. Composite formulations with the same uppercase letter/s above the bars were not significantly different at $p < 0.05$.

3.2. Live/Dead S.Mutans

Confocal microscopy images showed primarily dead bacteria with 8% PLS but live bacteria with 0% and 4% PLS levels. The 6% PLS samples had both live and dead bacteria (Figure 2). Quantification of live versus dead stain confirmed that formulae containing 6% and 8% PLS had significantly more dead *S. mutans* and significantly less live *S. mutans* than the 4% and the control formulations (Figure 3). Additionally, live and dead percentages gave linear trends versus concentration between 4% and 8% PLS (Figure 3). Additionally, live and dead percentages gave linear trends versus concentration between 4% and 8% PLS (Figure 3).

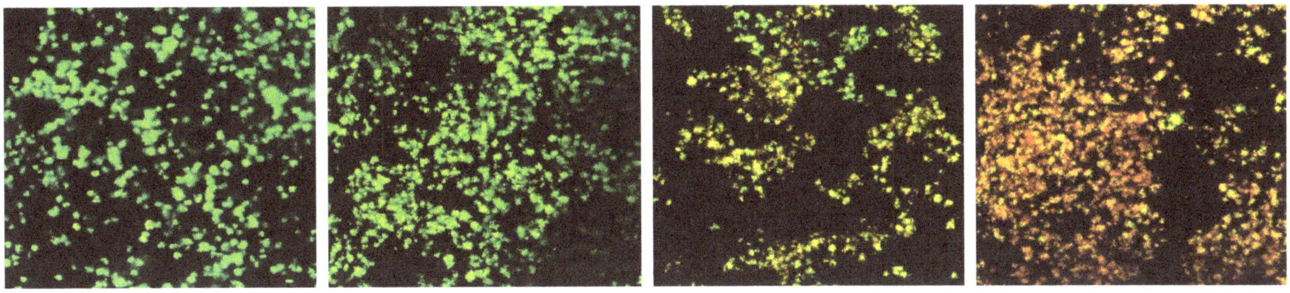

Figure 2. Example confocal microscopy images of live/dead stained biofilms formed on composite formulations containing different percentages of PLS added to the filler phase. Live bacteria stain green whereas dead bacteria are red.

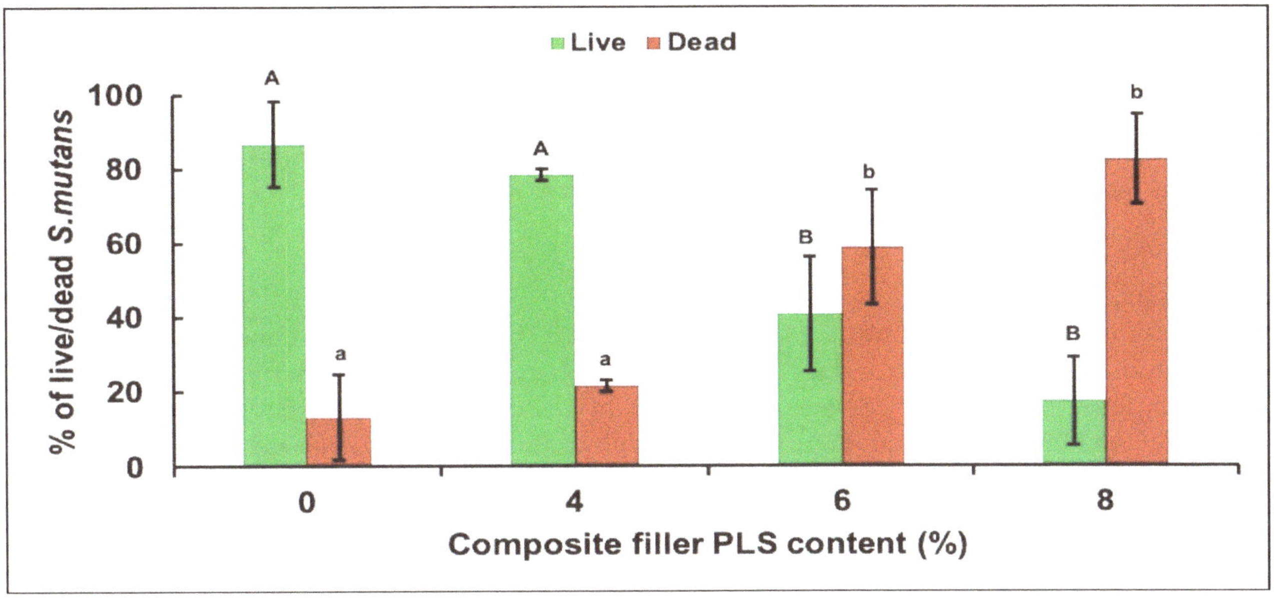

Figure 3. Mean ± (95%CI, $n = 3$) percentage of live and dead *S. mutans* in biofilm formed on discs of the four composite formulations with 0, 4, 6, or 8 wt% PLS in filler phase at 24 h (error bars are for 3 repetitions on different days with 1 specimen per formulation per day). Composite formulations with the same uppercase/lowercase letter/s were not significantly different at $p < 0.05$.

3.3. Biofilm Thickness

Due to the variability in biofilm thickness arising from day to day, the data were normalised by biofilm thickness of the control on the given day. All PLS-containing formulations (4, 6, and 8%) then showed significantly reduced normalised biofilm thickness compared to the control (Figure 4). In addition, the formula containing 8% PLS had significantly less biofilm thickness compared to that containing 4% PLS. Additionally, a linear decline in biofilm thickness was observed with increasing PLS concentration (Figure 4).

When biofilm mass and biofilm thickness were both normalised by results for the control, the data within experimental error overlapped. Additionally, both showed a linear decline in normalised mean with increasing PLS concentration (Figure 4). Linear declines of up to 28% and 33% in the biofilm mass and the biofilm thickness, respectively, were observed with increasing PLS concentration to 8% (Figure 4).

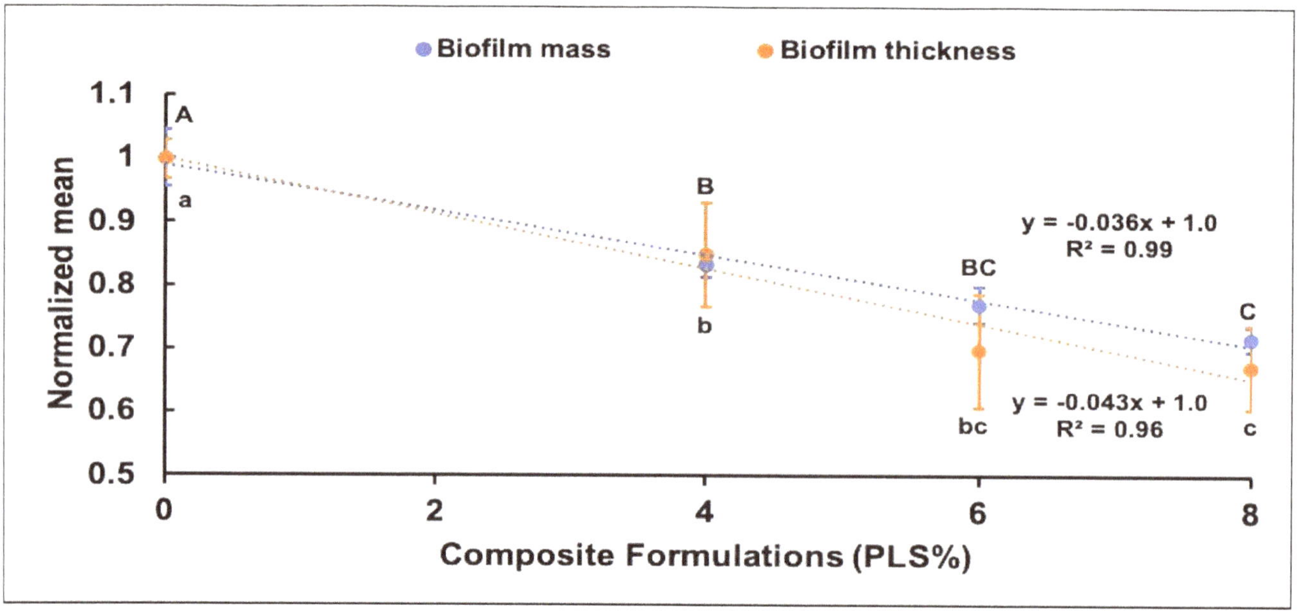

Figure 4. Scatter graph showing the relationship between normalised mean ± (95%CI) biofilm thickness (n = 3) and biofilm mass (n = 4) (Y-axis) for different composite formulations (X-axis). For biofilm mass and thickness, the formulations with the same uppercase letters above and lowercase letters below the bars, respectively, were not significantly different at $p < 0.05$.

3.4. Polylysine Release

Percentage PLS release was proportional to the square root of time up to 1, 2, or 3 months with 4%, 6%, and 8% PLS, respectively, but then levelled (Figure 5). The overall general linear model revealed a significant difference in the percentage of PLS released between different composite formulations at every time point. Cumulative release in µg/disc at 24 h and final percentage release both increased with raising the PLS filler content (Figure 6). Within error, final percentage release was 60/350 times the 24 h µg/disc release for all formulations (Figure 6). Final percentage releases were 42%, 28%, and 13% with 8%, 6%, and 4% PLS in the filler phase, respectively. Release at 24 h was 241, 163 and 85 µg/disc, respectively (Figure 6). At 6 h, the release was half these values.

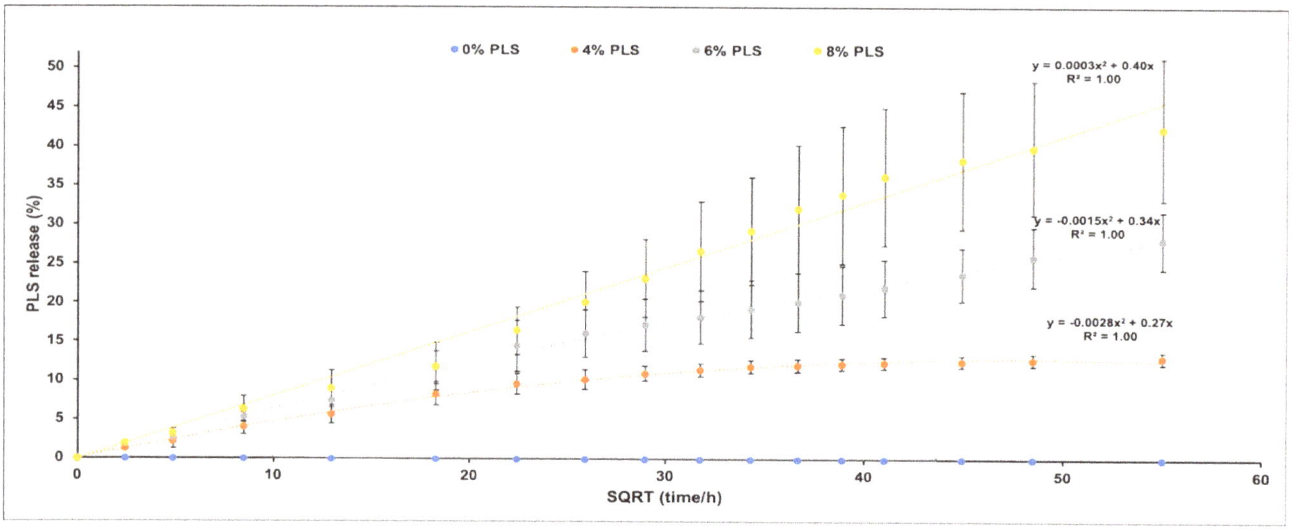

Figure 5. Scatter graph of mean ± (95%CI, n = 3) percentage PLS release (Y-axis) versus the square root of time/hours (X-axis) for each composite formula up to 18 weeks (the legend shows the composite filler PLS %). All final release values were significantly different for different PLS levels at $p < 0.05$.

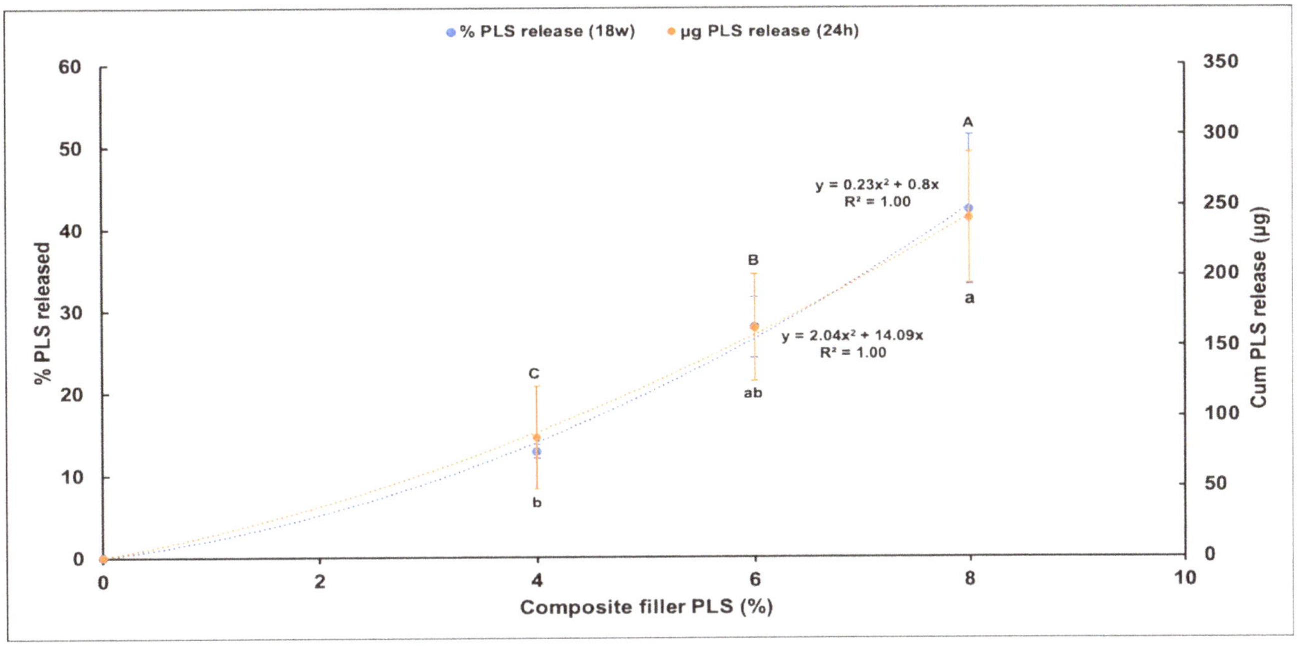

Figure 6. Scatter graph of mean ± (95%CI, $n = 3$) cumulative percentage PLS release at 18 weeks (left Y-axis) and mean ± (95%CI) cumulative PLS release in (µg/disc) at 24 h (right Y-axis) for different composite formulations (X-axis). The formulations with the same uppercase letter/s above or lowercase letter/s below the bars that indicate 18 week and 24 h data, respectively, were not significantly different at $p < 0.05$.

4. Discussion

In the current study, the antibacterial effects of composites formulated with simultaneously increasing levels of antibacterial PLS and remineralising MCPM was evaluated. MCPM/PLS weight ratio was fixed at 2. From relative densities and molecular weights, this gave approximately comparable volumes of the two components and the moles of MCPM and the lysine monomer units in all formulations. Previous studies have shown that, in composites, these may work synergistically at promoting surface mineralizing properties [22]. The aim of this study, however, was to assess how formulations with these two components affect *S. mutans* biofilm deposition and survival on the composite surface. Subsequent polylysine release rates were used to explain the large differences observed between materials with different PLS and MCPM levels.

Polylysine is effective against a wide range of bacteria, although concentrations required tend to be much higher than for conventional antibiotics or agents such as chlorhexidine. A recent study showed that increase in PLS concentration above 250 ppm caused reduction in survival rate, enzymatic activity, and adenosine triphosphate (ATP) levels of *Staphylococcus aureus*. It also increased cell collapse and membrane permeability. Additionally, it destroyed the peptidoglycan component of the cell wall and caused changes in the levels of several metabolites [23]. Another study compared the action of PLS of 750 and 74 ppm on Gram-positive and Gram-negative bacteria, *Listeria innocua*, and *E. coli*, respectively. In both cases, PLS exerted its activity by binding to negatively charged phospholipid head groups in the lipid bilayer of bacterial membranes and destabilized them, thus increasing permeability. In the case of *E. coli*, PLS also binds to and destroys the lipopolysaccharide component of the outer membrane [30].

The minimum inhibitory concentration of PLS against *S. mutans* with the standard initial inoculum level of 5.5×10^5 CFU/mL was found to be 20 µg/mL [31], but this increases with the higher bacterial levels seen in the oral cavity. *S. mutans* is a Gram-positive facultative anaerobic bacterium that was first identified as a cariogenic bacterium in 1924 [32]. A previous longitudinal study reported that 96.6% of patients aged between 6–30 have *S. mutans* present in their oral cavity [33]. In a recent study, composite formulations that released 93 ppm PLS upon the first 24 h of water immersion were able to reduce an initial inoculum level of 8×10^5 CFU/mL down to 10^2 CFU/mL [25]. In this present study, the formulation with 4% PLS with a similar level of PLS release, however, was unable to prevent *S. mutans* biofilm growth. This was likely due to the addition of sucrose enhancing the rate of bacterial growth in addition to enabling production of a protective extracellular matrix (ECM) [34]. The observed linear decline in biofilm mass with increasing PLS suggests it may have been causing a linear decline in the numbers of viable bacteria in the surrounding medium. Alternatively, this effect could have been independent of PLS bactericidal activity and due instead to biofilm matrix disruption caused by PLS [35].

Since CV may stain the ECM in addition to the bacterial cell wall, it provides a measure of the combined live and dead bacteria. In the present study, a live/dead stain was additionally used to determine the fraction of the bacterial population that were live. In regard to the live/dead stain, propidium iodide staining (red) revealed a damaged cell membrane. A statistically significant increase in the percentage of dead *S. mutans* was apparent with the composites containing 6% and 8% PLS compared to the 4% and the control formulations. This study, in conjunction with the previous work [25], suggests that the concentrations of PLS and MCPM in the filler need to be increased significantly to be effective when sucrose is added.

Considerable variation in biofilm thickness detected by confocal microscopy was observed between experiments, although this was not apparent in the biofilm mass measured by CV staining. This may reflect differences in biofilm structural organization between experiments. Nonetheless, when the data were normalised to the control in individual experiments, a consistent decline in both biofilm mass and thickness with increasing PLS concentration was evident.

The most widely used antibacterial agent in dental composites has been chlorhexidine (CHX). Previous studies, however, showed development of antibacterial resistance toward CHX [36] as well as severe [37] and sometimes fatal hypersensitivity reactions [38]. Furthermore, release from hydrophobic composites [39,40] can be restricted and can require addition of hydrophilic components to promote water sorption, which decreases strength. Whilst, in standard tests, minimum inhibitory concentrations of PLS are generally much higher (20 ppm) [31] than those of CHX (<1 ppm), the new studies suggest its very much higher aqueous solubility enables faster release from the composite surface.

In order to quantify the kinetics of PLS release from each formulation, a ninhydrin assay was used. Ninhydrin is used for the detection of ammonia, primary or secondary amines, amino acids, peptides, and proteins [41]. The reaction between NH_2-group present in protein, peptide, or amino acid with ninhydrin (originally yellow color) produces a coloured ninhydrin chromophore (deep purple colour) (Ruhemann's purple λ_{max} 570 nm) [41]. PLS is one of the peptides that can be detected by the ninhydrin reaction. Under appropriate conditions, the intensity of the purple colour is proportional to the NH_2-group (PLS concentration). Ninhydrin reaction is extremely sensitive to low concentrations of protein, peptide, or amino acid [41].

Unlike previous studies [22], there was no initial burst release of PLS in this new study. This may have been a consequence of higher filler content in the earlier work (80 wt%) leading to particles making more direct contact with the surface. In the current study, the percentage of PLS released was instead proportional to the square root of time. This is expected from the Higuchi equation for drug release from thin layers [42].

$$\frac{P_t}{P_\infty} = \frac{4}{L}\sqrt{\frac{Dt}{\pi}} \tag{2}$$

P_t and P_∞ are the percentage *PLS release* at time t and at infinity, respectively. D is a diffusion coefficient and L the thickness of the layer top and bottom of the sample from which the drug is released. If all the PLS is released from this layer but none is released from the remaining material bulk, layer thickness would be expected to be given by:

$$L = \frac{P_\infty h}{100} \tag{3}$$

where h is half the sample thickness and is equal to 0.5 mm. As maximum percentage polylysine releases are 13%, 28%, and 42%, the top and the bottom surface layers depleted of PLS are expected from this expression to be 65, 140 and 210 μm with 4%, 6%, and 8% PLS in the filler, respectively. These are approximately 2, 4, and 6 times the diameters of the PLS and the MCPM particles. The increase in thickness is likely due to higher levels of these hydrophilic components upon their release, generating pores in the surface that enable PLS release from deeper within the specimens. Doubling the concentration of PLS in the filler therefore more than doubles the release from the composite.

Combining Equations (2) and (3) gives:

$$P_t = \frac{400}{h}\sqrt{\frac{Dt}{\pi}} \tag{4}$$

At 24 h, this becomes:

$$P_{24} = \frac{2000}{h}\sqrt{\frac{D}{\pi}} \tag{5}$$

Additionally, from Figure 6:

$$P_{24} = 100\frac{w_{24}}{w_c} = \frac{[14+2c]}{100mf} \tag{6}$$

w_{24} and w_c are the weight of PLS released at 24 h in micrograms and total PLS in the composite disc. m, c, and f are mass of disc in grams (0.13 g), percentage of PLS in the filler, and filler fraction (0.75) in the composite. This equation shows that, upon doubling the PLS concentration in the filler, the early release in micrograms more than doubles. h, m, and f are all constants. Comparing Equations (5) and (6) therefore suggests that, upon increasing c, the diffusion coefficient for PLS increases, enabling faster release. This may be a consequence of higher c increasing PLS, MCPM, and water sorption. Further studies would be required to separate the effects of PLS and MCPM variables. The results, however, show that doubling both PLS and MCPM filler content more than doubles early PLS release mass.

When the composite is in direct contact with the dentine, release of PLS would be restricted. Release could occur, however, upon composite/dentine interface damage creating a water filled gap. These gaps may occur due poor bonding technique generated through composite shrinkage upon placement or formed at a later time due to cyclic stress on the bond. Rapid release of PLS into this gap could help to prevent biofilm formation initiating recurrent caries. The caries could, at early times after restoration, arise due to residual bacteria, or, if the gap is larger than a few microns, may be initiated by bacteria penetrating from the oral cavity. Additional diffusion of nutrients from the oral cavity would accelerate the bacterial growth within the gap.

If release of PLS is sufficiently fast to enable the minimum inhibitory concentration to be reached in the medium before exponential bacterial growth, then biofilm formation should be prevented. Alternatively, as occurred in this study, if release is not sufficiently fast to prevent biofilm initiation, longer-term release may kill the bacteria that are adherent on the composite surface. This study suggests that higher MCPM and PLS are required to achieve this mechanism of biofilm destruction. This antibacterial action would enable reduced risk with partial caries removal and possibly allow less affected dental hard tissue removal. In addition, it might increase the survival rate of the restoration and decrease the prevalence of recurrent caries. Excessive release of surface PLS, however, would have a negative effect on the top surface roughness and hardness. High levels could additionally reduce mechanical properties. This, however, could be addressed through use of the composite with high levels of MCPM and PLS beneath the control composite. This would likely block release of PLS from the top surface into the oral cavity.

5. Conclusions

Composites were prepared with PLS added to the filler phase at levels of 0, 4, 6, and 8 wt% and with monocalcium phosphate added simultaneously at double these levels. Upon incubating set composite discs with *S. mutans* and sucrose, a linear decline in surface biofilm mass and thickness occurred with increasing PLS level. Conversely, an abrupt increase in dead bacteria within the biofilm was observed with PLS levels above 4 wt%. Release studies suggest this was a consequence of 24 h PLS release needing to be above a critical level to kill bacteria within the surface biofilms. Early PLS release from the composite was proportional to the square root of time, as expected for a diffusion controlled process. Release levelled below 100%, suggesting it was from surface layers, which increased in thickness with raising PLS level. Upon damage of the composite restoration/tooth interface, either through polymerization shrinkage during placement or upon cyclic loading, a new composite surface was generated that was in contact with fluid. With rapid and sufficient PLS release from this new surface, risk of recurrent caries within the microgaps formed could potentially be reduced.

Author Contributions: Conceptualization, W.X., P.A., E.A., and A.M.Y.; Data curation, R.B.Y., W.X., and A.M.Y.; Formal analysis, R.B.Y. and A.M.Y.; Funding acquisition, R.B.Y., E.A., and A.M.Y.; Investigation, R.B.Y.; Methodology, W.X., E.A., and A.M.Y.; Project administration, E.A. and A.M.Y.; Resources, P.A., E.A., and A.M.Y.; Software, R.B.Y.; Supervision, P.A., E.A., and A.M.Y.; Validation, R.B.Y., W.X., P.A., E.A., and A.M.Y.; Visualization, R.B.Y.; Writing—original draft, R.B.Y.; Writing—review & editing, P.A., E.A., and A.M.Y. All authors have read and agreed to the published version of the manuscript.

Acknowledgments: Authors would like to acknowledge Nicola J. Mordan for providing technical support.

References

1. WHO. Sugars and Dental Caries. Available online: https://apps.who.int/iris/bitstream/handle/10665/259413/WHO-NMH-NHD-17.12-eng.pdf;jsessionid=32E391ADF801ABA40F4C08F06FAB6382?sequence=1 (accessed on 29 June 2020).
2. WHO. Data and Statistics. Available online: http://www.euro.who.int/en/health-topics/disease-prevention/oral-health/data-and-statistics (accessed on 29 June 2020).
3. Bourguignon, D. Briefing EU Legislation in Progress Mercury Aligning EU legislation with Minamata. Available online: http://www.europarl.europa.eu/RegData/etudes/BRIE/2017/595887/EPRS_BRI%282017%29595887_EN.pdf (accessed on 29 June 2020).
4. Heintze, S.D.; Rousson, V. Clinical effectiveness of direct class II restorations-a meta-analysis. *J. Adhes. Dent.* **2012**, *14*, 407–431. [CrossRef] [PubMed]
5. Sunnegardh-Gronberg, K.; van Dijken, J.W.; Funegard, U.; Lindberg, A.; Nilsson, M. Selection of dental materials and longevity of replaced restorations in Public Dental Health clinics in northern Sweden. *J. Dent.* **2009**, *37*, 673–678. [CrossRef] [PubMed]
6. Beck, F.; Lettner, S.; Graf, A.; Bitriol, B.; Dumitrescu, N.; Bauer, P.; Moritz, A.; Schedle, A. Survival of direct resin restorations in posterior teeth within a 19-year period (1996–2015): A meta-analysis of prospective studies. *Dent. Mater.* **2015**, *31*, 958–985. [CrossRef] [PubMed]
7. Alvanforoush, N.; Palamara, J.; Wong, R.H.; Burrow, M.F. Comparison between published clinical success of direct resin composite restorations in vital posterior teeth in 1995–2005 and 2006–2016 periods. *Aust. Dent. J.* **2017**, *62*, 132–145. [CrossRef] [PubMed]
8. Kopperud, S.E.; Tveit, A.B.; Gaarden, T.; Sandvik, L.; Espelid, I. Longevity of posterior dental restorations and reasons for failure. *Eur. J. Oral. Sci.* **2012**, *120*, 539–548. [CrossRef] [PubMed]
9. Bourbia, M.; Ma, D.; Cvitkovitch, D.G.; Santerre, J.P.; Finer, Y. Cariogenic bacteria degrade dental resin composites and adhesives. *J. Dent. Res.* **2013**, *92*, 989–994. [CrossRef]
10. Marsh, P.D. Dental plaque as a microbial biofilm. *Caries Res.* **2004**, *38*, 204–211. [CrossRef]
11. Seneviratne, C.J.; Zhang, C.F.; Samaranayake, L.P. Dental plaque biofilm in oral health and disease. *Chin. J. Dent. Res.* **2011**, *14*, 87–94.
12. Keijser, B.J.; Zaura, E.; Huse, S.M.; van der Vossen, J.M.; Schuren, F.H.; Montijn, R.C.; ten Cate, J.M.; Crielaard, W. Pyrosequencing analysis of the oral microflora of healthy adults. *J. Dent. Res.* **2008**, *87*, 1016–1020. [CrossRef]

13. Dewhirst, F.E.; Chen, T.; Izard, J.; Paster, B.J.; Tanner, A.C.; Yu, W.H.; Lakshmanan, A.; Wade, W.G. The human oral microbiome. *J. Bacteriol.* **2010**, *192*, 5002–5017. [CrossRef]
14. Aas, J.A.; Griffen, A.L.; Dardis, S.R.; Lee, A.M.; Olsen, I.; Dewhirst, F.E.; Leys, E.J.; Paster, B.J. Bacteria of dental caries in primary and permanent teeth in children and young adults. *J. Clin. Microbiol.* **2008**, *46*, 1407–1417. [CrossRef] [PubMed]
15. Munson, M.A.; Banerjee, A.; Watson, T.F.; Wade, W.G. Molecular analysis of the microflora associated with dental caries. *J. Clin. Microbiol.* **2004**, *42*, 3023–3029. [CrossRef] [PubMed]
16. Takahashi, N.; Nyvad, B. Ecological Hypothesis of Dentin and Root Caries. *Caries Res.* **2016**, *50*, 422–431. [CrossRef] [PubMed]
17. Ge, Z.Y.; Yang, L.M.; Xia, J.J.; Fu, X.H.; Zhang, Y.Z. Possible aerosol transmission of COVID-19 and special precautions in dentistry. *J. Zhejiang Univ. Sci. B* **2020**, *21*, 361–368. [CrossRef]
18. Odeh, N.D.; Babkair, H.; Abu-Hammad, S.; Borzangy, S.; Abu-Hammad, A.; Abu-Hammad, O. COVID-19: Present and Future Challenges for Dental Practice. *Int. J. Environ. Res. Public Health* **2020**, *17*, 3151. [CrossRef]
19. Schwendicke, F.; Frencken, J.E.; Bjorndal, L.; Maltz, M.; Manton, D.J.; Ricketts, D.; Van Landuyt, K.; Banerjee, A.; Campus, G.; Domejean, S.; et al. Managing Carious Lesions: Consensus Recommendations on Carious Tissue Removal. *Adv. Dent. Res.* **2016**, *28*, 58–67. [CrossRef]
20. Frencken, J.E.; Leal, S.C.; Navarro, M.F. Twenty-five-year atraumatic restorative treatment (ART) approach: A comprehensive overview. *Clin. Oral Investig.* **2012**, *16*, 1337–1346. [CrossRef]
21. Ye, R.; Xu, H.; Wan, C.; Peng, S.; Wang, L.; Xu, H.; Aguilar, Z.P.; Xiong, Y.; Zeng, Z.; Wei, H. Antibacterial activity and mechanism of action of ε-poly-L-lysine. *Biochem. Biophys. Res. Commun.* **2013**, *439*, 148–153. [CrossRef]
22. Panpisut, P.; Liaqat, S.; Zacharaki, E.; Xia, W.; Petridis, H.; Young, A.M. Dental Composites with Calcium/Strontium Phosphates and Polylysine. *PLoS ONE* **2016**, *11*, e0164653. [CrossRef]
23. Tan, Z.; Shi, Y.; Xing, B.; Hou, Y.; Cui, J.; Jia, S. The antimicrobial effects and mechanism of ε-poly-lysine against Staphylococcus aureus. *Bioresour. Bioprocess.* **2019**, *6*, 11. [CrossRef]
24. Kangwankai, K.; Sani, S.; Panpisut, P.; Xia, W.; Ashley, P.; Petridis, H.; Young, A.M. Monomer conversion, dimensional stability, strength, modulus, surface apatite precipitation and wear of novel, reactive calcium phosphate and polylysine-containing dental composites. *PLoS ONE* **2017**, *12*, e0187757. [CrossRef] [PubMed]
25. Nikolaos, N.N.; Allan, E.; Xia, W.; Ashley, P.F.; Young, A.M. Early polylysine release from dental composites and its effects on planktonic Streptococcus mutans growth. *J. Funct. Biomater.* **2020**, *11*, 53. [CrossRef]
26. Davies, D. Understanding biofilm resistance to antibacterial agents. *Nat. Rev. Drug. Discov.* **2003**, *2*, 114–122. [CrossRef] [PubMed]
27. ISO 4049:2019 Dentistry—Polymer-Based Restorative Materials. Available online: https://www.iso.org/standard/67596.html (accessed on 30 July 2020).
28. Astasov-Frauenhoffer, M.; Glauser, S.; Fischer, J.; Schmidli, F.; Waltimo, T.; Rohr, N. Biofilm formation on restorative materials and resin composite cements. *Dent. Mater.* **2018**, *34*, 1702–1709. [CrossRef] [PubMed]
29. Amrita. Quantitative Estimation of Amino Acids by Ninhydrin. Available online: http://vlab.amrita.edu/?sub=3&brch=63&sim=156&cnt=2 (accessed on 29 June 2020).
30. Hyldgaard, M.; Mygind, T.; Vad, B.S.; Stenvang, M.; Otzen, D.E.; Meyer, R.L. The antimicrobial mechanism of action of epsilon-poly-l-lysine. *Appl. Environ. Microbiol.* **2014**, *80*, 7758–7770. [CrossRef]
31. Badaoui Najjar, M.; Kashtanov, D.; Chikindas, M.L. Natural Antimicrobials epsilon-Poly-L-lysine and Nisin A for Control of Oral Microflora. *Probiotics Antimicrob. Proteins* **2009**, *1*, 143. [CrossRef]
32. Clarke, J.K. On the Bacterial Factor in the Ætiology of Dental Caries. *Br. J. Exp. Pathol.* **1924**, *5*, 141–147.
33. Oda, Y.; Hayashi, F.; Okada, M. Longitudinal study of dental caries incidence associated with Streptococcus mutans and Streptococcus sobrinus in patients with intellectual disabilities. *BMC Oral Health* **2015**, *15*, 102. [CrossRef]
34. Limoli, D.H.; Jones, C.J.; Wozniak, D.J. Bacterial Extracellular Polysaccharides in Biofilm Formation and Function. *Microbiol. Spectr.* **2015**, *3*. [CrossRef]
35. Feldman, M.; Sionov, R.; Smoum, R.; Mechoulam, R.; Ginsburg, I.; Steinberg, D. Comparative Evaluation of Combinatory Interaction between Endocannabinoid System Compounds and Poly-L-lysine against Streptococcus mutans Growth and Biofilm Formation. *Biomed. Res. Int.* **2020**, *2020*, 7258380. [CrossRef]

36. Kulik, E.M.; Waltimo, T.; Weiger, R.; Schweizer, I.; Lenkeit, K.; Filipuzzi-Jenny, E.; Walter, C. Development of resistance of mutans streptococci and Porphyromonas gingivalis to chlorhexidine digluconate and amine fluoride/stannous fluoride-containing mouthrinses, in vitro. *Clin. Oral Investig.* **2015**, *19*, 1547–1553. [CrossRef] [PubMed]
37. Calogiuri, G.; Di Leo, E.; Trautmann, A.; Nettis, E.; Ferrannini, A.; Vacca, A. Chlorhexidine hypersensitivity: A critical and updated review. *J. Allergy Ther.* **2013**, *4*, 10.4172.
38. Pemberton, M.N.; Gibson, J. Chlorhexidine and hypersensitivity reactions in dentistry. *Br. Dent. J.* **2012**, *213*, 547–550. [CrossRef]
39. Aljabo, A.; Abou Neel, E.A.; Knowles, J.C.; Young, A.M. Development of dental composites with reactive fillers that promote precipitation of antibacterial-hydroxyapatite layers. *Mater. Sci. Eng. C Mater. Biol. Appl.* **2016**, *60*, 285–292. [CrossRef] [PubMed]
40. Zhang, J.F.; Wu, R.; Fan, Y.; Liao, S.; Wang, Y.; Wen, Z.T.; Xu, X. Antibacterial Dental Composites with Chlorhexidine and Mesoporous Silica. *J. Dent. Res.* **2014**, *93*, 1283–1289. [CrossRef]
41. Friedman, M. Applications of the ninhydrin reaction for analysis of amino acids, peptides, and proteins to agricultural and biomedical sciences. *J. Agric. Food Chem.* **2004**, *52*, 385–406. [CrossRef]
42. Siepmann, J.; Peppas, N.A. Higuchi equation: Derivation, applications, use and misuse. *Int. J. Pharm.* **2011**, *418*, 6–12. [CrossRef]

10

Cerium Dioxide Particles to Tune Radiopacity of Dental Adhesives: Microstructural and Physico-Chemical Evaluation

Isadora Martini Garcia [1], Vicente Castelo Branco Leitune [1], Antonio Shigueaki Takimi [2], Carlos Pérez Bergmann [3], Susana Maria Werner Samuel [1], Mary Anne Melo [4,5,*] and Fabrício Mezzomo Collares [1,*]

1. Dental Materials Laboratory, School of Dentistry, Federal University of Rio Grande do Sul, Rua Ramiro Barcelos 2492, Rio Branco, Porto Alegre, RS 90035-003, Brazil; isadora.garcia@ufrgs.br (I.M.G.); vicente.leitune@ufrgs.br (V.C.B.L.); susana.samuel@ufrgs.br (S.M.W.S.)
2. Laboratory for Electrochemical Processes and Corrosion, Engineering School, Federal University of Rio Grande do Sul, Bento Gonçalves, 9500, Prédio 43427, Sala 216, Porto Alegre, RS 91501-970, Brazil; antonio.takimi@gmail.com
3. Laboratory of Ceramic Materials, Federal University of Rio Grande do Sul, Avenida Osvaldo Aranha 99, Porto Alegre, RS 90035-003, Brazil; bergmann@ufrgs.br
4. Division of Operative Dentistry, Department of General Dentistry, University of Maryland School of Dentistry, Baltimore, MD 21201, USA
5. Ph.D. Program in Biomedical Sciences, University of Maryland School of Dentistry, Baltimore, MD 21201, USA

* Correspondence: mmelo@umaryland.edu (M.A.M.); fabricio.collares@ufrgs.br (F.M.C.)

Abstract: The insufficient radiopacity of dental adhesives applied under composite restorations makes the radiographic diagnosis of recurrent caries challenging. Consequently, the misdiagnosis may lead to unnecessary replacement of restorations. The aims of this study were to formulate experimental dental adhesives containing cerium dioxide (CeO_2) and investigate the effects of different loadings of CeO_2 on their radiopacity and degree of conversion for the first time. CeO_2 was characterized by X-ray diffraction analysis, Fourier transforms infrared spectroscopy, and laser diffraction for particle size analysis. Experimental dental adhesives were formulated with CeO_2 as the inorganic filler with loadings ranging from 0.36 to 5.76 vol.%. The unfilled adhesive was used as a control. The studied adhesives were evaluated for dispersion of CeO_2 in the polymerized samples, degree of conversion, and radiopacity. CeO_2 presented a monoclinic crystalline phase, peaks related to Ce-O bonding, and an average particle size of around 16 µm. CeO_2 was dispersed in the adhesive, and the addition of these particles increased the adhesives' radiopacity ($p < 0.05$). There was a significant decrease in the degree of conversion with CeO_2 loadings higher than 1.44 vol.%. However, all materials showed a similar degree of conversion in comparison to commercially available adhesives. CeO_2 particles were investigated for the first time as a promising compound to improve the radiopacity of the dental adhesives.

Keywords: dental materials; dentistry; adhesives; light-curing of dental adhesives; composite resins; methylmethacrylate; oxides; cerium; polymers; dentine bonding agents

1. Introduction

Currently, resin composites and dental adhesive systems are used in restorative dentistry as primary direct restorative materials [1]. The failure of resin composites is mainly due to recurrent caries and fractures [2]. The diagnosis of recurrent caries underneath resin composite is a challenge for dentists [3]. Recurrent carious lesions may not always be seen during a clinical examination at the interface between the resin composite, and it requires radiographic evaluation for diagnosis [4,5].

Further, the application of adhesive systems can be seen radiographically as a radiolucent area, which mimics the radiographic appearance of carious lesions [6]. The radiolucency of dental adhesives can contribute to the misinterpretation of radiographic images [4,7,8]. Based on it, dentists may intervene surgically in existing composite restorations, replacing the resin [9].

A previous report has assessed and demonstrated the lack of radiopacity on many restorative dental materials [10]. In their results, all assessed materials were radiolucent and required alterations to their composition to facilitate their detection using radiographic images. The radiopacity of dental adhesives depends on their filler content, and it can be enhanced by incorporating elements with a high atomic weight as inorganic fillers [11].

Cerium dioxide (CeO_2), a rare-earth oxide found in the lanthanide series of the periodic table, has been increasingly used as a nanotherapeutic material [12]. The numerous commercial applications for CeO_2 also called ceria, include glass and glass polishing, phosphors, ceramics, catalysts, and metallurgy [13]. Cerium is found in various minerals, and its primary deposits are located in the United States (Florida and Idaho) and Brazil [14]. Interesting biological properties have been observed for both nanometric and micrometric CeO_2 [15]. Thus, as further advancement in CeO_2's applications, this compound has gained substantial interest in several innovative applications, mainly due to its redox property and catalytic activity [15,16]. In the dental field, CeO_2 was primarily used for dental ceramics since this compound stimulates the natural fluorescence found in human dental enamel [11]. The high atomic number 58 of cerium suggests that it can promote considerable attenuation of a dental X-ray beam [17,18]. The incorporation of CeO_2 in adhesives can be a valuable strategy to promote radiopacity and improve the detection of dental adhesives underneath resin composites. Therefore, the aims of this study were to formulate experimental dental adhesives containing CeO_2 and investigate the effects of different loadings of CeO_2 on their radiopacity and degree of conversion for the first time.

2. Results

Figure 1 shows the results of CeO_2 particles' characterization. In Figure 1A, the X-ray diffraction analysis of the powder shows the crystallinity pattern of a monoclinic phase of CeO_2 (powder diffraction file, ICDD-PDF 37-1468). In Figure 1B, the chemical composition analyzed by Fourier Transform Infrared Spectroscopy (FTIR) displays the peaks related to Ce–O bonds at 400 cm^{-1}. Figure 1C,D presents the results of size distribution analysis. The histogram shows a non-normal distribution of size (Figure 1C). The 10th percentile showed a particle diameter of 1.15 μm. The median (50th percentile) was 14.98 μm, the 90th percentile was 31.32 μm, and the mean particle size was around 16 μm (Figure 1D).

Figure 2 presents the qualitative assessment via micro-Raman of the materials' surfaces containing 0.36 (A) and 0.76 (B) vol.% of CeO_2. The image consists of a 2-D array of measured spectra, which means that the distribution of the chemical composition can be investigated. After mapping the polymer's surfaces, the integration of the corresponding CeO_2 peak (464 cm^{-1}) was used for analysis and graphs generation. In the graphs, from blue to yellow, more CeO_2 is identified. It was observed that the higher the load of CeO_2 in the resin, the larger the area under the curve (peak) in micro-Raman spectra for this oxide, generating more yellow regions in the graph. In these analyses, more areas in yellow were presented in the adhesive with 0.76 vol.% of CeO_2 in comparison to the group with 0.36 vol.%.

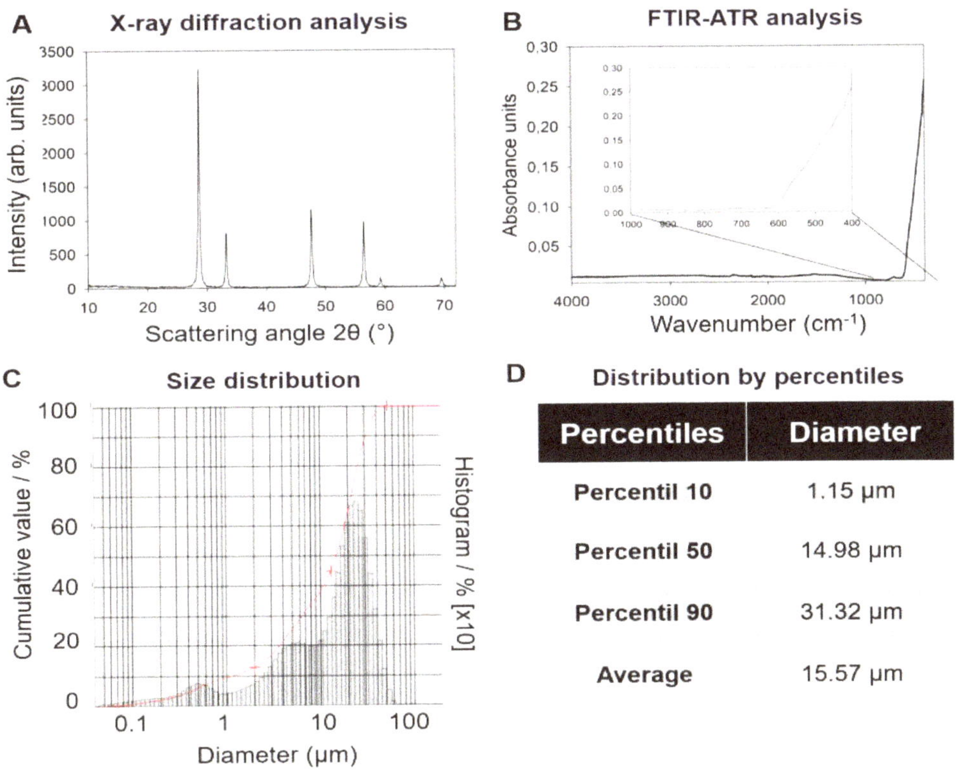

Figure 1. CeO_2 particles' characterization: (**A**) X-ray diffraction analysis shows the pattern of the monoclinic phase of crystallinity for CeO_2; (**B**) FTIR analysis displays the peaks related to Ce-O bonds at 400 cm^{-1}; (**C**) and (**D**) show the non-normal distribution size of CeO_2 and the values of size distribution.

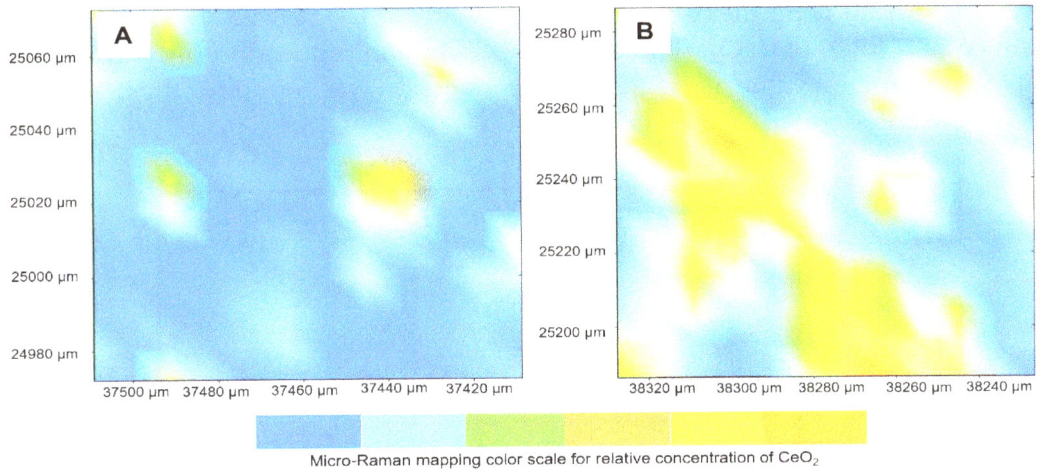

Figure 2. Micro-Raman analysis of the dental adhesive surfaces containing 0.36 (**A**) and 0.76 (**B**) vol.% of CeO_2. Both images display the intensity of the CeO_2 peak at 464 cm^{-1}. The higher the load of CeO_2 in the dental adhesive, the more areas in yellow are observed.

Figure 3 indicates the results of the radiopacity of each experimental adhesive resin containing a different percentage of volume fraction of CeO_2. In Figure 3A, an illustrative radiograph displays the location of the dental adhesive layer underneath the composite restorative material. The arrows indicate the radiolucent areas corresponding to the adhesive layer. The difference of radiopacity between the composite resin and the adhesive layer can be clearly observed. In Figure 2B, the mean and standard deviation of radiopacity is expressed in mm of aluminum. The control group, which is an unfilled adhesive, showed the lower mean value of radiopacity, without statistical difference for the groups with 0.36 vol.% and 0.72 vol.% of CeO_2. From the addition of 1.44 vol.% of CeO_2, there was increased radiopacity of the adhesive in comparison to the control group ($p < 0.05$). The group with 5.76 vol.% of CeO_2 showed the highest value of radiopacity among all groups ($p < 0.05$). The incorporation of 4.32 vol.% and 5.76 vol.% presented values of more than 1 mm of aluminum.

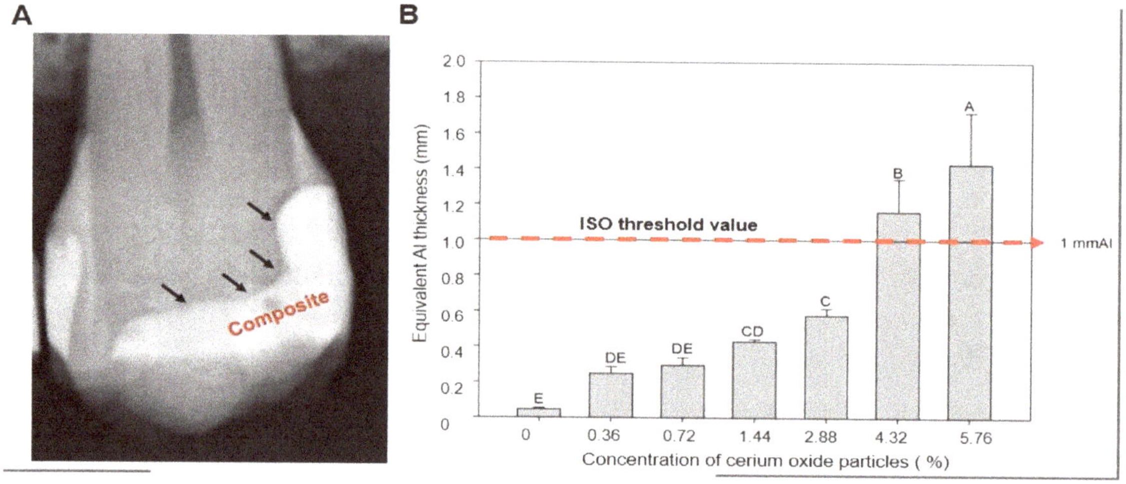

Figure 3. The dental radiograph displays the layer of dental adhesive applied under the composite resin (**A**) The arrows guide the visualization of the radiolucent adhesive layer. (**B**) The radiopacity of the experimental dental adhesives according the to the increasing concentration of cerium oxide. Different letters indicate statistical differences among groups ($p < 0.05$).

Figure 4 shows the results of the degree of conversion analysis of the experimental dental adhesives. The uncured adhesive samples were directly dispensed on the attenuated total reflection (ATR) device of FTIR to analyze the conversion of carbon-carbon double bonds in the aliphatic chain. The values ranged from 61.52 (±0.33) % for the control group to 47.90 (±1.64) % for 5.76 vol.% of CeO_2. From the incorporation of 2.88 vol.% of CeO_2, the degree of conversion reduced in comparison to the control group ($p < 0.05$). The lowest value of the degree of conversion was found for the highest load of CeO_2 incorporated in the adhesive ($p < 0.05$).

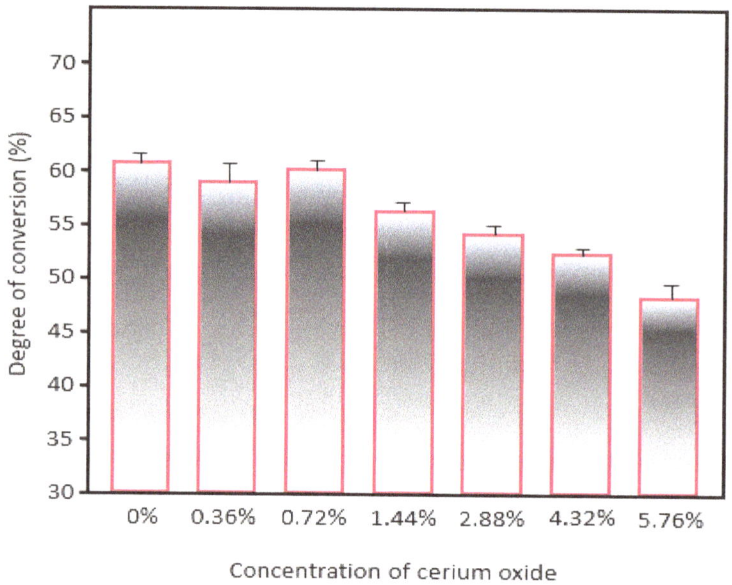

Figure 4. Degree of conversion of the experimental dental adhesives containing CeO_2. Different letters indicate statistical differences among groups ($p < 0.05$).

3. Discussion

In this in vitro study, CeO_2 particles were explored as potential radiopacifier for dental adhesives since high atomic weight and density can provide a suitable level of radiopacity. CeO_2 was first chemically characterized by XRD, Raman, and FTIR to be incorporated for the first time in a dental adhesive resin. In the current investigation, CeO_2 successfully increased the radiopacity of the adhesive, maintaining a suitable degree of monomer conversion.

CeO_2 particles used in this study presented a monoclinic crystalline phase with particular chemical groups and the average particle size of around 16 μm. This oxide was incorporated in an experimental adhesive resin formulated as previously reported, with conventional dental methacrylate monomers [19,20]. The presence of a radiopacifying agent is essential to enable the identification of restorative materials and dissimilarity from pathological processes in the adjacent areas [21]. Recurrent caries and marginal gaps are very often the reasons for the replacement of composite restorations [22]. The misdiagnosis and treatment decision for unnecessary replacement of restorations lead to additional loss of sound tooth tissue, with an increased cost and discomfort for the patient [23]. Therefore, the restorative materials should have optimal radiopacity for accurate radiographic differentiation for existing restorations and recurrent dental caries, supporting clinical follow-ups. Substantial changes in radiopacity are compulsory by the International Organization for Standardization (ISO) for dental restorative materials [24]. The compliance with the ISO 4049 requires a minimum radiopacity of restorative materials higher than that of dentin and greater or equivalent thickness of aluminum (with ≥98% purity) [24]. In the present study, the increased load of CeO_2, by the percentage of volume, was added to an experimental dental adhesive, providing a material with proper radiopacity. Our results have shown that CeO_2 at 4.32 vol.% had radiopacity higher than 1 mm of Al.

Besides the increase of radiopacity, the addition of inorganic fillers in monomeric blends may improve polymers properties, such as the elastic modulus, tensile strength, fracture toughness, Knoop hardness, and stability against solvents [25]. However, the higher filler addition can also decrease the degree of monomer's conversion [19]. The degree of conversion is a valuable chemical property for polymers, and it may be associated with the stability of the restoration over time [20]. Therefore, a reliable polymerization is desired for adhesive resins to reduce hydrolytic degradation in the clinical setting [26,27]. Here, we observed that the incorporation of CeO_2 at a load that reaches the high radiopacity level reduced the degree of conversion of the dental polymer. Previous studies have reported similar outcomes in the investigations of radiopacifying agents containing different kinds of heavy metals [28]. Marins et al. [29] evaluated the addition of niobium pentoxide (Nb_2O_5) nanoparticles to the dental adhesive as radiopacifiers and observed that the degree of conversion decreased with the addition of particles at percentage mass fraction equal or greater than 10%. In other studies, Nb_2O_5 and Ta_2O_5 showed a decrease in the degree of conversion up to 5 wt.% [19,20]. Our results are also in agreement with those of Amirouche-Korichi et al. [28], where progressive decreases of the degree of conversion were linearly related to the filler contents.

The outcome observed for the degree of conversion may be attributed to the high refractive index of CeO_2 (approx. $\eta = 2.2$ to 2.8) [30], which may have decreased the accessibility of light energy inside the polymer. The limited mobility of monomer chains by the incorporation of the opaque fillers has also been considered as a contributing factor for the decrease in the monomer's conversion [31]. Another consideration for observed decay in the degree of conversion with regard to the dental adhesive with loadings higher than 2.88 vol.% relies on particle size. The fillers used in our study are micro fillers with an average size of around 16 μm. Previous reports support the effect of particle size in microns and highlight that the volume occupied by the particles may compromise the polymerization rates of the material [32–34]. Further evaluation of the polymerization behavior of nanosized CeO_2 could be interesting to address this subject. Moreover, it would be noteworthy to evaluate the effect of micro-sized CeO_2 in the adhesive with thinner samples or in situ in dentin.

Moreover, we suggest further biological studies on dental adhesives containing CeO_2 in micro and nanoscale, since this oxide has emerged as a noteworthy agent for bioactive (such as scaffolds and bioglasses) and antimicrobial materials [35–37]. In this context, a dental adhesive with such properties could be a promising strategy to assist in decreasing the incidence of recurrent caries and improving the remineralization process after selective removal of carious dentin. In this study, despite the decreased degree of conversion observed by increasing CeO_2 addition, all groups showed values around 50%, which is in accordance with commercial dental adhesives [38]. Therefore, CeO_2 may be a promising alternative filler for biopolymers.

4. Materials and Methods

4.1. X-ray Diffraction Analysis of CeO_2

CeO_2 particles purchased were analyzed via X-ray diffraction to detect the crystalline phases of the powder. diffractometer (PW 1730/1 model, Philips, Santa Clara, CA, USA) was operated at 40 kV and 40 mA with CuKa radiation. The scanning rate used was 0.058/min, with 2 s of time-steps at 0.02° each, from 5° to 60° [18].

4.2. FTIR Analysis of CeO_2

Fourier Transform Infrared Spectroscopy (FTIR) was used to chemically characterize the powder of CeO_2. The analysis was performed using the spectrophotometer Vertex 70 (Bruker Optics, Ettlingen, Germany) with an attenuated total reflectance device (ATR). CeO_2 powder was placed on the ATR, and the analysis performed using 20 scans, 4 cm^{-1} of resolution in 5000 to 400 cm^{-1}, and Opus 6.5 software (Bruker Optics, Ettlingen, Germany).

4.3. Particle Size Distribution of CeO_2

CeO_2 particles were dispersed in water with sonication for 60 s. Then, particle size was analyzed via laser diffraction particle size analyzer (CILAS 1180, Cilas, Orleans, France) according to a previous study [18].

4.4. Preparation of Dental Adhesives

The adhesive resins were formulated by mixing 50 wt.% bisphenol A glycol dimethacrylate (BisGMA), 25 wt.% triethylene glycol dimethacrylate (TEGDMA), and 25 wt.% 2-hydroxyethyl methacrylate (HEMA). As a photoinitiator system, camphorquinone and ethyl 4-dimethylaminobenzoate were added at 1 mol%, each one in the base resin. As polymerization inhibition, 0.01 wt.% of butylated hydroxytoluene was incorporated. CeO_2 was added at 0.36, 0.72, 1.44, 2.88, 4.32, and 5.76 vol.%. The resins adhesives were hand-mixed for 5 min, sonicated during 180 s, and hand-mixed again for 5 min. One group without CeO_2 was used as control.

4.5. Qualitative Analysis of CeO_2 into Dental Adhesives

To identify the presence of CeO_2 in dental adhesives, two groups containing this filler were evaluated via micro-Raman Spectroscopy (Senterra, Bruker Optics, Ettlingen, Germany). One sample from the group with 0.36 vol.% and another from the group with 5.76 vol.% were prepared using a polyvinylsiloxane mold. The samples were photoactivated for 20 s on each side using a light-emitting diode dental curing unit (Radii Cal, SDI, Melbourne, Australia) with 1200 mW/cm^2. An area of 110 μm × 110 μm of the surfaces was analyzed via Opus 7.5 software (Opus 7.5, Bruker Optics, Ettlingen, Germany). The analyses were performed with a wavelength of 785 nm, with 5 s and two co-additions. The peak correspondent to CeO_2 (464 cm^{-1}) was used for integration.

4.6. Radiopacity Evaluation

The adhesive resins were evaluated for their radiopacity, according to the International Organization of Standardization (ISO) 4049/2009 guidelines [24]. Five samples per group ($n = 5$) with disc-shaped were prepared with 10.0 mm (±0.5 mm) in diameter and 1.0 mm (±0.1 mm) in thickness with photoactivation for 20 s on each side. The images were made using a phosphor plate for the digital system (VistaScan; Dürr Dental GmbH & Co. KG, Bietigheim-Bissingen, Germany) at 70 kV, 8 mA, and 0.4 s of exposure time. A focus-film distance of 400 mm was used in the assays. One specimen per group was positioned on the film for each X-ray exposition. An aluminum step-wedge (99.12 wt.% of aluminum, thickness from 0.5 mm to 5.0 mm, in increments of 0.5 mm) was exposed with the samples for each image specimens in all images. The images were saved in TIFF, analyzed using Photoshop software (Adobe Systems Incorporated, San Jose, CA, USA), and the mean and standard deviation of the grey levels (pixel density) were measured.

4.7. Degree of Conversion

To analyze the degree of conversion of the adhesives, FTIR-ATR was used according to a previous study [39]. Three drops per group (n = 3, 3 µL each one) were directly dispensed on ATR diamond crystal. An adjustable holder stand was used to fix the light-curing unit and to standardize the distance between its tip and the top of the samples. Two spectra were acquired per group from 4000 to 400 cm^{-1} with a resolution of 4 cm^{-1}. The first spectrum was obtained before the photoactivation. Then, the samples were photoactivated for 20 s and analyzed again. To calculate the monomer conversion, the peak related to the carbon-carbon (C=C) double bond in the aromatic ring of BisGMA (1610 cm^{-1}) was used as an internal standard. The peak related to C=C in the aliphatic chains (1640 cm^{-1}) was used along with the C=C at 1610 cm^{-1} according to the following equation:

$$\textbf{Degree of conversion}\ (\%) = 100 \times \left(\frac{I\_\ 1640 - cured/I\_\ 1610 - cured}{I\_\ 1640 - uncured/I\_1610 - uncured} \right)$$

4.8. Statistical Analysis

CeO_2 characterization was descriptively analyzed, as well as the identification of CeO_2 in the polymerized adhesives. Shapiro-Wilk test was used to evaluate the data normality. The data of radiopacity was evaluated via ANOVA on ranks and Dunn's test. The data of the degree of conversion was analyzed via one-way ANOVA and Tukey's post-hoc test. Both analyses were performed at 0.05 level of significance ($p < 0.05$).

5. Conclusions

CeO_2 was investigated for the first time as a promising filler to improve the radiopacity of dental adhesives. The particles were chemically analyzed and then used in experimental adhesives formulation. Through of incorporation of CeO_2 particles at 1.44 vol.%, the dental adhesives were able to show increased radiopacity and a proper degree of conversion. The restorative materials here proposed could be a reliable strategy to assist clinicians diagnose recurrent caries.

Author Contributions: I.M.G., contributed to data analysis, data interpretation, and drafted the manuscript; V.C.B.L., contributed to design, data acquisition, data analysis, and data interpretation; A.S.T., contributed to data analysis and data interpretation; C.P.B., contributed to data analysis and data interpretation; S.M.W.S., contributed to design and data interpretation; M.A.M., contributed to data interpretation, drafted the manuscript, and critically revised the manuscript; F.M.C., contributed to conception, design, data acquisition, analysis, and interpretation, and drafted and critically revised the manuscript. All authors gave final approval and agreed to be accountable for all aspects of the work.

Acknowledgments: This study was financed in part by the Coordenação de Aperfeiçoamento de Pessoal de Nível Superior—Brasil (CAPES)—Finance Code 001 (scholarship).

References

1. Alzraikat, H.; Burrow, M.F.; Maghaireh, G.A.; Taha, N.A. Nanofilled Resin Composite Properties and Clinical Performance: A Review. *Oper. Dent.* **2018**, *43*, E173–E190. [CrossRef] [PubMed]
2. Rodrigues, S.A.; Scherrer, S.S.; Ferracane, J.L.; Della Bona, A. Microstructural Characterization and Fracture Behavior of a Microhybrid and a Nanofill Composite. *Dent. Mater.* **2008**, *24*, 1281–1288. [CrossRef] [PubMed]
3. Oztas, B.; Kursun, S.; Dinc, G.; Kamburoglu, K. Radiopacity evaluation of composite restorative resins and bonding agents using digital and film x-ray systems. *Eur. J. Dent.* **2012**, *6*, 115–122. [CrossRef] [PubMed]
4. Keenan, J.R.; Keenan, A.V. Accuracy of dental radiographs for caries detection. *Evid. Based Dent.* **2016**, *17*, 43–49. [CrossRef] [PubMed]
5. Pekkan, G.; Ozcan, M. Radiopacity of different shades of resin-based restorative materials compared to human and bovine teeth. *Gen. Dent.* **2012**, *60*, e237–e243. [PubMed]
6. Raitz, R.; Moruzzi, P.D.; Vieira, G.; Fenyo-Pereira, M. Radiopacity of 28 Composite Resins for Teeth Restorations. *J. Contemp. Dent. Pract.* **2016**, *17*, 136–142. [CrossRef]
7. Brouwer, F.; Askar, H.; Paris, S.; Schwendicke, F. Detecting Secondary Caries Lesions: A Systematic Review and Meta-analysis. *J. Dent. Res.* **2016**, *95*, 143–151. [CrossRef]
8. Aoyagi, Y.; Takahashi, H.; Iwasaki, N.; Honda, E.; Kurabayashi, T. Radiopacity of experimental composite resins containing radiopaque materials. *Dent. Mater. J.* **2005**, *24*, 315–320. [CrossRef]
9. Schwendicke, F.; Tzschoppe, M.; Paris, S. Radiographic caries detection: A systematic review and meta-analysis. *J. Dent.* **2015**, *43*, 924–933. [CrossRef]
10. Melo, M.A.S.; Guedes, S.F.F.; Xu, H.H.K.; Rodrigues, L.K.A. Nanotechnology-based restorative materials for dental caries management. *Trends Biotechnol.* **2013**, *31*, 459–467. [CrossRef]
11. Espelid, I.; Tveit, A.B.; Erickson, R.L.; Keck, S.C.; Glasspoole, E.A. Radiopacity of restorations and detection of secondary caries. *Dent. Mater. Off. Publ. Acad. Dent. Mater.* **1991**, *7*, 114–117. [CrossRef]
12. Melo, M.A.S.; Weir, M.D.; Rodrigues, L.K.A.; Xu, H.H.K. Novel calcium phosphate nanocomposite with caries-inhibition in a human in situ model. *Dent. Mater.* **2013**, *29*, 231–240. [CrossRef]
13. Younis, A.; Chu, D.; Li, S. Cerium Oxide Nanostructures and their Applications. *Funct. Nanomater.* **2016**, *32*, 521–529.
14. Scire, S.; Palmisano, L. Cerium Oxide (CeO_2): Synthesis, Properties and Applications—1st Edition. Available online: https://www.elsevier.com/books/cerium-oxide-ceo2-synthesis-properties-and-applications/scire/978-0-12-815661-2 (accessed on 13 December 2019).
15. Hosseini, A.; Sharifi, A.M.; Abdollahi, M.; Najafi, R.; Baeeri, M.; Rayegan, S.; Cheshmehnour, J.; Hassani, S.; Bayrami, Z.; Safa, M. Cerium and yttrium oxide nanoparticles are neuroprotective. *Biol. Trace Elem. Res.* **2015**, *164*, 80–89. [CrossRef]
16. Rajeshkumar, S.; Naik, P. Synthesis and biomedical applications of Cerium oxide nanoparticles—A Review. *Biotechnol. Rep.* **2017**, *17*, 1–5. [CrossRef]
17. Akça, B.; Erzeneoğlu, S.Z. The Mass Attenuation Coefficients, Electronic, Atomic, and Molecular Cross Sections, Effective Atomic Numbers, and Electron Densities for Compounds of Some Biomedically Important Elements at 59.5 keV. Available online: https://www.hindawi.com/journals/stni/2014/901465/ (accessed on 14 January 2020).
18. Mullan, B.F.; Madsen, M.T.; Messerle, L.; Kolesnichenko, V.; Kruger, J. X-ray attenuation coefficients of high-atomic-number, hexanuclear transition metal cluster compounds: A new paradigm for radiographic contrast agents. *Acad. Radiol.* **2000**, *7*, 254–259. [CrossRef]
19. Leitune, V.C.B.; Collares, F.M.; Takimi, A.; de Lima, G.B.; Petzhold, C.L.; Bergmann, C.P.; Samuel, S.M.W. Niobium pentoxide as a novel filler for dental adhesive resin. *J. Dent.* **2013**, *41*, 106–113. [CrossRef]
20. Garcia, I.M.; Leitune, V.C.B.; Ferreira, C.J.; Collares, F.M. Tantalum oxide as filler for dental adhesive resin. *Dent. Mater. J.* **2018**, *37*, 897–903. [CrossRef]
21. Gu, S.; Rasimick, B.J.; Deutsch, A.S.; Musikant, B.L. Radiopacity of dental materials using a digital X-ray system. *Dent. Mater. Off. Publ. Acad. Dent. Mater.* **2006**, *22*, 765–770. [CrossRef]
22. Demarco, F.F.; Collares, K.; Correa, M.B.; Cenci, M.S.; de Moraes, R.R.; Opdam, N.J. Should my composite restorations last forever? Why are they failing? *Braz. Oral Res.* **2017**, *31*, e56. [CrossRef]
23. Kanzow, P.; Wiegand, A.; Schwendicke, F. Cost-effectiveness of repairing versus replacing composite or amalgam restorations. *J. Dent.* **2016**, *54*, 41–47. [CrossRef]

24. 14:00–17:00 ISO 4049:2009. Available online: http://www.iso.org/cms/render/live/en/sites/isoorg/contents/data/standard/04/28/42898.html (accessed on 16 January 2020).
25. Belli, R.; Kreppel, S.; Petschelt, A.; Hornberger, H.; Boccaccini, A.R.; Lohbauer, U. Strengthening of dental adhesives via particle reinforcement. *J. Mech. Behav. Biomed. Mater.* **2014**, *37*, 100–108. [CrossRef]
26. Abdalla, A.I.; Feilzer, A.J. Four-year water degradation of a total-etch and two self-etching adhesives bonded to dentin. *J. Dent.* **2008**, *36*, 611–617. [CrossRef]
27. Malacarne, J.; Carvalho, R.M.; de Goes, M.F.; Svizero, N.; Pashley, D.H.; Tay, F.R.; Yiu, C.K.; de Oliveira Carrilho, M.R. Water sorption/solubility of dental adhesive resins. *Dent. Mater. Off. Publ. Acad. Dent. Mater.* **2006**, *22*, 973–980. [CrossRef]
28. Amirouche-Korichi, A.; Mouzali, M.; Watts, D.C. Effects of monomer ratios and highly radiopaque fillers on degree of conversion and shrinkage-strain of dental resin composites. *Dent. Mater. Off. Publ. Acad. Dent. Mater.* **2009**, *25*, 1411–1418. [CrossRef]
29. Marins, N.H.; Meereis, C.T.W.; Silva, R.M.; Ruas, C.P.; Takimi, A.S.; Carreño, N.L.V.; Ogliari, F.A. Radiopaque dental adhesive with addition of niobium pentoxide nanoparticles. *Polym. Bull.* **2018**, *75*, 2301–2314. [CrossRef]
30. Debnath, S.; Islam, M.R.; Khan, M.S.R. Optical properties of CeO2 thin films. *Bull. Mater. Sci.* **2007**, *30*, 315–319. [CrossRef]
31. Garoushi, S.; Vallittu, P.K.; Watts, D.C.; Lassila, L.V.J. Effect of nanofiller fractions and temperature on polymerization shrinkage on glass fiber reinforced filling material. *Dent. Mater. Off. Publ. Acad. Dent. Mater.* **2008**, *24*, 606–610. [CrossRef]
32. Ordinola-Zapata, R.; Bramante, C.M.; García-Godoy, F.; Moldauer, B.I.; Gagliardi Minotti, P.; Tercília Grizzo, L.; Duarte, M.A.H. The effect of radiopacifiers agents on pH, calcium release, radiopacity, and antimicrobial properties of different calcium hydroxide dressings. *Microsc. Res. Tech.* **2015**, *78*, 620–625. [CrossRef]
33. Martins, G.C.; Reis, A.; Loguercio, A.D.; Zander-Grande, C.; Meier, M.; Mazur, R.F.; Gomes, O.M.M. Does Making An Adhesive System Radiopaque by Filler Addition Affect Its Bonding Properties? *J. Adhes. Dent.* **2015**, *17*, 513–519.
34. Collares, F.M.; Ogliari, F.A.; Lima, G.S.; Fontanella, V.R.C.; Piva, E.; Samuel, S.M.W. Ytterbium trifluoride as a radiopaque agent for dental cements. *Int. Endod. J.* **2010**, *43*, 792–797. [CrossRef]
35. Farias, I.A.P.; Dos Santos, C.C.L.; Sampaio, F.C. Antimicrobial Activity of Cerium Oxide Nanoparticles on Opportunistic Microorganisms: A Systematic Review. *BioMed Res. Int.* **2018**, *2018*, 1923606. [CrossRef]
36. Varini, E.; Sánchez-Salcedo, S.; Malavasi, G.; Lusvardi, G.; Vallet-Regí, M.; Salinas, A.J. Cerium (III) and (IV) containing mesoporous glasses/alginate beads for bone regeneration: Bioactivity, biocompatibility and reactive oxygen species activity. *Mater. Sci. Eng. C Mater. Biol. Appl.* **2019**, *105*, 109971. [CrossRef]
37. Walkey, C.; Das, S.; Seal, S.; Erlichman, J.; Heckman, K.; Ghibelli, L.; Traversa, E.; McGinnis, J.F.; Self, W.T. Catalytic Properties and Biomedical Applications of Cerium Oxide Nanoparticles. *Environ. Sci. Nano* **2015**, *2*, 33–53. [CrossRef]
38. Gaglianone, L.A.; Lima, A.F.; Gonçalves, L.S.; Cavalcanti, A.N.; Aguiar, F.H.B.; Marchi, G.M. Mechanical properties and degree of conversion of etch-and-rinse and self-etch adhesive systems cured by a quartz tungsten halogen lamp and a light-emitting diode. *J. Mech. Behav. Biomed. Mater.* **2012**, *12*, 139–143. [CrossRef]
39. Maktabi, H.; Ibrahim, M.; Alkhubaizi, Q.; Weir, M.; Xu, H.; Strassler, H.; Fugolin, A.P.P.; Pfeifer, C.S.; Melo, M.A.S. Underperforming light curing procedures trigger detrimental irradiance-dependent biofilm response on incrementally placed dental composites. *J. Dent.* **2019**, *88*, 103110. [CrossRef]

11

Understanding the Role of Shape and Composition of Star-Shaped Polymers and their Ability to Both Bind and Prevent Bacteria Attachment on Oral Relevant Surfaces

Hamid Mortazavian [1], Guillaume A. Picquet [2], Jānis Lejnieks [1], Lynette A. Zaidel [2], Carl P. Myers [2,*] and Kenichi Kuroda [1,*]

1 Department of Biologic and Materials Sciences & Prosthodontics, School of Dentistry, University of Michigan, Ann Arbor, MI 48109, USA; mortazavian.hamid@gmail.com (H.M.); jaanislejnieks@gmail.com (J.L.)

2 Oral Care Early Research, Colgate-Palmolive Company, Piscataway, NJ 08855, USA; guillaume_picquet@colpal.com (G.A.P.); Lynette_Zaidel@colpal.com (L.A.Z.)

* Correspondence: carl_myers@colpal.com (C.P.M.); kkuroda@umich.edu (K.K.)

Abstract: In this study, we have prepared a series of 4- and 6-arm star-shaped polymers with varying molecular weight and hydrophobicity in order to provide insight into the role and relationship that shape and composition have on the binding and protecting of oral relevant surfaces (hydroxyapatite, HAP) from bacteria colonization. Star-shaped acrylic acid polymers were prepared by free-radical polymerization in the presence of chain transfer agents with thiol groups, and their binding to the HAP surfaces and subsequent bacteria repulsion was measured. We observed that binding was dependent on both polymer shape and hydrophobicity (star vs. linear), but their relative efficacy to reduce oral bacteria attachment from surfaces was dependent on their hydrophobicity only. We further measured the macroscopic effects of these materials to modify the mucin-coated HAP surfaces through contact angle experiments; the degree of angle change was dependent on the relative hydrophobicity of the materials suggesting future in vivo efficacy. The results from this study highlight that star-shaped polymers represent a new material platform for the development of dental applications to control bacterial adhesion which can lead to tooth decay, with various compositional and structural aspects of materials being vital to effectively design oral care products.

Keywords: polymer; dental; antibacterial; antifouling; hydroxyapatite; star-shaped; hydrophobicity; acrylic acid; oral; composition

---

1. Introduction

The control and reduction of oral biofilm formation [1], initiated by bacterial species living in polymicrobial, pathogenic colonies at or below the gingival margin [2], are critical steps toward the prevention of dental caries and periodontal diseases [3–5]. While many methods have been proposed to prevent or treat these biofilms [6–10], one promising strategy is the use of synthetic polymer additives that bind to the tooth surface to act as a barrier or deterrent to the deposition of planktonic bacteria through either lethal [11–13] or non-lethal [14,15] mechanisms. Dental materials, especially those delivered from common over the counter products such as toothpaste or mouthwash, must effectively be multifunctional materials in that they must (1) deposit and stick to a tooth surface, (2) act as a barrier against bacteria attachment, (3) be robust against external challenges such as food and drink in order to not require constant reapplication, and (4) perform steps 1–3 in the presence of the salivary pellicle. Conventional polymers used for this strategy include poly (methyl vinyl ether/maleic acid) (Gantrez) and cross-linked micron-sized polyacrylic acid particles (carbopol). Additional polymers such as polyaspartate adhered to hydroxyapatite (HAP) and reduced the attachment of *Streptococcus sanguinis* [16]. While these materials do show the ability to reduce bacterial attachment to the tooth surface, the relationship between a polymer's structure and composition to maximize efficacy, i.e., to bind to an enamel surface and provide anti-attachment properties, remains disconnected.

We have previously shown that star-shaped polymers with pre-assembled poly(hydroxyethyl methacrylate) (HEMA) chains formed stable polymer coatings on polyethylene terephthalate surfaces [17]. Consistent with similar reports [18–32], these star-shaped architectures provided brush-like structures of highly packed polymer chains that could physically repel bacteria to result in a significant reduction of attached bacteria. While this approach using water-insoluble polymers was suitable for hydrophobic resin surfaces, those potentially delivered from common oral care products are required to have significant water solubility. Materials, such as poly(acrylic acid) (PAA) are indeed water soluble, and have been known to bind to the tooth or HAP surfaces through interactions between the anionic carboxylate (COO-) groups in the polymer side chains and cationic calcium ions at the enamel surface [33–35].

As illustrated in Figure 1, we have prepared a small library of linear and star-shaped water-soluble polymers comprising of acrylic acid (AA) and methyl acrylate (MA) in order to draw a relationship between polymer structure (linear vs. 4-arm vs. 6-arm) and polymer composition (variable hydrophobicity) with their ability to bind to oral-relevant surfaces and provide bacterial anti-attachment in model systems. The specific goal of this report is to increase fundamental understanding of polymer-tooth surface interactions toward the development of new polymer platforms and products for anti-bacterial attachment activity.

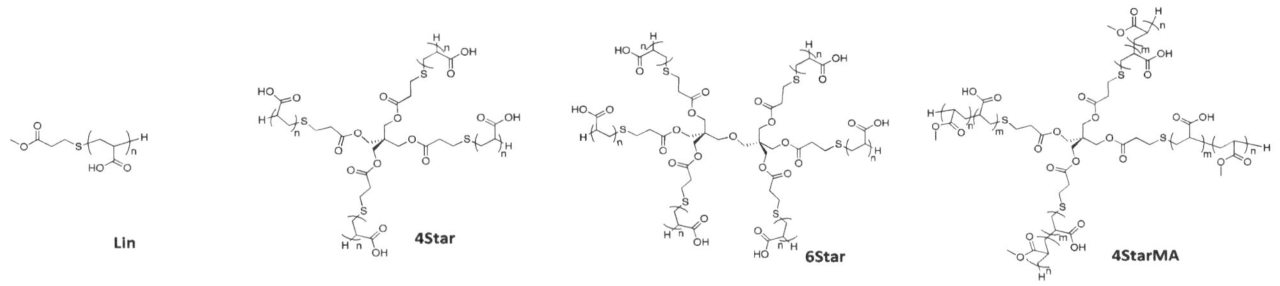

Figure 1. Star-shaped and linear poly(acrylic acid)s used in this study. The chemical structures of linear poly(acrylic acid) polymers (Lin), 4-arm (4Star) and 6-arm (6Star) star-shaped poly(acrylic acid), and 4-arm star-shaped copolymers with methyl acrylate (4StarMA).

2. Results and Discussion

2.1. Synthesis of 4- and 6-Arm Star-Shaped Polymers and Characterization

We wanted to test the free-radical polymerization in the presence of chain transfer agents (CTAs) as a facile synthetic strategy to prepare star-shaped polymers (Figure 2A) (See Tables S1–S6 in Supplementary Materials for polymerization conditions). In this polymerization, the thiol of a CTA reacts (R-SH) with the radical at the polymer chain and terminates the chain propagation by transferring the hydrogen atom (Figure S1). At the same time, the thiyl radical (R-S•) is generated and initiates new polymerization with the remaining monomers. This chain transfer cycle continues to consume all the remaining monomers, and the molecular weight of polymers can be determined by the relative reactivity of the radicals to CTAs compared to the monomers (chain transfer coefficient, C_{tr} in Equation (2)) (See Section 3.5. Analysis of Polymerization Process in Materials and Methods for Equation (2)) and the molar ratio of CTA to monomers ([SH]/[monomer]). We have previously prepared star-shape polymers with 10–12 polymer chain arms by crosslinking the end groups of pre-existing polyHEMA polymer chains [17]. However, this preparation method required multiple synthesis and purification steps. To that end, we synthesized a series of polymers with a range of molecular weights by altering the ratio of CTA to monomers to determine if this synthetic method can provide star-shaped polymers with sufficient size control. In general, star-shaped polymers have been synthesized by living radical polymerization methods, which provided well-defined polymers [36]. However, we chose free-radical polymerization with thiol CTAs because we are interested in a facile approach, potentially capable of large-scale production.

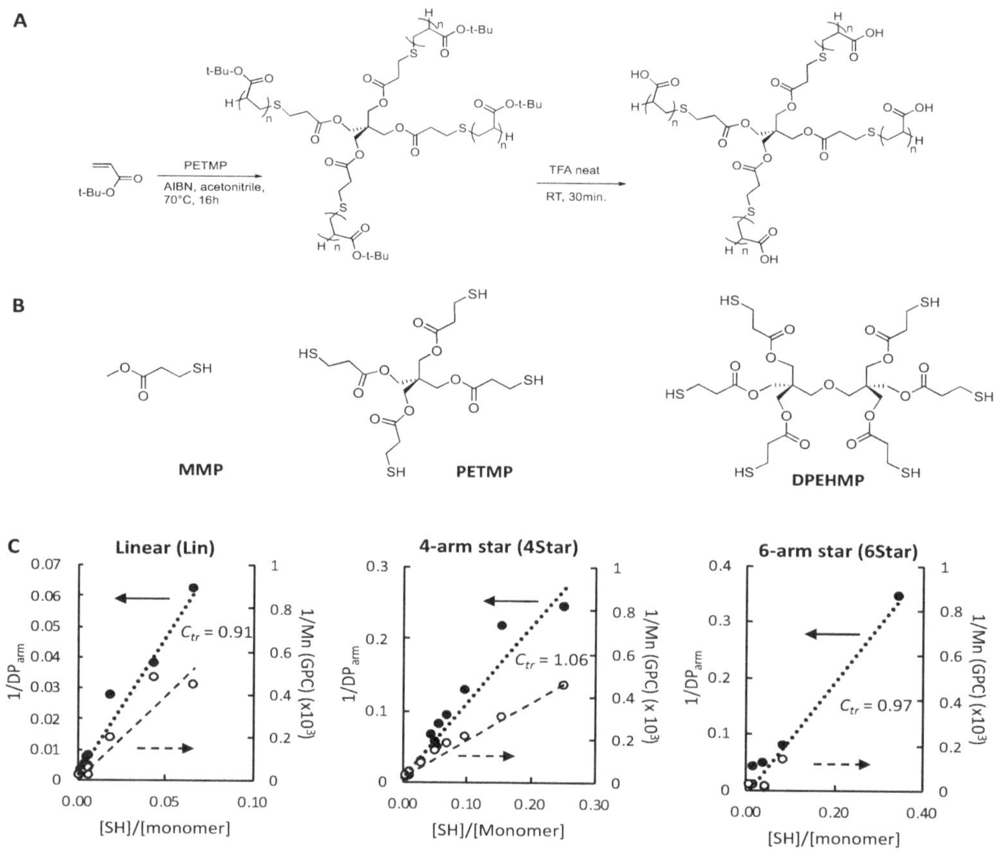

Figure 2. Synthesis of star-shaped polymers. (**A**) Synthesis of 4-arm star-shaped polymers, (**B**) Chemical structures of chain transfer agents. MMP: methyl 3-mercaptopropionate, PETMP: pentaerythritol tetrakis(3-mercaptopropionate), DPEHMP: dipentaerythritol hexakis(3-mercaptopropionate). (**C**) Mayo plots. The broken lines present the results of line fitting. C_{tr} was determined from the slope of the line. [SH]/[monomer] = (The number of thiol groups in a CTA) × [CTA]/[monomer].

The CTAs are small compounds with 4 or 6 thiol groups (PETMP and DPEHMP) (Figure 2B), which serve as core molecules to initiate propagation of polymer chains and yield star-shaped polymer structures. The mono-thiol chain transfer agent MMP provided linear polymers. We used *tert*-butyl acrylate (tBuA) as a protecting group of acrylic acid to facilitate polymer synthesis, and characterization through GPC and NMR spectroscopy. The average degree of polymerization of each arm (DP_{arm}) was determined by comparing the integrated peak area from the polymer backbone to that of CTAs in the ^{1}H NMR spectrum (See Experimental for details). As the ratio of CTA to monomers was increased, the molecular weight of polymers decreased, giving a series of star-shaped and linear polymers with M_n of ~2000 to 200,000 g/mole (See Table S7 for the molecular weight of polymers). It should be noted that the molecular weights of polymers were further measured by size exclusion chromatography (SEC), which separates materials of various masses by the hydrodynamic volume of polymer chains. In general, the hydrodynamic volume of star-shaped polymer is smaller than that of linear polymer with same absolute molecular weight [37]. Therefore, the comparison of molecular weights between the linear and star-shaped polymers by SEC alone would not be sufficient.

To probe the chain transfer polymerization, we examined the relationship between the ratio of the thiol groups to monomers and the polymer chain length. The Mayo plots (1/DP or 1/Mn (GPC) vs. [SH]/[monomer] based on Equation (2) for linear, 4-arm, and 6-arm star-shaped polymers showed linear correlations (Figure 2C), and the C_{tr} value of each CTA was determined as the slope of fitted lines in the Mayo plots (C_{tr} = 0.91 (Lin), 1.06 (4Star), 0.97, (6Star)). In addition, the plots of $1/M_n$ (determined by GPC) against [SH]/[Monomer] also showed linear correlations (Figure 2C). These results suggested that the polymerization was driven by independent chain transfer processes initiated by each thiol group of the CTAs. This further suggested that a polymer chain grew from each CTA arm (formation of star-shaped polymers), and the average polymer chain arm length could be controlled by varying the ratio of CTA to monomers.

The protected t-BuA polymers were treated with TFA to yield acrylic acid polymers (Figures 1 and 2). Because the resultant acrylic acid polymers were no longer soluble in GPC solvent (THF), the molecular weights and distribution of polymers were not determined. The DP of resultant acrylic acid polymers could also not be relatively determined by ^{1}H NMR analysis because the signals from the CTA agents were very small or not detected, which is likely due to low solubility of polymers in solvent. The linear, 4-arm, and 6 arm star-shaped polymers are denoted as Lin-X, 4Star-X, and 6Star-X, respectively, where X indicates the DP of each arm determined for the protected t-BuA polymers.

We also extended the synthetic approach to the preparation of hydrophobic random copolymers. tert-Bu acrylate (tBuA) was co-polymerized with methyl acrylate (MA) to give random copolymers with acidic carboxylic and methyl (ester) groups in the side chains (4StarMA) (Table S8). The mole percentages of MA in the polymers were close to the initial feed ratios, indicating that the MA monomers were quantitatively incorporated to the polymer chains. The copolymers are denoted as 4StarMAY-X, where X and Y indicates the DP of each arm and mole percentage of MA in a polymer, respectively.

2.2. Binding of Star-Shaped Polymers to HAP

We first investigated the binding behaviors of star-shaped polymers onto HAP as a tooth surface model as it has a similar chemical composition to enamel [38,39]. The intrinsic binding properties of polymers can provide useful insights into the relationship between polymer structure and surface activity. Specifically, the binding constant of the polymers and the maximum amount of binding sites on hydroxyapatite surfaces would represent the polymers binding properties. Such information would be helpful to predict polymer activity and design new polymers for subsequent improvements.

We synthesized rhodamine-labeled polymers (Figure 3A and Table S9) for the fluorescence-based binding assay described below. The assay used HAP powder dispersed in an aqueous solution as a model for HAP surfaces for polymer binding [40,41]. This assay provided a facile high-throughput method to determine the amounts of polymers that remained free in supernatant at equilibrium (C_{eq}) and adsorbed onto the HAP surface (q) (Figure 3B). The amount of polymers adsorbed onto the HAP surface was increased as the polymer concentration was increased and appears to level off at high concentrations (Figure 3B). The adsorption isotherms may be represented by the following equation for the Langmuir adoption model:

$$\frac{C_{eq}}{q} = \frac{C_{eq}}{q_{max}} + \frac{K_d}{q_{max}} \quad (1)$$

where q_{max} and K_d are the maximum amount of adsorbed polymers and dissociation constant, respectively [42–44]. The data were well fitted by Equation (1) (Figure 3C). The q_{max} and K_d values were calculated from the slope and intercept of each plot (Table S10). To compare the molecular behaviors of the star-shaped and linear polymers with different molecular sizes, we use the q_{max} and K_d values given in molar concentrations (μmol/g HAP and μM) for discussion, which present the binding behaviors of each polymer molecule. It should be noted that we used the DP of protected tBu polymers to calculate the M_n values of de-protected polymers because of the difficulty to determine the DP of de-protected polymers by ^{1}H NMR as described above. The M_n values were used to convert the q_{max} and K_d values given in weight-based concentrations to molar concentrations.

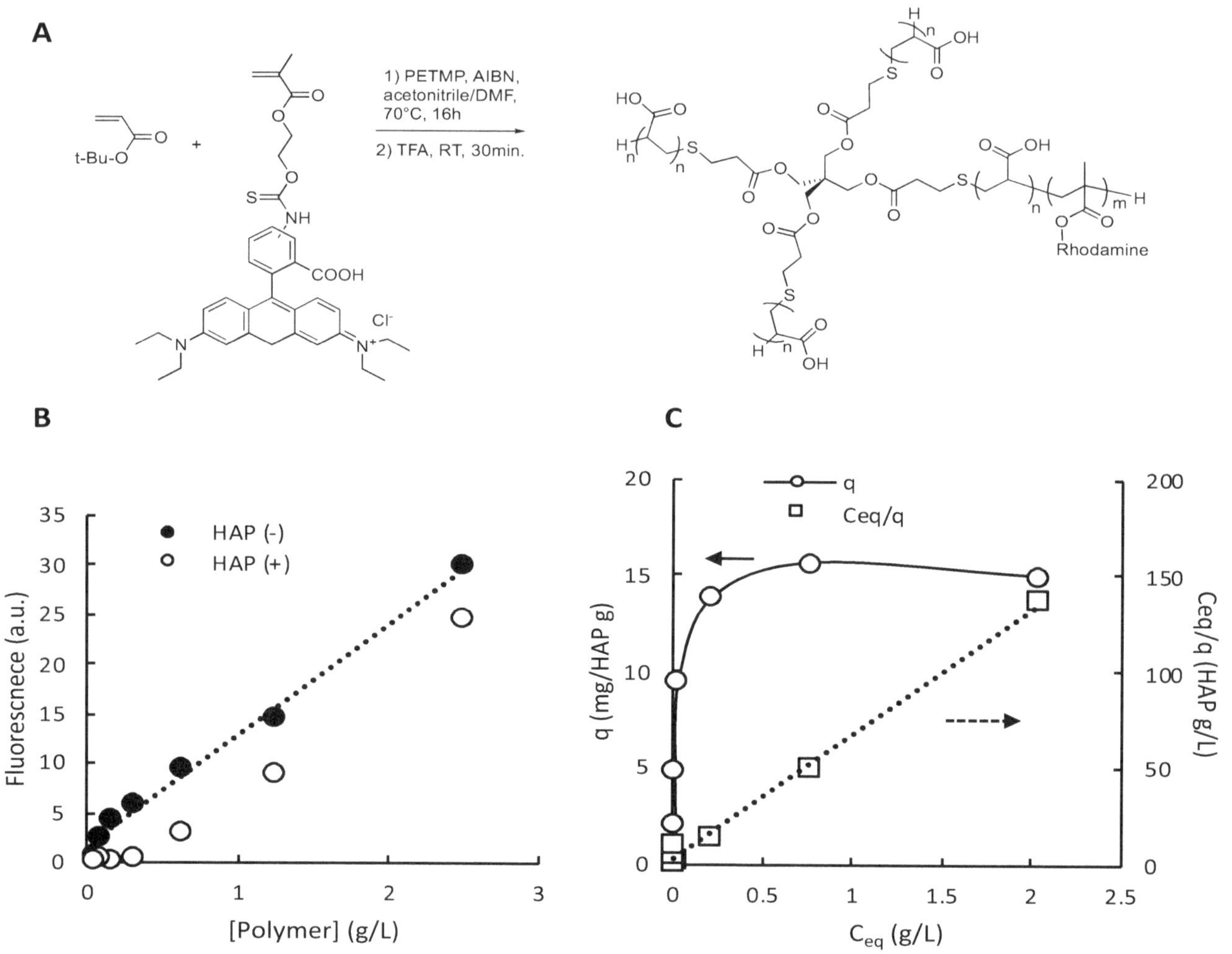

Figure 3. Synthesis of fluorescent dye-labeled polymers and their adsorption on hydroxyapatite powder (HAP). (**A**) Synthesis of rhodamine-labeled 4-arm star-shaped polymers. The rhodamine monomer (0.1 mol.% to the total number of monomers) was polymerized with t-Bu methacrylate. (**B**) Adsorption of 4-arm star-shaped polymer F-4Star-192 on HAP surfaces. Fluorescence intensities from supernatants of polymer assay solutions with and without HAP. (**C**) Adsorption isotherm and linear Langmuir plot. q: the amounts of polymers adsorbed onto the HAP surface. C_{eq}: the polymer concentration of supernatant at equilibrium.

First, we examined the binding properties of star-shaped and linear polymers which have a range of DPs of each polymer arm in order to evaluate the effects of assembly of polymer chains on their HAP binding as well as the effect of polymer arm length (DP) on their binding behavior. In general, the q_{max} values for 4- and 6-arm star-shaped polymers were smaller than that of the linear polymer (Figure 4A). This is likely because of the larger molecular sizes of star-shaped polymers, which occupy larger areas on the hydroxyapatite surface than the linear polymer, such that fewer star-shaped polymers could be bound to the hydroxyapatite surface. On the other hand, the dissociation constant K_d values of star-shaped polymers were smaller than that of the linear polymer (Figure 4B), indicating that the star-shaped polymers adsorbed on the hydroxyapatite surface more strongly than the linear polymer. This can be explained by the large polymer sizes of star-shaped polymers which have more contact points on the hydroxyapatite surface for binding. The 4- and 6-arm star-shaped polymers with DP~120 showed the similar q_{max} and K_d, indicating that these polymers occupy similar areas on the HAP surfaces and have similar binding.

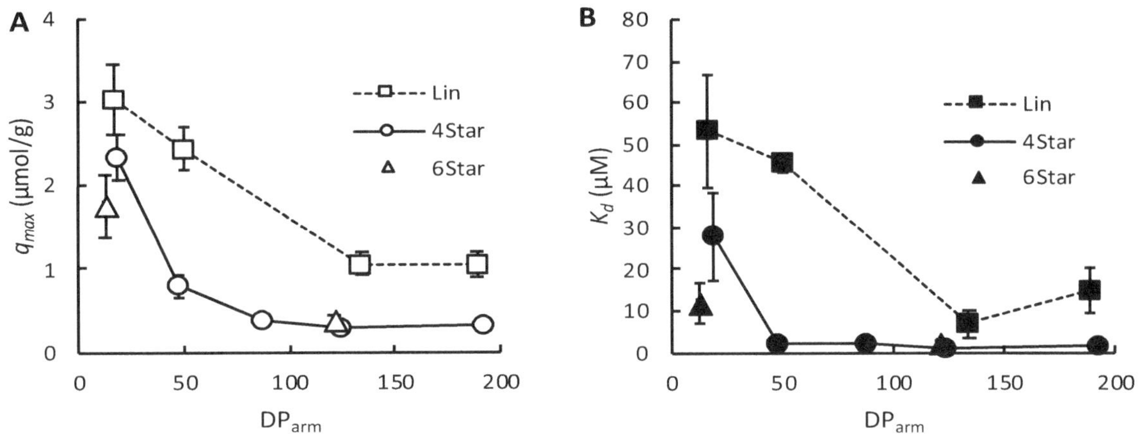

Figure 4. HAP adsorption of linear and 4-ram star-shaped polymers. (**A**) q_{max} and (**B**) K_d were determined by the Langmuir plot.

Regarding the effect of polymer arm length (DP) on their binding behavior, the q_{max} and K_d value of 4-arm star-shaped polymers decreased as the DP of arms increased and leveled off at large DPs (Figure 4A). On the other hand, the K_d value also leveled off for the polymers with large DPs (Figure 4B). The q_{max} and K_d values of linear polymers also decreased and appeared to level off at large DPs. These results suggest that the maximum number of adhered polymers and their binding affinity did not increase once the size of polymers became sufficiently large. This leveling-off of HAP binding behavior of the polymers may be explained by the following model. The anionic carboxylic groups of the polymer side chains are the binding ligand to HAP surfaces through electrostatic interactions. Therefore, as the polymer chains become longer, having more carboxylic side chains, the binding affinity of polymers for HAP would increase. However, the binding of carboxylic side chains to HAP surfaces requires the polymer chains to be flattened and/or stretched on the HAP surface, which is not favorable because of the large entropic penalty. Therefore, the binding of polymers would be determined by the balance between the two driving forces to maximize the number of binding sites by carboxylic groups on the HAP surface (enthalpy gain) and minimize the strain on polymer chains (entropic penalty). As the DP of the polymers increase, the number of carboxylic side chain groups increase, thus increasing their binding. However, once the polymers are long enough, the polymer chains would be difficult to be constrained on the HAP surface because of the entropic penalty, resulting in the leveling of q_{max} and K_d.

The effect of hydrophobic side chains on polymers binding to HAP surfaces was also examined. The random copolymers with hydrophobic monomer MA showed maximum points in the q_{max} and K_d values as the composition of MA was increased (Figure 5). This binding behavior with maximum points may be explained by the interplay between the electrostatic binding of carboxylate groups to HAP and the intramolecular and intermolecular associations of MA groups. Increasing the MA composition reduces the number of carboxylic side chains, which may in turn reduce the binding affinity of polymers (higher K_d). On the other hand, the hydrophobic groups may associate intramolecularly (within the same star-shaped polymer), which may prevent the extension of polymer chains for binding, resulting in low binding affinity (higher K_d). Based on this model, the increase in the K_d values for the low percentage of MA may indicate that the intramolecular association and/or reduced number of acidic groups are dominant, but low K_d value for the polymer with 55% MA indicates the intermolecular hydrophobic association between star-shaped polymers may play an important role to stabilize the polymer layer. On the other hand, the q_{max} also slightly increased, indicating the conformation of bound polymer chains are more compact (smaller occupied surface area). The polymers with 55% MA showed lower q_{max}, indicating the polymer chains are more expanded likely because of increased intermolecular associations of MA groups between the star-shaped polymers, which is in good agreement with the low K_d value. These results suggest that the binding behaviors of polymers to HAP surfaces can be controlled by their hydrophobicity, but is a less contributing factor than the overall shape (linear vs. star) of the polymer.

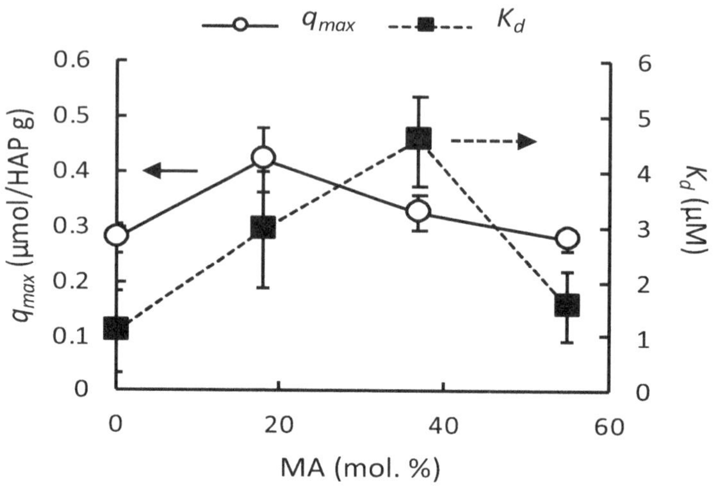

Figure 5. Effect of hydrophobic monomer composition on HAP adsorption of 4-arm star-shaped polymers.

2.3. *Anti-Bacterial Attachment Activity of Linear and Star-Shaped Polymers*

We have shown that shape significantly impacts the binding constant of polymers to HAP surfaces and that higher DPs are required for linear polymers than star-shaped in order to reach minimum K_d values. As such, we selected a subset of linear, star-shaped, and hydrophobic polymers based on their respective DP values that were similar to their tightly-binding fluorescent counterparts (DP = 100–200) in order to choose those materials with the strongest affinity to the HAP surface (Figure 6 and Table 1). In this way, we have effectively normalized to the polymers' K_d such that any differences in anti-attachment or contact angle measurements could be ascribed to the shape and composition of the polymers rather than simply their lack of presence through dissociation from the HAP surface. Table 1 lists the non-fluorescent polymers chosen for further evaluation. Additionally, we have intentionally chosen materials that do not kill bacteria but instead repel. Surface modifications that reduce bacteria deposition and colonization through contact kill or simple cell repulsion will ultimately appear the same, i.e., both surfaces will have a sufficiently reduced amount of living bacteria. We acknowledge that a combination of mechanisms, that is, kill + repel, would likely have the greatest efficacy, however by using materials known to not kill, but rather repel, we can isolate the mechanism to a single mode, subsequently making for more easily understood results. Consumer product constraints surrounding materials that reduce bacteria population through bactericidal mechanisms will inherently certain elicit regulatory restrictions. It is therefore important to have an understanding on materials that act as a non-lethal, almost mechanical, barrier only.

HAP-coated substrates were used as an enamel surface model to test the attachment of a mixture of oral bacteria *Actinomyces viscosus* and *Streptococcus oralis*. These bacteria are known as early colonizers of the oral biofilm formation [45,46], so significant reductions of these species are suggestive of efficacy on full healthy oral biofilms. In general, all of the polymers reduced the attachment of the bacteria onto the HAP surfaces by 17–54% relative to untreated control. However, what is immediately clear is that the six samples separated into two distinct groupings based on their relative hydrophobicity (Figure 6). Among the acrylic acid homopolymers, the linear (Lin-211) and 6-arm (6Star-129) star-shaped polymers showed a 30–32% reduction, while the 4-arm star (4Star-165) had only a 17% reduction. In contrast, all hydrophobic random copolymers gave higher percent reductions regardless of their shape. The linear copolymer (LinMA48-194), and 4-arm star-shaped copolymers (4StarMA56-215 and 4StarMA34-171) showed percent reductions of 43–54%, and were statistically superior to their homopolymer counterparts.

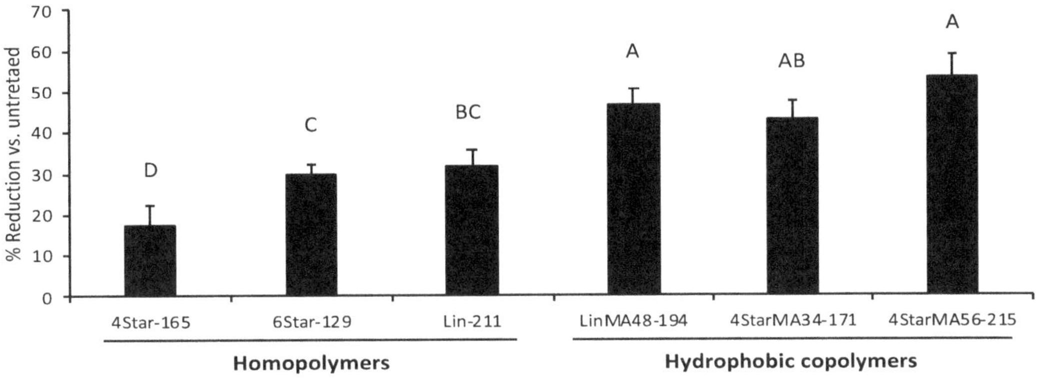

Figure 6. Anti-bacterial attachment activity of linear and star-shaped polymers. The activity of polymers was assessed by the percent reduction in bacterial attachment relative to control (untreated HAP surface). The data and error bars represent the average of 12 replicates with 95% confidence limits. The alphabetical letters on the bars present statistical grouping.

Table 1. Polymers selected for anti-bacterial adhesion assay and contact angle experiments and analogue polymers for HAP-binding assay.

Polymers Selected for Anti-Bacterial Adhesion and Contact Angle Experiments				Polymer Analogues for HAP-Binding Assay				
Polymer	DP_{arm}	M_n [a]	% Reduction	Polymer	DP_{arm}	M_n [a]	q_{max} (μmol/HAP g)	K_d (μM)
Lin-211	211	15,300	31.7 ± 4.2	F-Lin-189	189	13,700	1.05 ± 0.14	14.8 ± 5.5
4Star-165	165	48,000	17.6 ± 5.0	F-4Star-192	192	55,800	0.33 ± 0.06	1.4 ± 0.4
6Star-129	129	56,600	29.9 ± 2.5	F-6Star-121	121	53,100	0.38 ± 0.07	2.1 ± 0.6
LinMA48-194	194 [b]	15,400	46.3 ± 4.3	F-LinMA51-189	189 [b]	15,100	2.83 ± 0.11	14.0 ± 2.0
4StarMA34-171	171	53,000	43.2 ± 4.2	F-4StarMA37-185	185	57,700	0.33 ± 0.03	4.6 ± 0.8
4StarMA56-215	215	69,200	53.5 ± 5.5	F-4StarMA55-149	149	48,000	0.28 ± 0.02	1.6 ± 0.6

[a] The Mn (the number average molecular weight) of the polymers was calculated based on the DP of protected tBu polymers and molecular weights of chain transfer agent and acrylic acrylate; [b] The theoretical DP calculated based on the Mayo equation using the C_{tr} value and [SH]/[monomer].

This data is suggestive of several points in regard to the material characteristics required for anti-attachment properties. First, while there may be small differences between the efficacies of various shapes within the homo vs. copolymer families, their effect is diminished by the presence of hydrophobic monomers within the random polymer chain. This is to say that bacteria are less able to attach themselves to the HAP surface when that surface is coated with a hydrophobic polymer, regardless of whether that polymer is linear or star-shaped. Second, the statistical groupings of the star-shaped hydrophobic polymers were near equivalent, with 34 and 56 mol.% of methyl acrylate providing similar effects. This implies that a "hydrophobic" polymer provides better anti-attachment, but no significant increases in this effect were observed over the ranges evaluated. In the future, we will explore this facet more closely as it may be possible to draw a true correlation here. In addition, the maximum amount of adsorbed polymers q_{max} and dissociation constant K_d of the homopolymer and hydrophobic copolymer with the same shape (linear, 4-, 6-arm star-shape) are very similar (Table 1). This suggests that the enhanced effect of anti-bacterial adhesion by the hydrophobicity of copolymers is not due to the difference in their inherent binding properties (the amount of polymers adhered) to HAP surfaces, but it could be related to the physicochemical properties of polymers or polymer conformations on the surface. It has been previously reported that random, block, cross-linked amphiphilic copolymers effectively prevent protein adhesion and bacterial adhesion [47–54]. The proposed mechanism is that these polymers form phase separated nano-scale domains, which reduce protein adsorption and subsequent bacterial attachment [48]. These domains are smaller than the hydrophobic/hydrophilic domains of proteins so that it is difficult for proteins to adopt their conformations to match with the surface domains. While it is not clear at this point, we speculate that the copolymers in our study may also form such segregated microdomains by association of hydrophobic side chains, which may be a more dominant factor for bacterial attachment than polymer shapes.

The ability for a polymer to provide anti-attachment effects to an oral surface can only happen if the material sufficiently first binds to the surface. The data above has demonstrated that the chemistries needed to bind and repel are not the same. A multi-arm star-shaped polymer had significantly better binding to HAP, but in contrast composition played no such dominant role. Hydrophobicity did not dramatically decrease K_d, however its presence significantly decreased bacteria attachment. Taken together, a hydrophobic star-shaped material would be the ideal polymer system to both bind to enamel and repel bacteria in our model systems.

2.4. Water Contact Angle

The polymer binding isotherms combined with bacteria anti-attachment clearly indicate the tunability and functionality of these polymer systems. However, these materials would need to perform in the presence of the salivary pellicle that coats all oral surfaces in order to provide sufficient effects in-vivo. The pellicle is a complex mixture of proteins, deposited to the surface of enamel by salivary flow [52], and fundamentally examining and predicting the interactions of star-shaped polymers with a pellicle surface is a sufficient and ongoing challenge for our group. Polymers will interact with a pellicle layer in different ways, depending on the dominate chemistry. For example, a recent publication [55] showed that polyanions and polycations interacted differently with the pellicle, which included their penetration depth relative to the HAP-pellicle interface. Another described changes in pellicle thickness as well as antimicrobial functionality as a function of polymer deposition and interaction with pellicle-coated HAP surfaces [12]. This effect can be rationally extended to variations in hydrophobicity and shape. While the presence of a pellicle would add significant complexity, and is outside of the scope of our current study, we did choose to examine how these polymers affected the *macroscopic* properties of HAP through contact angle measurements after pre-treatment with artificial saliva in order to demonstrate a small facet of in-vivo activity. Mucin-based artificial saliva has been a substitute for human saliva in dental research [56], and we found that HAP discs first treated with artificial saliva produced sufficient surfaces allowing for consistent measurements. Significant changes in surface energies, exhibited by major differences in water droplet contact angle, would indicate positive interactions between polymers and mucin-coated surfaces. This experiment represents our first bridging data between fundamental studies and practical applications.

We generally observed that following treatment with polymer solutions, an increase in CA was observed for most samples by >7°, indicating that the polymer-treated surfaces were more hydrophobic than the untreated control (Figure 7). The magnitude of this difference also reflected the compositional changes within the polymers themselves. 4StarMA56-171, for example, had the highest contact angle of 87.6°, an effect attributed to the 56% MA concentration within the star shaped material. Example images of the droplets can be seen in Figure 7, illustrating that these materials are effective at altering the surface characteristics of HAP.

Within this series, however, the linear hydrophobic polymer LinMA48-194, exhibited a lower CA than the untreated control, even though the polymer contains 48% methyl acrylate. The hydrophobic side chains might stabilize the polymer coatings on the HAP surface by the hydrophobic interactions with HAP and/or between the polymer chains. Such polymer network anchored on the HAP surface might retain more water and therefore exhibit higher hydrophilicity, as compared to homopolymer Lin-211 which increased CA. On the other hand, the hydrophobic star-shaped polymers exhibited larger contact angles than LinMA48-194. It may be possible that linear polymer chains can adopt a conformation on the surface such that the hydrophobic side chains face down toward the HAP, and the hydrophilic (carboxylate) face up. The formation of such amphiphilic polymer conformation would be more efficient than the star-shaped polymers which have denser polymer chains, giving more constraints to conformational change. Because of the difference in the HAP pre-treatment (mucin-coated or non-coated), we cannot directly compare these results to those of binding and anti-bacterial attachment. However, the results suggest that the polymers are capable of altering the surface properties of HAP even in the presence of a protein layer.

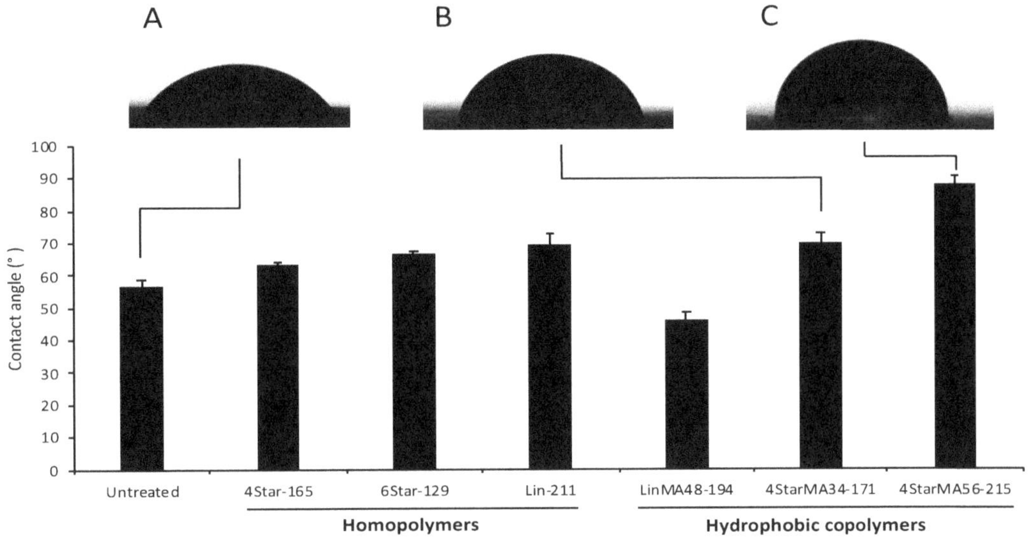

Figure 7. Water contact angle of polymer treated HAP surfaces pre-treated with artificial saliva. Example contact angle images of treated HAP surfaces: (**A**) untreated; (**B**) 4StarMA34-171; (**C**) 4StarMA56-215.

3. Materials and Methods

3.1. Materials

2,2′-azobisisobutyronitrile (AIBN) and pentaerythritol tetrakis(3-mercaptopropionate) (PETMP) was purchased from Sigma-Aldrich Co. LLC. (St. Louis, MO, USA). Dipentaerythritol hexakis(3-mercaptopropionate) (DPEHMP) was purchased from TCI America (Montgomeryville, PA, USA). Methacryloxyethyl thiocarbamoyl rhodamine B was purchased from Polysciences (Warrington, PA, USA). Trifluoroacetic acid (TFA) and solvents were purchased from Thermo Fisher Scientific, Inc. (Waltham, MA, USA). *tert*-Butyl acrylate, methyl acrylate, and methyl mercaptopropionate (MMP) were purchased from Acros Organics (Morris County, NJ, USA). The inhibitors of these monomers were removed by passing through alumina before use. Other chemicals and solvents were used without further purification. 1H NMR was performed using a Varian MR400 (400 MHz, Agilent Scientific Instruments, Santa Clara, CA, USA) and analyzed using VNMRJ 3.2 (Agilent Scientific Instruments, Santa Clara, CA, USA) and MestReNova. Gel permeation chromatography (GPC) analysis was performed using a Waters 1515 HPLC instrument (Milford, MA, USA) using THF as an eluent, equipped with Waters Styragel (7.8 × 300 mm) HR 0.5, HR 1, and HR 4 columns in sequence and detected by a differential refractometer (RI). Sintered HAP discs (0.5 cm in diameter) were purchased from Himed, Inc. (Old Bethpage, NY, USA).

3.2. Synthesis of tBu PAA Homopolymers

tert-Butyl acrylate (t-BuA), AIBN, and chain transfer agent (CTA) (MMP, PETMP, or DPEHMP) in acetonitrile were mixed in a flask (See Table S1 for the polymerization conditions). The oxygen of the reaction mixture was removed by bubbling nitrogen gas for 10 min, and the reaction solution was stirred at 70 °C for 16 h. The reaction was cooled to room temperature. The solvent was removed by evaporation under reduced pressure. The resultant residue was dissolved in diethyl ether, and the polymer was isolated by precipitation in a methanol:water [50:50 (v/v)] mixture. The yield of purification was >90% for most cases. The polymer arm length (DP) was calculated by comparing the integrated peaks of -OCH2- group of chain transfer agent to the -CH- polymer backbone. The number average molecular weight (Mn) was calculated using the DP and molecular weights of monomers and

CTAs. Gel permeation chromatography molecular mass results were determined using a calibration curve based on the standard samples of polystyrene. 1H NMR ($CDCl_3$, 400 MHz) δ: 4.21–4.06 (s, 2H, $-OCH_2-$ of PETMP), 2.85–2.51 (brs, 4H, $-SCH_2CH_2-$), 2.37-2.07 (brs, 1H, –CH–,), 1.97–1.14 (brs, 11H, $-CH_3$ and $-CH_2-$).

The tBu groups of polymers were then removed by the addition of trifluoroacetic acid (TFA) (5 mL to 1 g of polymer). After stirring for 30 min, TFA was removed by blowing with nitrogen gas in a closed container, and the gas was passed through a base (NaOH) aqueous solution to trap TFA. The residue was dissolved in methanol, and deprotected polymers were isolated by precipitating in excess diethyl ether. Subsequently, the precipitate was dissolved in distilled water and lyophilized to yield a powdery product. 1H NMR (DMSO, 400 MHz) 2.4-2.0 (brs, 1H, –CH–,), 1.8-1.2 (brs, 2H, $-CH_2-$).

3.3. Synthesis of Random Copolymers with MA

The PAA random copolymers with methacrylate (MA) were synthesized by the same method with the tBu PAA homopolymers as described above. See Table S2 in Supporting Information for the monomer feed compositions and reaction conditions.

3.4. Synthesis of Rhodamine B-Labeled Polymers

The rhodamine B-labeled copolymers were synthesized using methacryloxyethyl thiocarbamoyl rhodamine B (0.1 mol.% to the total amount of monomers) by the same method as described above with the tBu PAA homopolymers. See Supporting Information for the detailed procedure, polymerization conditions, and monomer feed compositions (Tables S3–S6). The Mayo plots showed linear correlations, and the Ctr values of each thiol group of linear and 4-arm polymers are 0.91 and 0.97 (Figure S2 and Table S11).

3.5. Analysis of Polymerization Process

In general, DP_{arm} of polymer prepared in the presence of thiol groups as a CTA may be presented by the Mayo equation [38]:

$$\frac{1}{DP_{arm}} = \frac{1}{DP_0} + C_{tr}\frac{[SH]}{[Monomer]} \tag{2}$$

where DP_0, C_{tr}, [CTA] and [Monomer] represent the DP of each polymer arm in the absence of CTA, chain transfer coefficient, initial mole concentration of thiol groups, and mole concentration of monomers, respectively. According to the Mayo equation, the plot of 1/DP would be proportional to [SH]/[Monomer], and the slop presents C_{tr}.

3.6. HAP Binding Assay

Fluorescence spectroscopy was used to evaluate the binding capacity of rhodamine-labeled polymers onto HAP powder. The polymer solutions in 10 mM phosphate buffer with 150 mM NaCl with different concentrations (pH = 7, adjusted by NaOH aq., 0.5 mL, 0.04, 0.08, 0.16, 0.31, 0.63, and 1.25 g/L) were mixed with HAP (30 mg/mL) in a 1.5 mL tube. The solution was gently shaken using a mechanical shaker for 2 h at room temperature and then centrifuged at 10,000 rpm for 10 min. The fluorescence emission intensities of the supernatant were measured (excitation wavelength = 553 nm, emission wavelength = 627 nm) and compared with those for samples with same concentration of polymers without HAP.

3.7. Anti-Bacterial Adhesion Assay

HAP coated MBECTM lids were treated by polymer solutions in MilliQ water (1 wt.%, pH 6.5 adjusted with NaOH or HCl) and allowed to shake in the incubator at 37 °C for 1 h. Following treatment, excess polymer solution was removed from the MBECTM lids by submerging in Trypticase soy broth (TSB) for 10–15 s for three cycles, replacing the TSB broth for each new cycle. The MBECTM lids were then incubated with freshly prepared overnight cultures of mixed *Actinomyces viscosus* (ATCC#43146, American Type Culture Collection, Manassas, VA, USA) and *Streptococcus oralis* (ATCC#35037, American Type Culture Collection, Manassas, VA, USA) for 3 h at 37 °C. After incubation the MBECTM lids were submerged in TSB and sonicated two times for 2 min each time in order to detach the HAP-bound bacteria into the TSB. The BacTiter-Glo Microbial Cell Viability Assay was utilized on the re-suspended TSB to determine the percent reduction in the cell viability. The percent reduction was calculated by the following equation based on the luminescent output of bacteria removed from untreated surfaces and polymer-treated surfaces: % reduction = 100 × (bacteria attached on untreated surface—bacteria attached on polymer-treated surface)/bacteria on untreated surface.

Bartlett's test ($p = 0.265$) suggested that any variations are not significant, and the samples have equal variances. Therefore one-way analysis of variance (ANOVA) was used to assess the treatment effect and determine the statistical differences between the various sets. A Tukey multiple comparison test was used to assess pairwise treatment differences. A $p < 0.05$ was used to indicate significant statistical differences.

3.8. Contact Angle Measurements

Contact angle was performed on an Attension Theta instrument from Biolin Scientific (Stockholm, Sweden). Data was analyzed using One Attension software v 2.9. Briefly, 1.0 wt.% polymer solutions in MilliQ water were prepared, and their pH adjusted to 6.5 with concentrated NaOH or HCl. Because of the immediate absorption of solution droplets into hydroxyapatite, surface modification was required prior to treatment with polymer solutions in order to obtain stable droplets for comparison. Sintered HAP was first treated with modified artificial saliva [39] for 1 h (see Supporting Information). After this time, the discs were soaked in 2 mL of polymer solution for three hours on an orbital shaker. The discs were removed and rinsed slightly to remove excess or loosely bound material, and then dried overnight. Contact angle measurements of a 3 μL droplet on four separate HAP discs were collected and averaged to provide statistical significance.

4. Conclusions

In summary of the present study, we synthesized linear, 4- and 6-arm star-shaped polymers based on acrylic acid using chain transfer agents with corresponding thiol groups in order to provide insight into the types of polymers that could both bind to HAP and repel bacteria from the surface. We have found that polymer shape was more important to HAP surface binding than polymer composition (hydrophobicity). However, polymer composition played a larger role than polymer shape (linear vs. star-shape) when providing anti-bacterial protection. This information will be important for targeted properties (binding, anti-bacterial attachment, wettability, etc.,) and further design polymers for dental applications. In this study, our focus was the synthesis of star-shaped polymers and initial evaluation of their physical and biological properties in order to test new polymer platforms for dental applications. The oral environment is quite dynamic and subject to continuously changing environments due to salivary flow, food and drink intake, and the resulting fluctuating pH. Therefore, the efficiency of dental materials to provide benefits, as delivered through common oral care products, must be investigated through delivery, substantivity, and efficacy. While limited to very simple systems here, this approach is critical to build an understanding of dental materials as it can more effectively isolate and identify specific modes of action in addition to chemical or physical barriers to the effectiveness of these materials. Our future research will focus on further developing an understanding of star-shaped polymers in reference to artificial-saliva and human-saliva-coated HAP surfaces, including binding activity and bacterial anti-attachment properties.

S3: Polymerization conditions for rhodamine-labeled tBu linear polymers. Table S4: Polymerization conditions for rhodamine-labeled tBu 4-arm star-shaped polymers. Table S5: Polymerization conditions for rhodamine-labeled tBu 6-arm star-shaped polymers. Table S6: Polymerization conditions of rhodamine-labeled tBu linear and 4-arm PAA/MA random copolymer. Table S7: Polymer characterization of tBu-protected polymers. Table S8: Polymer characterization of tBuA-MA random copolymers. Table S9: Polymer characterization of F-labeled polymers. Table S10: Polymer characterization and Langmuir constants. Table S11: Chain transfer constants for tBu polymers.

Author Contributions: Conceptualization, L.A.Z., C.P.M., and K.K.; investigation, H.M., G.A.P., J.L., and C.P.M.; writing—original draft preparation, C.P.M., and K.K.; writing—review and editing, C.P.M., and K.K.; supervision, C.P.M. and K.K.; project administration, C.P.M. and K.K.; funding acquisition, K.K.

Acknowledgments: We would like to thank Rehana Begum-Gafur and Mark Vandeven for their help with statistical analysis of anti-attachment microbial data, and Donghui Wu for helpful discussions.

References

1. Wu, H.; Moser, C.; Wang, H.-Z.; Høiby, N.; Song, Z.-J. Strategies for combating bacterial biofilm infections. *Int. J. Oral Sci.* **2014**, *7*, 1–7. [CrossRef] [PubMed]
2. Teles, R.; Teles, F.; Frias-Lopez, J.; Paster, B.; Haffajee, A. Lessons learned and unlearned in periodontal microbiology. *Periodontol 2000* **2013**, *62*, 162. [CrossRef]
3. Koo, H.; Falsetta, M.L.; Klein, M.I. The Exopolysaccharide Matrix: A Virulence Determinant of Cariogenic Biofilm. *J. Dental Res.* **2013**, *92*, 1065–1073. [CrossRef] [PubMed]
4. Sanz, M.; Beighton, D.; Curtis, M.A.; Cury, J.A.; Dige, I.; Dommisch, H.; Ellwood, R.; Giacaman, R.A.; Herrera, D.; Herzberg, M.C.; et al. Role of microbial biofilms in the maintenance of oral health and in the development of dental caries and periodontal diseases. Consensus report of group 1 of the Joint EFP/ORCA workshop on the boundaries between caries and periodontal disease. *J. Periodontol.* **2017**, *44*, S5–S11. [CrossRef] [PubMed]
5. Bowen, W.H.; Burne, R.A.; Wu, H.; Koo, H. Oral Biofilms: Pathogens, Matrix, and Polymicrobial Interactions in Microenvironments. *Trends Microbiol.* **2018**, *26*, 229–242. [CrossRef] [PubMed]
6. Chaves, P.; Oliveira, J.; Haas, A.; Beck, R.C.R. Applications of Polymeric Nanoparticles in Oral Diseases: A Review of Recent Findings. *Curr. Pharm. Des.* **2018**, *24*, 1377–1394. [CrossRef]
7. Fernandes, T.; Bhavsar, C.; Sawarkar, S.; D'Souza, A. Current and novel approaches for control of dental biofilm. *Int. J. Pharm.* **2018**, *536*, 199–210. [CrossRef]
8. Hu, X.Q.; Huang, Y.Y.; Wang, Y.G.; Wang, X.Y.; Hamblin, M.R. Antimicrobial Photodynamic Therapy to Control Clinically Relevant Biofilm Infections. *Front. Microbiol.* **2018**, *9*, 1299. [CrossRef]
9. Koo, H.; Allan, R.N.; Howlin, R.P.; Stoodley, P.; Hall-Stoodley, L. Targeting microbial biofilms: Current and prospective therapeutic strategies. *Nat. Rev. Microbiol.* **2017**, *15*, 740. [CrossRef]
10. Pleszczynska, M.; Wiater, A.; Bachanek, T.; Szczodrak, J. Enzymes in therapy of biofilm-related oral diseases. *Biotechnol. Appl. Biochem.* **2017**, *64*, 337–346. [CrossRef]
11. Gaffar, A.; Solis-Gaffar, M.C.; Tavss, E.; Marcussen, H.W.; Rustogi, K.N. Long-term Antiplaque, Anticalculus, and Antigingivitis Effects of Benzethonium/Polymer Complex in Beagle Dogs. *J. Dent. Res.* **1981**, *60*, 1897–1903. [CrossRef] [PubMed]
12. Lee, H.S.; Myers, C.; Zaide, L.; Nalam, P.C.; Caporizzo, M.A.; Daep, C.A.; Eckmann, D.M.; Masters, J.G.; Composto, R.J. Competitive Adsorption of Polyelectrolytes onto and into Pellicle-Coated Hydroxyapatite Investigated by QCM-D and Force Spectroscopy. *Acs Appl. Mater. Interfaces* **2017**, *9*, 13079–13091. [CrossRef] [PubMed]
13. Zhang, Q.M.; Serpe, M.J. Synthesis, Characterization, and Antibacterial Properties of a Hydroxyapatite Adhesive Block Copolymer. *Macromolecules* **2014**, *47*, 8018–8025. [CrossRef]
14. Cui, X.N.; Koujima, Y.; Seto, H.; Murakami, T.; Hoshino, Y.; Miura, Y. Inhibition of Bacterial Adhesion on Hydroxyapatite Model Teeth by Surface Modification with PEGMA-Phosmer Copolymers. *Acs Biomater. Sci. Eng.* **2016**, *2*, 205–212. [CrossRef]

15. Kang, S.; Lee, M.; Kang, M.; Noh, M.; Jeon, J.; Lee, Y.; Seo, J.-H. Development of anti-biofouling interface on hydroxyapatite surface by coating zwitterionic MPC polymer containing calcium-binding moieties to prevent oral bacterial adhesion. *Acta Biomater* **2016**, *40*, 70–77. [CrossRef]
16. Guan, Y.H.; Lath, D.L.; de Graaf, T.; Lilley, T.H.; Brook, A.H. Moderation of oral bacterial adhesion on saliva-coated hydroxyapatite by polyaspartate. *J. Appl. Microbiol.* **2003**, *94*, 456–461. [CrossRef]
17. Totani, M.; Ando, T.; Terada, K.; Terashima, T.; Kim, I.Y.; Ohtsuki, C.; Xi, C.; Kuroda, K.; Tanihara, M. Utilization of star-shaped polymer architecture in the creation of high-density polymer brush coatings for the prevention of platelet and bacteria adhesion. *Biomater. Sci.* **2014**, *2*, 1172–1185. [CrossRef]
18. Muszanska, A.K.; Rochford, E.T.J.; Gruszka, A.; Bastian, A.A.; Busscher, H.J.; Norde, W.; van der Mei, H.C.; Herrmann, A. Antiadhesive Polymer Brush Coating Functionalized with Antimicrobial and RGD Peptides to Reduce Biofilm Formation and Enhance Tissue Integration. *Biomacromolecules* **2014**, *15*, 2019–2026. [CrossRef]
19. Nejadnik, M.R.; van der Mei, H.C.; Norde, W.; Busscher, H.J. Bacterial adhesion and growth on a polymer brush-coating. *Biomaterials* **2008**, *29*, 4117–4121. [CrossRef]
20. Roest, S.; van der Mei, H.C.; Loontjens, T.J.A.; Busscher, H.J. Charge properties and bacterial contact-killing of hyperbranched polyurea-polyethyleneimine coatings with various degrees of alkylation. *Appl. Surf. Sci.* **2015**, *356*, 325–332. [CrossRef]
21. Swartjes, J.; Veeregowda, D.H.; van der Mei, H.C.; Busscher, H.J.; Sharma, P.K. Normally Oriented Adhesion versus Friction Forces in Bacterial Adhesion to Polymer-Brush Functionalized Surfaces Under Fluid Flow. *Adv. Funct. Mater.* **2014**, *24*, 4435–4441. [CrossRef]
22. Mi, L.; Jiang, S.Y. Integrated Antimicrobial and Nonfouling Zwitterionic Polymers. *Angew. Chem. -Int. Ed.* **2014**, *53*, 1746–1754. [CrossRef] [PubMed]
23. Shao, Q.; Jiang, S.Y. Molecular Understanding and Design of Zwitterionic Materials. *Adv. Mater.* **2015**, *27*, 15–26. [CrossRef] [PubMed]
24. Ibanescu, S.A.; Nowakowska, J.; Khanna, N.; Landmann, R.; Klok, H.A. Effects of Grafting Density and Film Thickness on the Adhesion of Staphylococcus epidermidis to Poly(2-hydroxy ethyl methacrylate) and Poly(poly(ethylene glycol)methacrylate) Brushes. *Macromol. Biosci.* **2016**, *16*, 676–685. [CrossRef]
25. Klok, H.A.; Genzer, J. Expanding the Polymer Mechanochemistry Toolbox through Surface-Initiated Polymerization. *Acs Macro Letters* **2015**, *4*, 636–639. [CrossRef]
26. Zoppe, J.O.; Ataman, N.C.; Mocny, P.; Wang, J.; Moraes, J.; Klok, H.A. Surface-Initiated Controlled Radical Polymerization: State-of-the-Art, Opportunities, and Challenges in Surface and Interface Engineering with Polymer Brushes. *Chem. Rev.* **2017**, *117*, 1105–1318. [CrossRef]
27. Gasteier, P.; Reska, A.; Schulte, P.; Salber, J.; Offenhausser, A.; Moeller, M.; Groll, J. Surface grafting of PEO-Based star-shaped molecules for bioanalytical and biomedical applications. *Macromol. Biosci.* **2007**, *7*, 1010–1023. [CrossRef]
28. Heyes, C.D.; Groll, J.; Moller, M.; Nienhaus, G.U. Synthesis, patterning and applications of star-shaped poly(ethylene glycol) biofunctionalized surfaces. *Mol. Biosyst.* **2007**, *3*, 419–430. [CrossRef]
29. Morgese, G.; Trachsel, L.; Romio, M.; Divandari, M.; Ramakrishna, S.N.; Benetti, E.M. Topological Polymer Chemistry Enters Surface Science: Linear versus Cyclic Polymer Brushes. *Angew. Chem. -Int. Ed.* **2016**, *55*, 15583–15588. [CrossRef]
30. Kim, D.-G.; Kang, H.; Choi, Y.-S.; Han, S.; Lee, J.-C. Photo-cross-linkable star-shaped polymers with poly(ethylene glycol) and renewable cardanol side groups: Synthesis, characterization, and application to antifouling coatings for filtration membranes. *Polym. Chem.* **2013**, *4*, 5065–5073. [CrossRef]
31. Kim, D.-G.; Kang, H.; Han, S.; Lee, J.-C. The increase of antifouling properties of ultrafiltration membrane coated by star-shaped polymers. *J. Mater. Chem.* **2012**, *22*, 8654–8661. [CrossRef]
32. Kim, D.G.; Kang, H.; Han, S.; Kim, H.J.; Lee, J.C. Bio- and oil-fouling resistance of ultrafiltration membranes controlled by star-shaped block and random copolymer coatings. *Rsc Advances* **2013**, *3*, 18071–18081. [CrossRef]
33. Fukuda, R.; Yoshida, Y.; Nakayama, Y.; Okazaki, M.; Inoue, S.; Sano, H.; Suzuki, K.; Shintani, H.; Meerbeek, B.V. Bonding efficacy of polyalkenoic acids to hydroxyapatite, enamel and dentin. *Biomaterials* **2003**, *24*, 1867. [CrossRef]
34. Yoshida, Y.; Van Meerbeek, B.; Nakayama, Y.; Snauwaert, J.; Hellemans, L.; Lambrechts, P.; Vanherle, G.; Wakasa, K. Evidence of Chemical Bonding at Biomaterial-Hard Tissue Interfaces. *J. Dental Res.* **2000**, *79*, 714. [CrossRef]

35. McConnell, M.D.; Liu, Y.; Nowak, A.P.; Pilch, S.; Masters, J.G.; Composto, R.J. Bacterial plaque retention on oral hard materials: Effect of surface roughness, surface composition, and physisorbed polycarboxylate. *J. Biomed. Mater. Res. Part A* **2010**, *92*, 1518–1527. [CrossRef]
36. Ren, J.M.; McKenzie, T.G.; Fu, Q.; Wong, E.H.H.; Xu, J.; An, Z.; Shanmugam, S.; Davis, T.P.; Boyer, C.; Qiao, G.G. Star Polymers. *Chem. Rev.* **2016**, *116*, 6836. [CrossRef]
37. Voit, B.I.; Lederer, A. Hyperbranched and Highly Branched Polymer Architectures—Synthetic Strategies and Major Characterization Aspects. *Chem. Rev.* **2009**, *109*, 5924–5973. [CrossRef]
38. Clark, W.B.; Bammann, L.L.; Gibbons, R.J. comparative estimates of bacterial affinities and adsorption sites on hydroxyapatite surfaces. *Infect. Immun.* **1978**, *19*, 846–853.
39. Hillman, J.D.; Vanhoute, J.; Gibbons, R.J. sorption of bacteria to human enamel powder. *Arch. Oral Biol.* **1970**, *15*, 899–903. [CrossRef]
40. Lei, Y.; Wang, T.; Mitchell, J.W.; Qiu, J.; Kilpatrick-Liverman, L. Synthesis of Carboxylic Block Copolymers via Reversible Addition Fragmentation Transfer Polymerization for Tooth Erosion Prevention. *J. Dental Res.* **2014**, *93*, 1264–1269. [CrossRef]
41. Lei, Y.D.; Wang, T.X.; Mitchell, J.W.; Zaidel, L.; Qiu, J.H.; Kilpatrick-Liverman, L. Bioinspired amphiphilic phosphate block copolymers as non-fluoride materials to prevent dental erosion. *Rsc Adv.* **2014**, *4*, 49053–49060. [CrossRef] [PubMed]
42. Misra, D.N. adsorption of LOW-molecular-weight poly(acrylic acid) on hydroxyapatite-role of molecular association and apatite dissolution. *Langmuir* **1991**, *7*, 2422–2424. [CrossRef]
43. Misra, D.N. Adsorption OF low-molecular-weight sodium polyacrylate on hydroxyapatite. *J. Dent. Res.* **1993**, *72*, 1418–1422. [CrossRef] [PubMed]
44. Misra, D.N. Adsorption of polyacrylic acids and their sodium salts on hydroxyapatite: Effect of relative molar mass. *J. Colloid Interface Sci.* **1996**, *181*, 289–296. [CrossRef]
45. Huang, R.; Li, M.; Gregory, R.L. Bacterial interactions in dental biofilm. *Virulence* **2011**, *2*, 444. [CrossRef] [PubMed]
46. Kolenbrander, P.E.; Andersen, R.N.; Blehert, D.S.; Egland, P.G.; Foster, J.S.; Palmer, R.J. Communication among Oral Bacteria. *Microbiol. Mol. Biol. Rev.* **2002**, *66*, 486–505. [CrossRef]
47. Gudipati Chakravarthy, S.; Greenlief, C.M.; Johnson Jeremiah, A.; Prayongpan, P.; Wooley Karen, L. Hyperbranched fluoropolymer and linear poly(ethylene glycol) based amphiphilic crosslinked networks as efficient antifouling coatings: An insight into the surface compositions, topographies, and morphologies. *J. Polym. Sci. Part A Polym. Chem.* **2004**, *42*, 6193–6208. [CrossRef]
48. Kerstetter, J.L.; Gramlich, W.M. Nanometer-scale self-assembly of amphiphilic copolymers to control and prevent biofouling. *J. Mater. Chem. B* **2014**, *2*, 8043–8052. [CrossRef]
49. Krishnan, S.; Ayothi, R.; Hexemer, A.; Finlay, J.A.; Sohn, K.E.; Perry, R.; Ober, C.K.; Kramer, E.J.; Callow, M.E.; Callow, J.A.; et al. Anti-Biofouling Properties of Comblike Block Copolymers with Amphiphilic Side Chains. *Langmuir* **2006**, *22*, 5075–5086. [CrossRef]
50. Martinelli, E.; Agostini, S.; Galli, G.; Chiellini, E.; Glisenti, A.; Pettitt, M.E.; Callow, M.E.; Callow, J.A.; Graf, K.; Bartels, F.W. Nanostructured Films of Amphiphilic Fluorinated Block Copolymers for Fouling Release Application. *Langmuir* **2008**, *24*, 13138–13147. [CrossRef]
51. Weinman, C.J.; Gunari, N.; Krishnan, S.; Dong, R.; Paik, M.Y.; Sohn, K.E.; Walker, G.C.; Kramer, E.J.; Fischer, D.A.; Ober, C.K. Protein adsorption resistance of anti-biofouling block copolymers containing amphiphilic side chains. *Soft Matter* **2010**, *6*, 3237–3243. [CrossRef]
52. Zhao, Z.; Ni, H.; Han, Z.; Jiang, T.; Xu, Y.; Lu, X.; Ye, P. Effect of Surface Compositional Heterogeneities and Microphase Segregation of Fluorinated Amphiphilic Copolymers on Antifouling Performance. *ACS Appl. Mater. Interfaces* **2013**, *5*, 7808–7818. [CrossRef] [PubMed]
53. Gudipati, C.S.; Finlay, J.A.; Callow, J.A.; Callow, M.E.; Wooley, K.L. The Antifouling and Fouling-Release Perfomance of Hyperbranched Fluoropolymer (HBFP)−Poly(ethylene glycol) (PEG) Composite Coatings Evaluated by Adsorption of Biomacromolecules and the Green Fouling Alga Ulva. *Langmuir* **2005**, *21*, 3044–3053. [CrossRef] [PubMed]
54. Imbesi, P.M.; Gohad, N.V.; Eller, M.J.; Orihuela, B.; Rittschof, D.; Schweikert, E.A.; Mount, A.S.; Wooley, K.L. Noradrenaline-Functionalized Hyperbranched Fluoropolymer–Poly(ethylene glycol) Cross-Linked Networks As Dual-Mode, Anti-Biofouling Coatings. *ACS Nano* **2012**, *6*, 1503–1512. [CrossRef]

55. Delvar, A.; Lindh, L.; Arnebrant, T.; Sotres, J. Interaction of Polyelectrolytes with Salivary Pellicles on Hydroxyapatite Surfaces under Erosive Acidic Conditions. *ACS Appl. Mater. Interfaces* **2015**, *7*, 21610–21618. [CrossRef]
56. Ionta, F.Q.; Mendonça, F.L.; de Oliveira, G.C.; de Alencar, C.R.B.; Honório, H.M.; Magalhães, A.C.; Rios, D. In vitro assessment of artificial saliva formulations on initial enamel erosion remineralization. *J. Dent.* **2014**, *42*, 175–179. [CrossRef]

12

Physicochemical, Mechanical and Antimicrobial Properties of Novel Dental Polymers Containing Quaternary Ammonium and Trimethoxysilyl Functionalities

Diane R. Bienek [1,*], Anthony A. Giuseppetti [1], Stanislav A. Frukhtbeyn [1], Rochelle D. Hiers [2], Fernando L. Esteban Florez [2], Sharukh S. Khajotia [2] and Drago Skrtic [1]

1 ADA Foundation, Research Division, Frederick, MD 21704, USA; giuseppettia@ada.org (A.A.G.); frukhtbeyns@ada.org (S.A.F.); dskrtic@verizon.net (D.S.)

2 College of Dentistry, University of Oklahoma Health Sciences Center, Oklahoma City, OK 73117, USA; Shelley-Hiers@ouhsc.edu (R.D.H.); fernando-esteban-florez@ouhsc.edu (F.L.E.F.); Sharukh-Khajotia@ouhsc.edu (S.S.K.)

* Correspondence: bienekd@ada.org

Abstract: The aims of this study were to evaluate the physicochemical and mechanical properties, antimicrobial (AM) functionality, and cytotoxic potential of novel dental polymers containing quaternary ammonium and trimethoxysilyl functionalities (e.g., N-(2-(methacryloyloxy)ethyl)-*N*,*N*-dimethyl-3-(trimethoxysilyl)propan-1-aminium iodide (AM_{sil1}) and N-(2-(methacryloyloxy)ethyl)-*N*,*N*-dimethyl-11-(trimethoxysilyl)undecan-1-aminium bromide (AM_{sil2})). AM_{sil1} or AM_{sil2} were incorporated into light-cured (camphorquinone + ethyl-4-*N*,*N*-dimethylamino benzoate) urethane dimethacrylate (UDMA)/polyethylene glycol-extended UDMA/ethyl 2-(hydroxymethyl)acrylate (EHMA) resins (hereafter, UPE resin) at 10 or 20 mass %. Cytotoxic potential was assessed by measuring viability and metabolic activity of immortalized mouse connective tissue and human gingival fibroblasts in direct contact with monomers. AM_{sil}–UPE resins were evaluated for wettability by contact angle measurements and degree of vinyl conversion (DVC) by near infra-red spectroscopy analyses. Mechanical property evaluations entailed flexural strength (FS) and elastic modulus (E) testing of copolymer specimens. The AM properties were assessed using *Streptococcus mutans* (planktonic and biofilm forms) and *Porphyromonas gingivalis* biofilm. Neither AM_{sil} exhibited significant toxicity in direct contact with cells at biologically relevant concentrations. Addition of AM_{sil}s made the UPE resin more hydrophilic. DVC values for the AM_{sil}–UPE copolymers were 2–31% lower than that attained in the UPE resin control. The mechanical properties (FS and E) of AM_{sil}–UPE specimens were reduced (11–57%) compared to the control. Compared to UPE resin, AM_{sil1}–UPE and AM_{sil2}–UPE (10% mass) copolymers reduced *S. mutans* biofilm 4.7- and 1.7-fold, respectively ($p \leq 0.005$). Although not statistically different, *P. gingivalis* biofilm biomass on AM_{sil1}–UPE and AM AM_{sil2}–UPE copolymer disks were lower (71% and 85%, respectively) than that observed with a commercial AM dental material. In conclusion, the AM function of new monomers is not inundated by their toxicity towards cells. Despite the reduction in mechanical properties of the AM_{sil}–UPE copolymers, AM_{sil2} is a good candidate for incorporation into multifunctional composites due to the favorable overall hydrophilicity of the resins and the satisfactory DVC values attained upon light polymerization of AM_{sil}-containing UDMA/PEG-U/EHMA copolymers.

Keywords: antimicrobial effect; biofilms; cytotoxicity; dental resins; physicochemical properties; mechanical properties; quaternary ammonium methacrylates

1. Introduction

As people live longer and retain more of their own teeth, the incidence of dental caries, especially root caries, increases. Currently, the prevalence of root caries in older adults ranges from 29% to 89% [1]. The expected aging of the population will further increase root caries occurrences. Therefore, implementing more effective prevention strategies and/or developing new treatments for root caries is prudent. Often, compromised integrity of the conventional restorative/tooth interface [2,3] ultimately results in bacterial microleakage and secondary caries. Class V restoratives may release fluoride ions which, at adequate concentrations, protect teeth from demineralization and possibly contribute to regeneration of mineral lost to caries. Fluoride release, however, does not provide an effective antimicrobial (AM) protection, although fluoride can have some AM properties [4,5]. The majority of the contemporary dental restoratives do not possess substantial AM properties [6] verifiable in clinical trials [7]. To improve the longevity of repair, the restorative material should be AM. Adding AM function to dental materials typically focuses on release/slow release of various low molecular weight AM agents [5,8–15]. However, mechanism(s) of their actions are elusive, and there are concerns about their toxicity to human cells, the development of tolerances (in the case of antibiotics), and long-term efficacies. Moreover, the release of these agents can compromise mechanical performance of the restoratives and, if the dose or release kinetics are not properly controlled, can induce toxicity to the surrounding tissues [16].

Antimicrobial polymeric materials with quaternary ammonium (QA) salts have been widely applied to a variety of antimicrobial-relevant areas (reviewed by [17,18]). QA methacrylates are known for their AM action against both Gram-positive and Gram-negative bacteria. Studies have indicated that QA compounds destroy bacterial cell membrane integrity and eventually lead to cell death [19–21]. The proposed mechanism of action is the electrostatic interaction between positively charged molecules and negatively charged microbial cell membranes. So far, QA methacrylates have not been successfully incorporated into dental restorative(s) to yield a sustained AM function [22]. Historically, the most attention has been given to methacryloyloxydodecyl pyrimidinium bromide (MDPB) and its acrylamide copolymer [6,23]. MDBP has been commercialized and suggested to be potentially applicable to various restoratives. However, due to their poor color stability, MDBP-based materials can only be used for aesthetically inferior restorations. To widen the utility of QAs in restorative dentistry, various QAs have been formulated into bonding agents and dental resin composites [20,24–26]. Successful incorporation of these new AM QAs into polymeric phases of composite materials would be a major step in creating new Class V restoratives that are clinically effective against secondary caries. We are advancing the development of Class V restorative materials by introducing bioactive amorphous calcium phosphate (ACP) filler into polymer-based restorative in parallel to the AM monomer, thus creating a multifunctional AM and remineralizing materials (hereafter AMRE). ACP has been indicated as a precursor to hydroxyapatite formation both in vitro and in vivo [27–33]. ACP also exhibited favorable in vivo osteoconductivity compared to hydroxyapatite [34]. Based on our group's knowledge of ACP chemistry and our understanding of structure/composition/property relationships existing in ACP polymeric systems [35–39], we have undertaken a task to formulate AMRE polymeric composites that maintain a desired state of supersaturation with respect to hydroxyapatite and efficiently restore mineral-depleted tooth structures while providing sustained AM protection. Prior to formulating AMRE composites, it is essential to evaluate the AM-containing resins (no ACP filler) to establish the effect of AM monomers on basic biological, physicochemical, and mechanical properties of copolymers.

AM_{sil} syntheses and subsequent validation protocols of novel dental monomers containing QA and trimethoxysilyl functionalities are described in detail by Okeke et al. (2019) [40]. The motivation for synthesizing AM_{sil1} and AM_{sil2} was to develop coupling agents capable of conferring the AM properties and coupling with both ACP phase and polymer phase of Class V resin-based composites. This study reports on the incorporation of these two polymerizable QA monomers with different alkyl chain lengths (e.g., N-(2-(methacryloyloxy)ethyl)-*N*,*N*-dimethyl-3-(trimethoxysilyl)propan-1-aminium iodide (AM_{sil1}) and N-(2-(methacryloyloxy)ethyl)-*N*,*N*-dimethyl-11-(trimethoxysilyl)undecan-1-aminium bromide (AM_{sil2})) (Figure 1) into UDMA/poly(ethylene glycol)-extended UDMA (PEG-U)/ethyl 2-(hydroxymethyl) acrylate (EHMA) resins (hereafter UPE resin) and the biological, physicochemical, and mechanical screening of AM–UPE copolymers. Working hypotheses were that AM_{sil} monomers will show minimal or no toxicity towards immortalized mouse subcutaneous connective tissue fibroblasts (CCL1) or human gingival fibroblasts (HGF) and that AM_{sil}–UPE copolymers will have similar physicochemical and mechanical properties compared to the parent UPE copolymers. AM_{sil1}– and AM_{sil2}–UPE copolymers were assessed for their AM activity against *Streptococcus mutans* and *Porphyromonas gingivalis,* which are model microorganisms for dental caries [41,42] and periodontal disease [43,44], respectively.

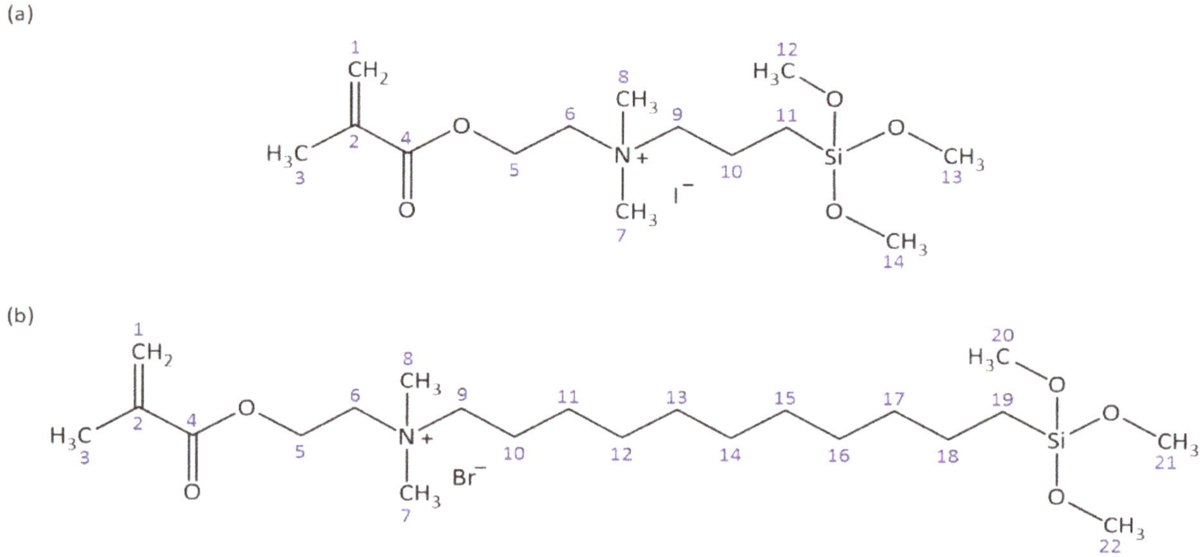

Figure 1. Skeletal structural formulas of AM_{sil1} (**a**) and AM_{sil2} (**b**) monomers.

2. Results

2.1. Structural Verification of AM_{sil}s

The AM_{sil} structures were verified by ^{1}H and ^{13}C NMR (Tables 1 and 2). In brief, both ^{1}H and ^{13}C NMR spectra of AM_{sil}s confirmed the successful quaternization of 2-(dimethylamino)ethyl methacrylate (DMAEMA) precursor. By performing the syntheses in chloroform, methoxy groups of (3-iodopropyl)trimethoxy silane (IPTMS) and (11-bromoundecyl)trimethoxy silane (BrUDTMS) were protected from hydrolysis to which they are prone in aqueous environment.

Table 1. Assignments of ^{13}C and ^{1}H NMR chemical shifts of AM_{sil1}.

Atom #	^{13}C Chemical Shift, ppm	^{1}H Chemical Shift, ppm	# of H's	Signal Splitting
1	126.6 (CH_2)	5.77, 6.09	1, 1	singlets
2	135.3 (C)		0	
3	17.8 (CH_3)	1.92	3	singlet
4	165.8 (C)		0	
5	58.0 (CH_2)	4.52	2	multiplet
6	61.7 (CH_2)	3.70	2	multiplet
7, 8	50.6 (CH_3)	3.09	6	singlet
9	65.9 (CH_2)	3.34	2	multiplet
10	15.6 (CH_2)	1.72	2	multiplet
11	5.2 (CH_2)	0.54	2	multiplet
12, 13, 14	50.1 (CH_3)	3.51	9	singlet

Atom numbering is illustrated in Figure 1.

Table 2. Assignments of ^{13}C and ^{1}H NMR chemical shifts of AM_{sil2}.

Atom #	^{13}C Chemical Shift, ppm	^{1}H Chemical Shift, ppm	# of H's	Signal Splitting
1	126.5 (CH_2)	5.76, 6.08	1, 1	singlets
2	135.3 (C)		0	
3	17.8 (CH_3)	1.91	3	singlet
4	165.8 (C)		0	
5	58.1 (CH_2)	4.52	2	multiplet
6	61.6 (CH_2)	3.70	2	multiplet
7, 8	50.4 (CH_3)	3.09	6	singlet
9	63.8 (CH_2)	3.36	2	multiplet
10	21.7 (CH_2)	1.67	2	multiplet
11–18	22.1, 25.7, 28.4, 28.6, 28.7, 28.8, 28.9, 32.3 (CH_2)	1.25	16	multiplet
19	8.6 (CH_2)	0.57	2	multiplet
20, 21, 22	49.9 (CH_3)	3.46	9	singlet

Atom numbering is illustrated in Figure 1.

2.2. *Biocompatibility Testing*

2.2.1. AM_{sil1}

AM_{sil1} concentration did not exert a statistically significant effect on the viability of CCL1 cells (Figure 2). However, the exposure time reduced the number (1.2-fold difference of mean, $p \leq 0.002$) of live cells. Similarly, AM_{sil1} concentration did not affect the metabolic activity of CCL1 cells. Time of exposure had a modest effect ($p \leq 0.02$) on CCL1 metabolic activity, although no significant paired comparisons (within each concentration) were observed.

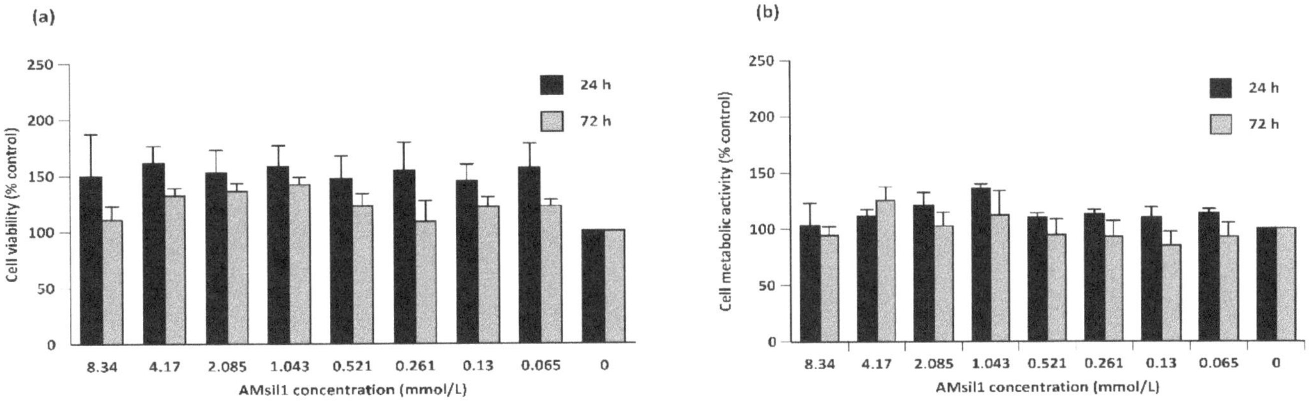

Figure 2. Percent control value of viability (**a**) and metabolic activity (**b**) of CCL1 cells exposed to 2-fold serial dilutions of AM_{sil1} ($\leq$8.34 mmol/L) for 24 or 72 h. Data represent mean ± standard error for five independent replicates tested in triplicate.

Independent of time, AM_{sil1} concentration exerted a main effect ($p \leq 0.001$) on the number of viable HGFs (Figure 3). Paired comparisons indicated that at lower AM_{sil1} concentrations ($\leq$0.13 mmol/L), the number of live HGFs decreased. Independent of AM_{sil1} concentration, exposure time reduced (19.73 difference of means, $p \leq 0.001$) HGF viability. Monomer concentration or time of exposure did not statistically affect the metabolic activity of HGF cells (data not shown).

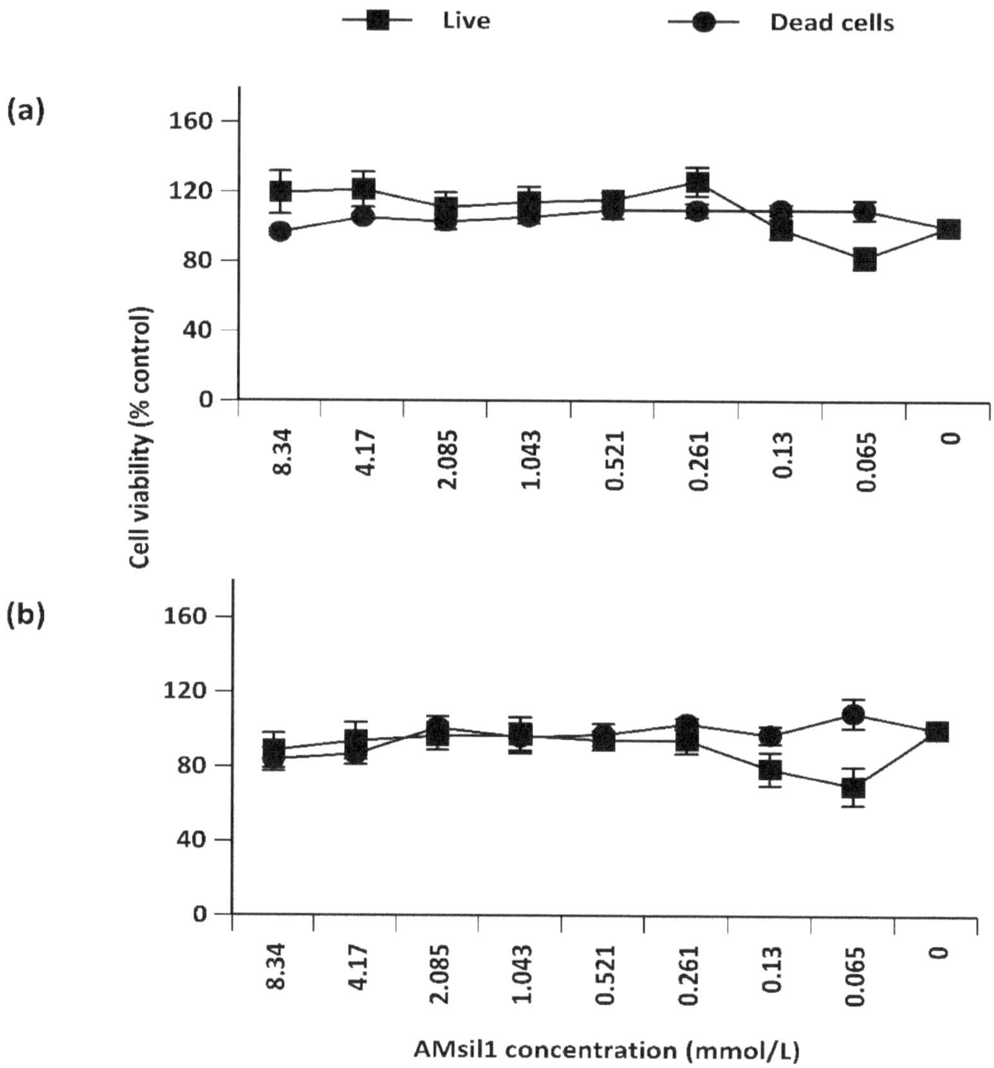

Figure 3. Percent control value of viability of human gingival fibroblast (HGF) cells exposed to 2-fold serial dilutions of AM_{sil1} (≤8.34 mmol/L) for (**a**) 24 h or (**b**) 72 h. Data represent mean ± standard error for five independent replicates tested in triplicate.

2.2.2. AM_{sil2}

Regardless of time, AM_{sil2} concentration exerted a main effect ($p \leq 0.001$) on the number of viable CCL1s (Figure 4). Paired comparisons indicated that at 24 h exposure, CCL1 cells exposed to ≥3.64 mmol/L were lower ($p \leq 0.05$) than the number of live cells exposed to all lower concentrations. At 72 h exposure, the percentage of live CCL1 cells exposed to ≥1.82 mmol/L AM_{sil2} was at least 3- to 4-fold lower ($p \leq 0.001$) compared to all concentrations ≤ 0.91 mmol/L.

Like cell viability, AM_{sil2} concentration exerted an effect ($p \leq 0.001$) on CCL1 metabolic activity. Viability and metabolic activity of CCL1 cells exposed to AM_{sil2} showed a strong positive linear correlation at 24 h ($R^2 = 0.91, p \leq 0.0005$) and 72 h ($R^2 = 0.93, p \leq 0.0005$) (data not shown).

AM_{sil2} exhibited a concentration effect ($p \leq 0.001$) on HGF cell viability (Figure 5). Paired comparisons indicated that exposure to ≥1.82 mmol/L AM_{sil2} reduced the number of live HGFs by more than 3-fold ($p \leq 0.05$) compared to the control group. When considering the effect of time regardless of AM_{sil2} concentration, the number of live cells was consistently lower (~23% difference of means). Like viability, AM_{sil2} concentration exhibited an effect ($p \leq 0.001$) on HGF metabolic activity. At 24 and 72 h, viability and metabolic activity of HGF cells exposed to AM_{sil2} showed a positive linear correlation ($R^2 = 0.94$; ($p \leq 0.0005$) and $R^2 = 0.77$; ($p \leq 0.001$), respectively) (data not shown).

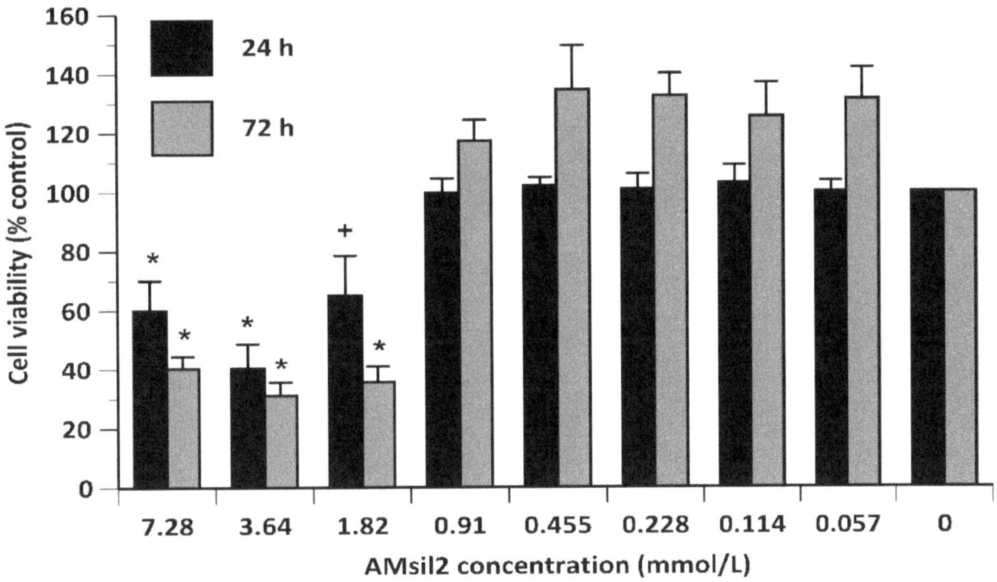

Figure 4. Percent control value of viability of CCL1 cells exposed to 2-fold serial dilutions of AM_{sil2} ($\leq$7.28 mmol/L) for 24 or 72 h. Data represent mean ± SEM for five independent replicates tested in triplicate. * indicates $p \leq 0.05$ when compared to concentrations $\leq$ 0.91 mmol/L within the same time period. + indicates $p \leq 0.05$ when compared to 0.455, 0.228, or 0.114 mmol/L concentrations within same time period.

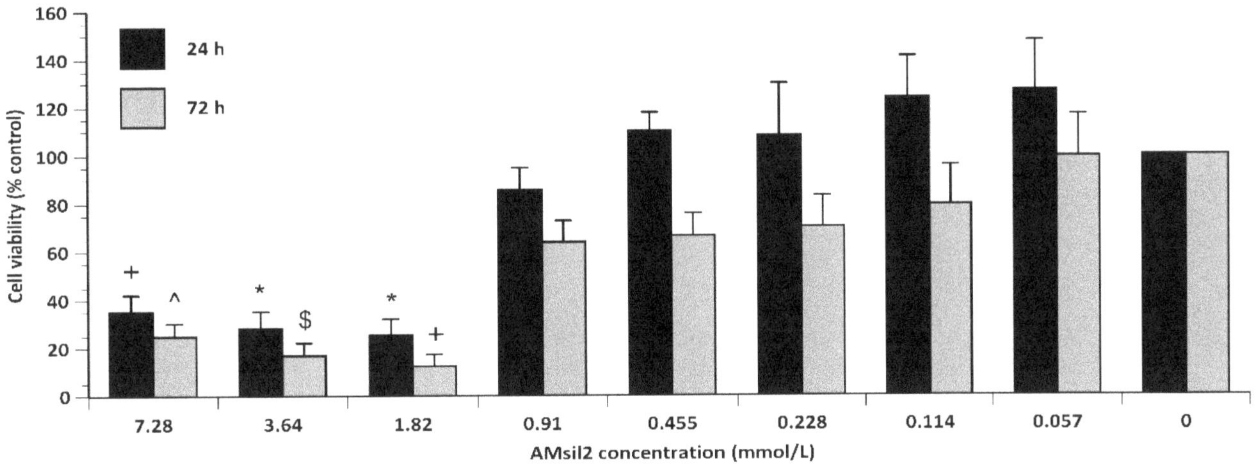

Figure 5. Percent control value of viability of HGF cells exposed to 2-fold serial dilutions of AM_{sil2} ($\leq$7.28 mmol/L) for 24 h or 72 h. Data represent mean ± SEM for five independent replicates tested in triplicate. + indicates $p \leq 0.05$ when compared to concentrations $\leq$ 0.455 mmol/L within same time period. * indicates $p \leq 0.05$ when compared to concentrations $\leq$ 0.91 mmol/L within same time period. ^ indicates $p \leq 0.05$ when compared to concentrations $\leq$ 0.114 mmol/L within same time period. $ indicates $p \leq 0.05$ when compared to concentrations $\leq$ 0.228 mmol/L within same time period.

For both AM_{sil}s, control wells (with or without cells) in which the tetrazolium salt reagent was omitted resulted in negligible optical density values. Positive control wells containing unexposed cells (i.e., no AM_{sil}s) that were given an equal volume of culture medium were not significantly different from cells that were previously treated with the viability stain (data not shown).

2.3. *Hydrophobicity/Hydrophilicity of the Resins*

Copolymers comprised of UPE resin with added AM_{sil}s generally exhibited lower contact angles (CAs) (Figure 6), suggesting change in their hydrophilic/hydrophobic balance toward more hydrophilic surfaces. At 10 mass % monomer in the resin, CAs of both AM_{sil1}–UPE and AM_{sil2}–UPE copolymers (46.9 ± 5.9° and 37.4 ± 9.2°, respectively) were significantly lower (23% and 38% reduction, respectively; $p \leq 0.01$) than the CA of the UPE control 60.8 ± 5.1°. The apparent increase in the CA in going from 10% to 20% AM_{sil} in the resin was significant only for AM_{sil2} ($p \leq 0.035$). The overall order of the decreasing relative hydrophilicity (evidenced by the increasing CA values) of the examined UPE-based copolymers was as follows: (10% AM_{sil2}–UPE ≥ 10% AM_{sil1}–UPE) > (20% AM_{sil2}–UPE = 20% AM_{sil1}–UPE) > UPE control.

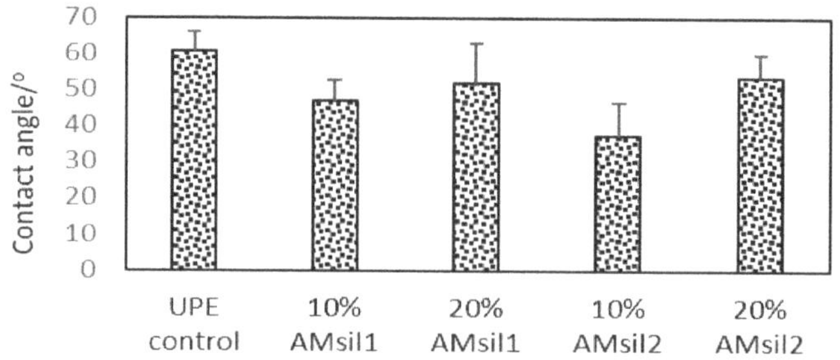

Figure 6. The contact angle (CA) values of AM_{sil}–UPE and UPE control indicative of the changes in resin's overall hydrophilicity/hydrophobicity upon introduction of AM_{sil} monomers at 10 and 20 mass % relative to UPE. Shown are mean values + standard deviation of four repetitive measurements in each experimental group.

2.4. *Effect of AM_{sil}s on Degree of Vinyl Conversion (DVC)*

Introduction of 10% and 20% AM_{sil1} into UPE reduced ($p \leq 0.05$) the mean vinyl moiety conversion upon photopolymerization by 31% and 20%, respectively (Figure 7). No significant effect was observed with the increasing levels of AM_{sil1} in the resin. Although reduced, the DVC observed amongst the AM_{sil2} groups was not statistically different from one another or the UPE control group.

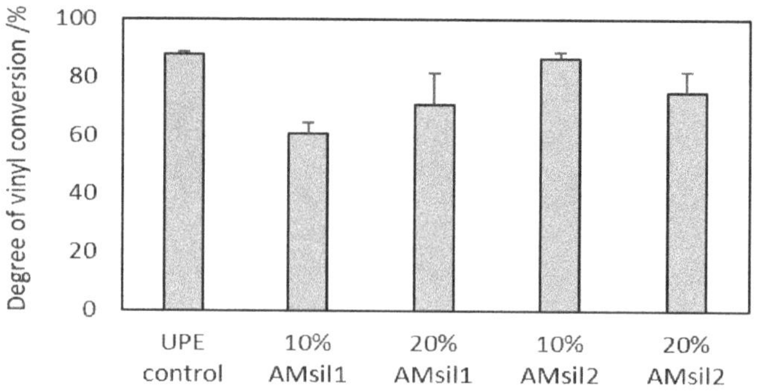

Figure 7. The values for degree of vinyl conversion (DVC) attained 24 h post-cure in AM_{sil}–UPE copolymers compared to no-AM UPE control. Shown are mean values + standard deviation of three repetitive measurements.

2.5. *Mechanical Properties of AM_{sil}–UPE Copolymers*

The FS and E of AM_{sil}–UPE copolymers were, generally, diminished compared to the UPE resin control (Figure 8). The extent of reduction in FS and E varied with the type and the concentration of AM_{sil}. In all AM_{sil}–UPE formulations, the FS values were significantly ($p \leq 0.05$) lower than the UPE control counterparts. In both 10 mass % AM_{sil} formulations, the E was reduced, although not statistically significant. At 20 mass %, the E of both AM_{sil} formulations were notably lower ($p \leq 0.0008$) than the UPE resin control. Both FS and E reductions ranged from moderate (11–13%) for 10 mass % AM_{sil} formulations to substantial (25–57%) for 20 mass % AM_{sil} formulations.

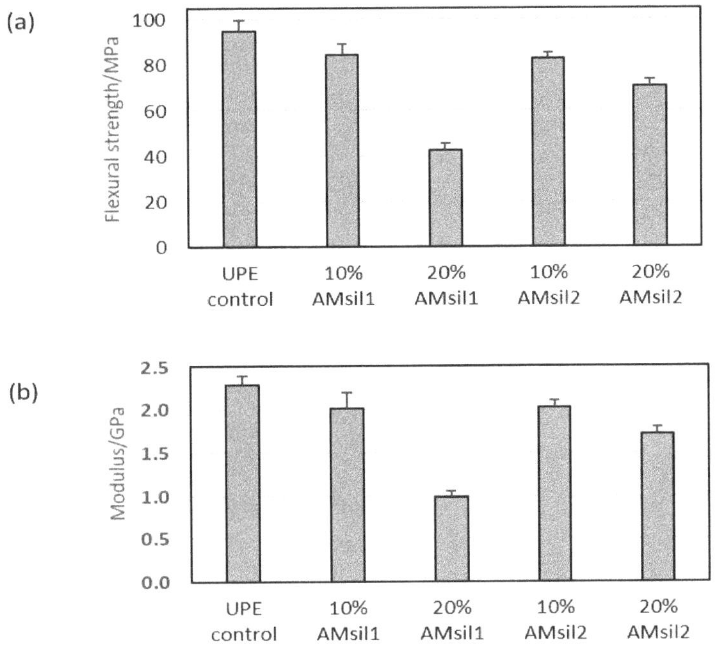

Figure 8. (**a**) Flexural strength and (**b**) tensile elasticity of AM_{sil}–UPE copolymers in comparison with the UPE control. Indicated are mean values + standard deviation of three specimens.

2.6. *Bacterial Testing*

For planktonic bacterial testing, the number of *S. mutans* colony-forming units/mL observed amongst the AM_{sil} groups were not statistically different from one another or the control groups (UPE only and commercial control). However, compared to UPE resin, AM_{sil1}–UPE and AM_{sil2}–UPE (10% mass) copolymers reduced the colonization of *S. mutans* biofilm 4.7- and 1.7-fold, respectively ($p \leq 0.002$) (Figure 9). *S. mutans* biofilms exposed to AM_{sil1}–UPE were at least 2.8-fold lower ($p \leq 0.005$) than that observed with AM_{sil2}–UPE.

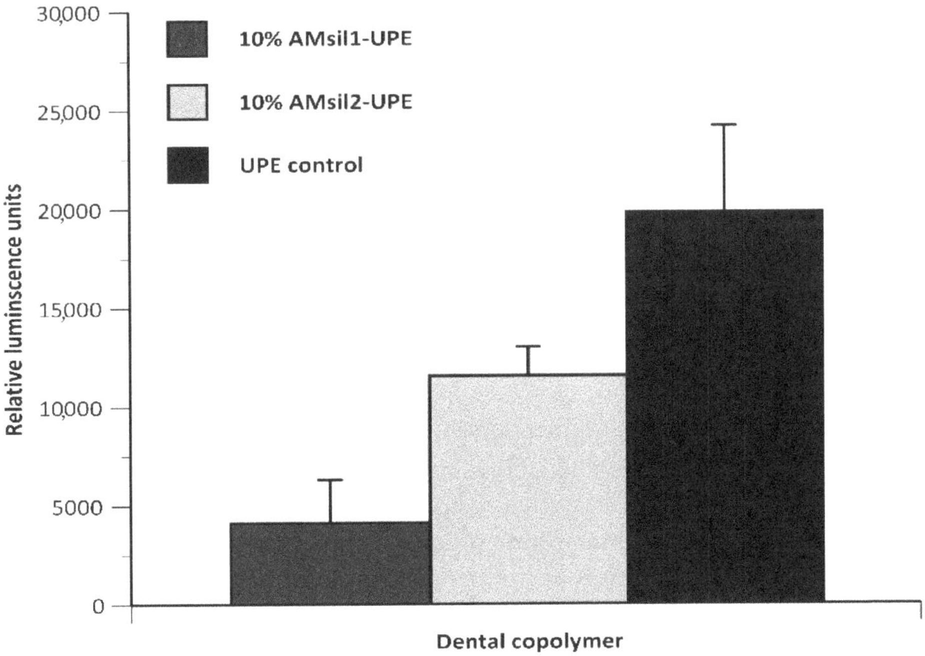

Figure 9. *Streptococcus mutans* biofilm growth inhibition by the experimental $AM_{sil}s$–UPE (10 mass %) copolymers compared to UPE control resin. Bar height indicates mean + standard deviation of 5 specimens/group.

P. gingivalis biofilm biomass on copolymer disks exposed to AM_{sil1}–UPE and AM_{sil2}–UPE were lower (71% and 85%, respectively) than that observed with the commercial control, albeit not statistically different ($p \leq 0.07$) (Figure 10).

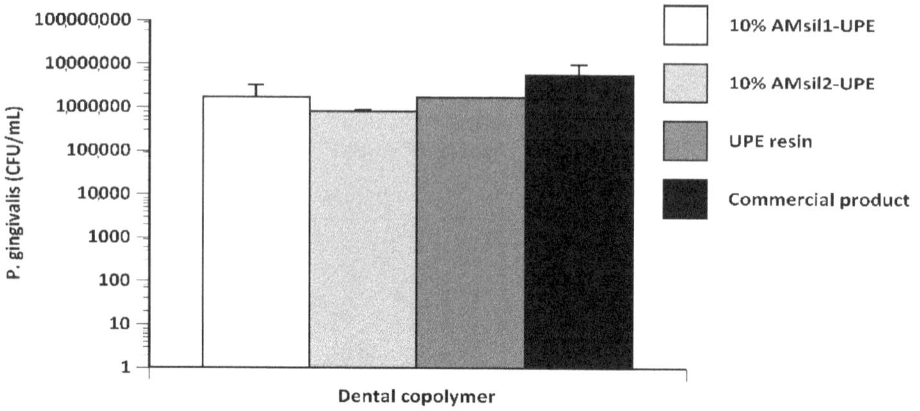

Figure 10. *Porphyromonas gingivalis* biofilm growth inhibition by the experimental AM_{sil}s–UPE (10 mass %) copolymers compared to UPE control resin. Bar height indicates mean + standard deviation of 5 specimens/group.

3. Discussion

We considered cytotoxicity of any AM monomer to be a major determinant of whether the materials that incorporate the monomer in their resin phase are worthy of further study. We believe that direct contact cellular testing of the new agent must be done at biologically relevant eluent concentrations. In this study, we employed conditions that reflect the accelerated leachability of UPH resins and included AM_{sil} concentrations that significantly exceed the upper thresholds established experimentally in the previous work [45]. The direct toxicity of AM_{sil}s towards CCL1 cells and/or HGFs was demonstrated to be marginal or undetectable, except at the higher concentrations of monomers tested. These high AM_{sil} levels correspond to unrealistically high levels of the unreacted monomers and are highly unlikely to ever be registered clinically. Our cytotoxicity results support the basic hypothesis of the study and suggest that, from a biotoxicity viewpoint, AM_{sil}s can be safely utilized in design of AM new materials. Leachability studies of AM–UPE formulations employing high-performance liquid chromatography are currently underway in our laboratory, and are expected to confirm the conclusions derived from the tests based on the accelerated UPH leachability study.

Upon introduction of AM_{sil} into the UPE resin, a shift towards lower CA values, consistent with the moderate increase in the overall hydrophilicity, was seen in all AM_{sil}–UPE formulations. The detected range of CAs in AM_{sil}–UPE resins (37.4–53.3°) correlates very well with the range of CAs typical for the commercial resin composites (37.4–53.3°) [46]. The lowest CAs detected in 10% AM_{sil2}–UPE formulation make this resin a good candidate for the incorporation of the ACP filler in future design of AMRE composites. ACP-filled composite requires sufficient water absorption to initiate water-catalyzed transformation of ACP during which the remineralizing calcium and phosphate ions are released, by diffusion, into surrounding mineral-deficient tooth structures. There, they regenerate these mineral-depleted structures via redeposition of hydroxyapatite [47]. Taken together, the enhanced wettability should ease a diffusion of water into AMRE composite and result in the subsequent release of calcium and phosphate ions from the composite needed for demineralization prevention and/or active remineralization at the restoration site.

The range of DVC values attained in AM_{sil}–UPE copolymers (60.7–86.7%), dependent on both the monomer type and its quantity in the resin, were higher or equal to the DVC reported for 2,2-bis[p-(2-hydroxy-3-methacryloxypropoxy)phenyl]propane (bis-GMA)-based resins/composites with incorporated QA ionic dimethacrylate (67.9–70.7%) [25]. AM_{sil2} copolymers reached significantly higher DVC values (75.2–86.7%) compared to their AM_{sil1} counterparts (60.7–70.9%). In AM_{sil2}–UPE formulations, the inclusion of AM monomer apparently did not affect the high levels of DVC typically seen in UDMA-based resins [35,36]. This phenomenon has been attributed to the chain transfer reactions caused by UDMA's –NH– groups, resulting in increased mobility of the resin network's radical sites [48]. The DVCs attained in AM_{sil2}–UPE copolymers suggest limited mobility of cross-linked polymer matrix, thus reducing the likelihood of unreacted monomers leaching out to a minimum. The observed DVC decrease in AM_{sil1}–UPE formulations compared to those of AM_{sil2}–UPE is yet to be explained.

The results of FS and E tests indicated a reduction of the copolymers' mechanical properties in going from the UPE control to 10% AM_{sil}–UPE to 20% AM_{sil}–UPE. The reduction was far more pronounced in AM_{sil1} series (50%) compared to the AM_{sil2} series (15%). This overall reduction in mechanical properties, particularly in AM_{sil2}–UPE copolymers, should not disqualify this monomer from further exploration, as AM agent in multifunctional AMRE composites. To compensate for the reduction in the mechanical properties, incorporation into composites of the reinforcing fillers in addition to ACP should be considered.

AM_{sil}s integrated into UPE resin were effective in reducing ($p \leq 0.002$) *S. mutans* biofilms. Compared to the commercial control, *P. gingivalis* biofilm biomass was notably lower (71–85%) on AM_{sil}s–UPE copolymer disks, however, not statistically different. As Gram-positive bacteria have peptidoglycan with long anionic polymers, called teichoic acids [49] (i.e., yielding a higher cell surface net negative charge than Gram-negative organisms), one could anticipate *S. mutans* to be more susceptible to AM_{sil}s. Notwithstanding, quaternary ammonium compound AM functionality can also be affected by the type of counter-ion [50], pendant active groups [51], molecular weight, and length of the alkyl chains [52].

AM_{sil}s show promise, as *S. mutans* planktonic and biofilm forms were reduced. Nonetheless, this reduction was only significant ($p \leq 0.002$) for biofilms. When comparing planktonic and biofilm responses, similar trends were observed with an endodontic sealer. For example, bacteria tested with a resin-based root canal sealer did not statistically reduce the planktonic forms, while notably decreasing bacteria in monospecies biofilms [53]. These authors attributed this to the release of substances during the setting process. This attribute is unlikely applicable to our material, as DVC was high and aqueous extraction was conducted for 72 h. In another report, *Staphylococcus aureus* biofilms were demonstrated to be more susceptible to killing than the planktonic form of the same strain [54].

Although AM functionality is observed, we believe that the full potential of the AM_{sil} monomers has not yet been realized. As reported for other quaternary ammonium compounds [47], the current AM_{sil}–UPE copolymer formulations are likely to have N^+ charges randomly distributed throughout the material. As the mechanism of AM action is contingent on contact, it would be advantageous to develop fabrication methods that would favor charge density at the materials surface. Further, others have demonstrated that proteins can diminish the AM capability of quaternary ammonium methacrylates (reviewed by [6]). Currently, there is insufficient information concerning the interaction of proteins with quaternary ammonium methacrylates. Elucidation of the protein–material interactions would yield valuable information to develop strategies to maximize AM efficacy of materials with a charge-based AM mechanism of action.

In conclusion, our novel AM dental monomers (AM_{sil1} and AM_{sil2}) exhibited minimal or no toxicity upon direct contact with biologically relevant concentrations, while reducing *S. mutans* and *P. gingivalis* biofilm forms. AM_{sil}s made the UDMA/PEG-U/EHMA resin more hydrophilic. This would be an advantageous feature in AMRE composites that require water to induce their remineralizing effects. At 10 mass % level of AM_{sil} monomer, DVC of the ensuing AM_{sil}–UPE copolymers was only marginally lower than in UPE control and still exceeded DVCs typically seen in the commercial composites based on bis-GMA/triethyleneglycol dimethacryalate (TEGDMA) resins. The mechanical properties of AM_{sil}–UPE copolymers were reduced (11–57%) compared with the UPE control. The extent of reduction depended on both the type and the concentration of AM_{sil} monomer in the resin. This finding should not disqualify the AM_{sil}–UPE resins from use in AMRE composites intended for Class V restorations where the mechanical stability is not a critical factor.

4. Materials and Methods

4.1. Monomer Synthesis

The synthesis and validation protocols for the AM_{sil}s are described in detail by Okeke et al. (2019) [40]. In brief, AM_{sil1} and AM_{sil2} were synthesized at 50–55 °C by reacting equimolar amounts of tertiary amine, DMAEMA, with IPTMS and BrUDTMS, respectively, in the presence of chloroform and butylated hydroxytoluene. DMAEMA, IPTMS, and butylated hydroxytoluene were purchased from Sigma, St. Louis, MO, USA. BrUDTMS was purchased from Gelest Inc., Morrisville, PA, USA. Reactants and solvents (chloroform, diethyl ether, hexane; Sigma, St. Louis, MO, USA) used during synthesis and the subsequent purification were used as received, without further purification. The reaction yields were 94.8% and 36.0% for AM_{sil1} and AM_{sil2}, respectively. Due to the generally hygroscopic nature of QA monomers, the AM_{sil}s were stored under vacuum (25 mm Hg) before being used for resin formulation and/or copolymer disk specimen preparation.

4.2. Structural Verification

Purified monomers were characterized by ^1H and ^{13}C NMR spectroscopy as described [40]. Briefly, spectra were obtained using a Bruker Advance II (600 MHz) spectrometer equipped with a Broadband Observe room temperature probe (Bruker, Corp., Billerica, MA, USA). Monomers were dissolved in deuterated dimethyl sulfoxide containing tetramethylsilane.

4.3. Experimental Resin Formulation

UPE resin was formulated from the commercially available monomers UDMA, PEG-U, and EHMA at 2.8:1.0:1.7 mass ratio (corresponds to the average mass ratio of the ternary UDMA-based formulations explored by our group so far). A conventional visible light initiator system comprised of camphorquinone and ethyl-4-*N,N*-dimethylamino benzoate (4EDMAB) was introduced to the resin at concentrations of 0.2 mass % camphorquinone and 0.8 mass % 4EDMAB. AM_{sil}s were blended into UPE resin to yield (AM_{sil1} or AM_{sil2})–UPE resin with 10 or 20 mass % of AM component. Addition of AM_{sil1} or AM_{sil2} to the light-activated UPE resin took place in the absence of blue light. The rationale for the chosen levels of AM monomers is based on the previously reported AM activities of similar QA methacrylates in camphorquinone /4EDMAB-activated bis-GMA/TEGDMA resins [25]. Once all components were introduced, the mixture was stirred magnetically (38 rad/s) at 22 °C until a uniform consistency was achieved. CLEARFIL SE Protect BOND (Kurary America, Inc., New York, NY, USA) was used as a comparative commercial AM material. This resin was prepared using equal quantities of primer (containing MDPB) and bonding (containing bis-GMA-HEMA) agent.

4.4. Biocompatibility Tests

Direct contact cytotoxicity of AM_{sil}s was determined following described protocols [55,56]. Briefly, immortalized mouse subcutaneous connective tissue fibroblasts (NCTC clone 929 [L-cell, L-929, Strain L derivative]; American Type Culture Collection (ATCC), Manassas, VA, USA) (CCL1) or HGF (Applied Biological Materials, Inc., Richmond, BC, Canada) were exposed to 2-fold serial dilutions (AM_{sil1}: ≤8.34 mmol/L; AM_{sil2}: ≤7.28 mmol/L). Chosen concentrations corresponded to approx. 7% mass fraction of AM_{sil1} or AM_{sil2} in the copolymer resin and a maximum of 2% leaching. To allow for the possibility of restoration multiplicity and variable size, a 2-fold greater dilution was also included in the testing. These calculations are based on the accelerated leachability study of UDMA/PEG-U/2-hydroxyethyl methacrylate (HEMA) resin (abbreviated UPH; a close analog to UPE resin used in this study) and ACP-UPH composites [57]. After 24 and 72 h incubation, cells were assessed for cell viability (LIVE/DEAD® Viability/Cytotoxicity kit, Life Technologies, Corp., Grand

Island, NY, USA) and metabolic activity (CellTiter® AQueous One Solution Reagent; Promega, Corp., Madison, WI, USA). Controls were without the AM_{sil}s and/or cells. The CCL1 cells and HGFs were maintained, at 37 °C and 5% CO_2, in 10% serum-supplemented Eagle's minimum essential medium (ATCC) and PriGrow III medium (Applied Biological Materials, Inc.), respectively. For experiments, cells were obtained from a subconfluent stock culture. Means were obtained from 5 independent replicates tested in duplicate.

4.5. Contact Angle (CA)

Changes in hydrophilicity/hydrophobicity of UPE resins due to the introduction of AM_{sil}s were assessed by CA measurements (drop shape analyzer DSA100, Krüss GmbH, Hamburg, Germany). Following the deposition of the sessile droplets of the resin on the substrate, they were imaged after 1 min resting time with a charge-coupled device camera at the points of intersection (three-phase contact points) between the drop contour and the projection of the surface (baseline). The CA water values were calculated employing the Krüss Advance software. Four repetitive measurements were performed in each group.

4.6. Copolymer Specimen Preparation

For biotesting, UPE and AM_{sil1}–UPE and $AMsi_{l2}$–UPE copolymer specimens were fabricated by filling circular openings of a flat stainless-steel molds (6 mm diameter, 0.5 mm thickness) with the resins. Each side of the mold was covered with Mylar film and a glass slide, firmly clamped, and then cured (2 min/side: Triad 2000; Dentsply International, York, PA, USA).

Specimens were subjected to extraction in Dulbecco's phosphate-buffered saline lacking both calcium and magnesium (Life Technologies, Grand Island, NY, USA) for 72 h, at 37 °C and 6.3 rad/s using an orbital shaker. After extraction, the disks were dried under vacuum (desiccator; ~22 °C) for 7 days. Specimens were sterilized for 12 h using an Anprolene gas sterilization chamber (Andersen Products, Inc., Haw River, NC, USA). Prior to bacterial testing, specimens were degassed for ≥5 days under vacuum (desiccator; ~22 °C).

4.7. Degree of Vinyl Conversion (DVC)

DVC of UPE and (AM_{sil1} or AM_{sil2})–UPE resins was determined by collecting the near-IR (NIR) spectra (Nexus; ThermoFisher, Madison, WI, USA) before and 24 h after the light cure and calculating the reduction in =C–H absorption band at 6165 cm^{-1} in the overtone region in going from monomers to polymers. By maintaining a constant specimen thickness, a need for an invariant internal standard was eliminated. The DVC was calculated as

$$\text{DVC (\%)} = [(\text{area}_{\text{monomer}} - \text{area}_{\text{polymer}})/\text{area}_{\text{monomer}}] \times 100 \quad (1)$$

where $\text{area}_{\text{polymer}}$ and $\text{area}_{\text{monomer}}$ correspond to the areas under 6165^{-1} absorption peak after and before the polymerization, respectively.

4.8. Mechanical Properties of Copolymers

Test specimens (2 mm × 2 mm × 25 mm) for flexural strength (FS) and elastic modulus (E) determinations were photopolymerized in the same manner as the copolymer disks for biological testing. Polymerized specimens did not undergo any additional treatment. The FS and E of UPE and (AM_{sil1} or AM_{sil2}) UPE copolymer specimens was tested employing the Universal Testing Machine (Instron 5500R, Instron Corp., Canton, MA, USA). The load was applied (crosshead speed of 1 mm/min) to the center of a specimen positioned on a test device with supports 20 mm apart. The FS and E of the specimens (three replicates/experimental group) were calculated as instructed in the ISO4049:2009 document.

4.9. Bacterial Testing

4.9.1. Planktonic

Testing of *Streptococcus mutans* UA-159 (ATCC® 700610) planktonic forms was according to described methods [47,58]. Briefly, bacterial cultures with an optical density of 1.2–1.3 at 600 nm (Unico® 1200 Spectrophotometer, United Products & Instruments, Inc., Dayton, NJ, USA) were diluted and seeded onto copolymer disks at a density of ~3×10^7 CFU/disk. Another disk was placed atop to maximize contact. After a 2 h incubation (37 °C, 5% CO_2) the samples were placed in 1 mL of Todd Hewitt broth, rigorously mixed, and utilized to prepare a 10-fold dilution series. A 100 μL aliquot of the resulting suspensions were spread onto the surface of THB agar plates. After incubation (~20 h at 37 °C, 5% CO_2), colony-forming units were enumerated using an IncuCount Colony Counter (Revolutionary Science, Shafer, MN, USA). UPE resin disks and HemCon® Dental Dressing (HemCon Medical Technologies, Inc., Portland, OR, USA) were used as negative and positive controls, respectively. Around 30 to 300 CFU per spread plate was the range considered countable. Notwithstanding, agar plates streaked with neat solutions of some groups yielded less than the lower limit of detection. Such data were reported as less than the limit of quantification. The number of CFU/mL was calculated as CFU number/(volume plated × dilution factor). Mean counts were obtained from five independently tested copolymer disk sandwiches.

4.9.2. Biofilm

A bioluminescent *S. mutans* strain JM 10 (derivative of wild type UA159 [59] was used to assess the AM properties of AM_{sil}s. Methods of the real-time bioluminescence assay were as described [41,58].

Porphyromonas gingivalis, strain FDC 381 (ATCC® BAA-1703) was propagated in Becton Dickinson BBL chopped meat carbohydrate, pre-reduced II broth, using a shaking incubator (37 °C, anaerobic conditions). Three-day cultures were diluted in broth to approximate 5×10^6 CFU/mL. Copolymer disks, vertically supported in a 24-well plate, were immersed in 1.6 mL of the bacterial suspension. In anaerobic conditions, the plate was incubated at 37 °C for 4 days. The copolymer disks were washed thrice in sterile 0.89% NaCl solution. Thereafter, the biofilm was displaced from the copolymer disks by transferring them to a sterile glass tube containing 1 mL of saline, vortexed (1 min), sonicated (10 min), and vortexed (1 min). Each disk was visually examined to ensure that the biomass was removed. The resulting suspensions were used to make 10-fold serial dilutions and subsequently spread onto the surface of Brucella agar with hemin and vitamin K1 (Sigma-Aldrich, St. Louis, MO, USA) plates. After incubation (3 days at 37 °C, anaerobic conditions), colony-forming units were enumerated.

4.10. Statistical Analyses

Analysis of variance and multiple paired comparisons (two-sided, 95% confidence interval) were used to analyze the experimental data as a function of material makeup and/or exposure/incubation time and establish a statistical significance of differences between the experimental groups. Correlation coefficient (r) was calculated to determine the functional dependence between cellular metabolic activity and viability. (SigmaPlot™, Systat Software, San Jose, CA, USA and/or Microsoft Office Excel 2016; Microsoft, Redmond, WA, USA). Graphics were created using Microsoft Office Excel 2016 and/or DeltaGraph6 for Windows® (Red Rock Software, Inc., Salt Lake City, UT, USA).

Author Contributions: D.R.B. conceptualized and conducted biotesting, fabricated copolymer specimens, and conducted statistical analyses. A.A.G. conducted biotesting, physicochemical/mechanical testing of copolymers. S.A.F. conducted monomer synthesis/validation, fabrication of copolymer resins, and measured their physicochemical/mechanical properties. S.S.K., F.L.E.F., and R.D.H. conducted S. mutans biofilm analyses. D.S. conceptualized the AM monomers, performed literature compilation, and statistical data interpretation. All authors contributed to the preparation/review of this manuscript. All authors have read and agreed to the published version of the manuscript.

Acknowledgments: Assistance of U.C. Okeke (formerly ADA Foundation) in monomer synthesis/characterization are gratefully acknowledged. Technical expertise of H. Kim (Integrated Pharma Services) to assess AM properties of *P. gingivalis* is appreciated. Authors gratefully acknowledge donation of UDMA and PEG-U from Esstech, Essington, PA, USA.

Disclaimer: The sole purpose of identifying certain commercial materials and equipment in this article was to adequately define the experimental protocols. Such identification, in no instance, implies recommendation or endorsement by the ADA or ADA Foundation, or means that the material/equipment specified is the best available for the purpose.

Abbreviations

ACP	amorphous calcium phosphate
AM	antimicrobial
AMRE	antimicrobial and remineralizing
AM_{sil1}	N-(2-(methacryloyloxy)ethyl-*N*,*N*-dimethyl-3-(trimethoxysilyl)propan-1-aminium iodide
AM_{sil2}	N-(2-(methacryloyloxy)ethyl-*N*,*N*-dimethyl-3-(trimethoxysilyl)undecan-1-aminium bromide
Bis-GMA	2,2-bis[p-(2-hydroxy-3-methacryloxypropoxy)phenyl]propane
BrUDTMS	(11-bromoundecyl)trimethoxy silane
CA	contact angle
CCL1	immortalized mouse subcutaneous connective tissue fibroblasts
CQ	camphorquinone
DMAEMA	2-(dimethylamino)ethyl methacrylate
DVC	degree of vinyl conversion
4EDMAB	ethyl-4-*N*,*N*-dimethylamino benzoate
EHMA	ethyl 2-(hydroxymethyl) acrylate
HGF	human gingival fibroblasts
IPTMS	(3-iodopropyl)trimethoxy silane
MDBP	methacryloyloxydodecyl pyrimidinium bromide
NMR	nuclear magnetic resonance
PEG-U	poly(ethylene glycol)-extended UDMA
QA	quaternary ammonium
TEGDMA	triethyleneglycol dimethacrylate
UDMA	urethane dimethacrylate
UPE	UDMA/PEG-U/EHMA resin

References

1. Gluzman, R.; Katz, R.V.; Frey, B.J.; McGowan, R. Prevention of root caries: A literature review of primary and secondary preventive agents. *Spec. Care Dentist.* **2013**, *33*, 133–140. [CrossRef] [PubMed]
2. Cramer, N.B.; Stansbury, J.W.; Bowman, C.N. Recent advances and developments in composite dental restorative materials. *J. Dent. Res.* **2011**, *90*, 402–416. [CrossRef] [PubMed]
3. Ferracane, J.L. Resin composite—state of the art. *Dent. Mater.* **2011**, *27*, 29–38. [CrossRef] [PubMed]
4. Moreau, J.L.; Xu, H.H. Fluoride releasing restorative materials: Effects of pH on mechanical properties and ion release. *Dent. Mater.* **2010**, *26*, e227–e235. [CrossRef] [PubMed]
5. Wiegand, A.; Buchalla, W.; Attin, T. Review on fluoride-releasing restorative materials–fluoride release and uptake characteristics, antibacterial activity and influence on caries formation. *Dent. Mater.* **2007**, *23*, 343–362. [CrossRef] [PubMed]
6. Imazato, S. Bio-active restorative materials with antibacterial effects: New dimension of innovation in restorative dentistry. *Dent. Mater. J.* **2009**, *28*, 11–19. [CrossRef] [PubMed]
7. Pereira-Cenci, T.; Cenci, M.S.; Fedorowicz, Z.; Marchesan, M.A. Antibacterial agents in composite restorations for the prevention of dental caries. *Cochrane Database Syst. Rev.* **2009**. [CrossRef]

8. Dallas, P.; Sharma, V.K.; Zboril, R. Silver polymeric nanocomposites as advanced antimicrobial agents: Classification, synthetic paths, applications, and perspectives. *Adv. Colloid Interface Sci.* **2011**, *166*, 119–135. [CrossRef]
9. Jedrychowski, J.R.; Caputo, A.A.; Kerper, S. Antibacterial and mechanical properties of restorative materials combined with chlorhexidines. *J. Oral Rehabil.* **1983**, *10*, 373–381. [CrossRef]
10. Kawahara, K.; Tsuruda, K.; Morishita, M.; Uchida, M. Antibacterial effect of silver-zeolite on oral bacteria under anaerobic conditions. *Dent. Mater.* **2000**, *16*, 452–455. [CrossRef]
11. Knetsch, M.L.; Koole, L.H. New strategies in the development of antimicrobial coatings: The example of increasing usage of silver and silver nanoparticles. *Polymers* **2011**, *3*, 340–366. [CrossRef]
12. Osinaga, P.W.; Grande, R.H.; Ballester, R.Y.; Simionato, M.R.; Delgado Rodrigues, C.R.; Muench, A. Zinc sulfate addition to glass-ionomer-based cements: Influence on physical and antibacterial properties, zinc and fluoride release. *Dent. Mater.* **2003**, *19*, 212–217. [CrossRef]
13. Syafiuddin, T.; Hisamitsu, H.; Toko, T.; Igarashi, T.; Goto, N.; Fujishima, A.; Miyazaki, T. In vitro inhibition of caries around a resin composite restoration containing antibacterial filler. *Biomaterials* **1997**, *18*, 1051–1057. [CrossRef]
14. Takahashi, Y.; Imazato, S.; Kaneshiro, A.V.; Ebisu, S.; Frencken, J.E.; Tay, F.R. Antibacterial effects and physical properties of glass-ionomer cements containing chlorhexidine for the ART approach. *Dent. Mater.* **2006**, *22*, 647–652. [CrossRef] [PubMed]
15. Yoshida, K.; Tanagawa, M.; Atsuta, M. Characterization and inhibitory effect of antibacterial dental resin composites incorporating silver-supported materials. *J. Biomed. Mater. Res.* **1999**, *47*, 516–522. [CrossRef]
16. Weng, Y.; Guo, X.; Chong, V.J.; Howard, L.; Gregory, R.L.; Xie, D. Synthesis and evaluation of a novel antibacterial dental resin composite with quaternary ammonium salts. *J. Biomed. Sci. Eng.* **2011**, *4*, 147. [CrossRef]
17. Makvandi, P.; Jamaledin, R.; Jabbari, M.; Nikfarjam, N.; Borzacchiello, A. Antibacterial quaternary ammonium compounds in dental materials: A systematic review. *Dent. Mater.* **2018**, *34*, 851–867. [CrossRef] [PubMed]
18. Xue, Y.; Xiao, H.; Zhang, Y. Antimicrobial polymeric materials with quaternary ammonium and phosphonium salts. *Int. J. Mol. Sci.* **2015**, *16*, 3626–3655. [CrossRef]
19. Gottenbos, B.; van der Mei, H.C.; Klatter, F.; Nieuwenhuis, P.; Busscher, H.J. In vitro and in vivo antimicrobial activity of covalently coupled quaternary ammonium silane coatings on silicone rubber. *Biomaterials* **2002**, *23*, 1417–1423. [CrossRef]
20. Lee, S.B.; Koepsel, R.R.; Morley, S.W.; Matyjaszewski, K.; Sun, Y.; Russell, A.J. Permanent, nonleaching antibacterial surfaces. 1. Synthesis by atom transfer radical polymerization. *Biomacromolecules* **2004**, *5*, 877–882. [CrossRef]
21. Lu, G.; Wu, D.; Fu, R. Studies on the synthesis and antibacterial activities of polymeric quaternary ammonium salts from dimethylaminoethyl methacrylate. *React. Funct. Polym.* **2007**, *67*, 355–366. [CrossRef]
22. Li, F.; Chen, J.; Chai, Z.; Zhang, L.; Xiao, Y.; Fang, M.; Ma, S. Effects of a dental adhesive incorporating antibacterial monomer on the growth, adherence and membrane integrity of Streptococcus mutans. *J. Dent.* **2009**, *37*, 289–296. [CrossRef] [PubMed]
23. Thome, T.; Mayer, M.P.; Imazato, S.; Geraldo-Martins, V.R.; Marques, M.M. In vitro analysis of inhibitory effects of the antibacterial monomer MDPB-containing restorations on the progression of secondary root caries. *J. Dent.* **2009**, *37*, 705–711. [CrossRef] [PubMed]
24. Antonucci, J.M. Polymerizable biomedical composition. U.S. Patent 8,217,081 B2, 10 July 2012.
25. Antonucci, J.M.; Zeiger, D.N.; Tang, K.; Lin-Gibson, S.; Fowler, B.O.; Lin, N.J. Synthesis and characterization of dimethacrylates containing quaternary ammonium functionalities for dental applications. *Dent. Mater.* **2012**, *28*, 219–228. [CrossRef]
26. Li, F.; Chai, Z.G.; Sun, M.N.; Wang, F.; Ma, S.; Zhang, L.; Fang, M.; Chen, J.H. Anti-biofilm effect of dental adhesive with cationic monomer. *J. Dent. Res.* **2009**, *88*, 372–376. [CrossRef]
27. Boskey, A.L. Amorphous calcium phosphate: The contention of bone. *J. Dent. Res.* **1997**, *76*, 1433–1436. [CrossRef]
28. Dorozhkin, S.V. Biocomposites and hybrid biomaterials based on calcium orthophosphates. *Biomatter* **2011**, *1*, 3–56. [CrossRef]
29. Dorozhkin, S.V. Calcium orthophosphates: Occurrence, properties, biomineralization, pathological calcification and biomimetic applications. *Biomatter* **2011**, *1*, 121–164. [CrossRef]

30. He, G.; Dahl, T.; Veis, A.; George, A. Nucleation of apatite crystals in vitro by self-assembled dentin matrix protein 1. *Nat. Mater.* **2003**, *2*, 552–558. [CrossRef]
31. Tsuji, T.; Onuma, K.; Yamamoto, A.; Iijima, M.; Shiba, K. Direct transformation from amorphous to crystalline calcium phosphate facilitated by motif-programmed artificial proteins. *Proc. Natl. Acad. Sci. USA* **2008**, *105*, 16866–16870. [CrossRef]
32. Weiner, S. Transient precursor strategy in mineral formation of bone. *Bone* **2006**, *39*, 431–433. [CrossRef] [PubMed]
33. Weiner, S.; Sagi, I.; Addadi, L. Structural biology. Choosing the crystallization path less traveled. *Science* **2005**, *309*, 1027–1028. [CrossRef] [PubMed]
34. Tadic, D.; Peters, F.; Epple, M. Continuous synthesis of amorphous carbonated apatites. *Biomaterials* **2002**, *23*, 2553–2559. [CrossRef]
35. Antonucci, J.M.; Skrtic, D. Fine-tuning of polymeric resins and their interfaces with amorphous calcium phosphate. A strategy for designing effective remineralizing dental composites. *Polymers* **2010**, *2*, 378–392. [CrossRef]
36. Skrtic, D.; Antonucci, J.M. Dental composites based on amorphous calcium phosphate - resin composition/physicochemical properties study. *J. Biomater. Appl.* **2007**, *21*, 375–393. [CrossRef]
37. Skrtic, D.; Antonucci, J.M.; Eanes, E.D. Amorphous calcium phosphate-based bioactive polymeric composites for mineralized tissue regeneration. *J. Res. Natl. Inst. Stan.* **2003**, *108*, 167–182. [CrossRef]
38. Skrtic, D.; Antonucci, J.M.; Eanes, E.D.; Eidelman, N. Dental composites based on hybrid and surface-modified amorphous calcium phosphates. *Biomaterials* **2004**, *25*, 1141–1150. [CrossRef]
39. Zhang, F.; Allen, A.J.; Levine, L.E.; Vaudin, M.D.; Skrtic, D.; Antonucci, J.M.; Hoffman, K.M.; Giuseppetti, A.A.; Ilavsky, J. Structural and dynamical studies of acid-mediated conversion in amorphous-calcium-phosphate based dental composites. *Dent. Mater.* **2014**, *30*, 1113–1125. [CrossRef]
40. Okeke, U.C.; Synder, C.R.; Frukhtbeyn, S.A. Synthesis, purification and characterization of polymerizable multifunctional quaternary ammonium compounds. *Molecules* **2019**, *24*, 1464. [CrossRef]
41. Esteban Florez, F.L.; Hiers, R.D.; Smart, K.; Kreth, J.; Qi, F.; Merritt, J.; Khajotia, S.S. Real-time assessment of Streptococcus mutans biofilm metabolism on resin composite. *Dent. Mater.* **2016**, *32*, 1263–1269. [CrossRef]
42. Forssten, S.D.; Bjorklund, M.; Ouwehand, A.C. Streptococcus mutans, caries and simulation models. *Nutrients* **2010**, *2*, 290–298. [CrossRef] [PubMed]
43. Fenesy, K.E. Periodontal disease: An overview for physicians. *Mt. Sinai J. Med.* **1998**, *65*, 362–369. [PubMed]
44. Rafiei, M.; Kiani, F.; Sayehmiri, K.; Sayehmiri, F.; Tavirani, M.; Dousti, M.; Sheikhi, A. Prevalence of Anaerobic Bacteria (P.gingivalis) as Major Microbial Agent in the Incidence Periodontal Diseases by Meta-analysis. *J. Dent.* **2018**, *19*, 232–242.
45. Antonucci, J.M.; Davis, C.H.; Sun, J.; O'Donnell, J.N.; Skrtic, D. Leachability and Cytotoxicity of an Experimental Polymeric ACP Composite. *PMSE Prepr. Am. Chem. Soc. Div. Polym. Mater. Sci. Eng. Meet.* **2011**, *104*, 250–252.
46. Da Silva, E.M.; Almeida, G.S.; Poskus, L.T.; Guimaraes, J.G. Relationship between the degree of conversion, solubility and salivary sorption of a hybrid and a nanofilled resin composite. *J. Appl. Oral Sci.* **2008**, *16*, 161–166. [CrossRef] [PubMed]
47. Bienek, D.R.; Giuseppetti, A.A.; Skrtic, D. Amorphous calcium phosphates as bioactive filler in polymeric dental composites. In *Calcium Phosphates-From Fundamentals to Applications*; Dutour-Sikiric, M., Furedi-Milhofer, H., Eds.; IntechOpen Limited: London, UK, 2019. [CrossRef]
48. Sideridou, I.; Tserki, V.; Papanastasiou, G. Effect of chemical structure on degree of conversion in light-cured dimethacrylate-based dental resins. *Biomaterials* **2002**, *23*, 1819–1829. [CrossRef]
49. Silhavy, T.J.; Kahne, D.; Walker, S. The bacterial cell envelope. *Cold Spring Harb. Perspect. Biol.* **2010**, *2*, a000414. [CrossRef]
50. Chen, C.Z.; Beck-Tan, N.C.; Dhurjati, P.; van Dyk, T.K.; LaRossa, R.A.; Cooper, S.L. Quaternary ammonium functionalized poly (propylene imine) dendrimers as effective antimicrobials: Structure–activity studies. *Biomacromolecules* **2000**, *1*, 473–480. [CrossRef]
51. Ikeda, T.; Hirayama, H.; Yamaguchi, H.; Tazuke, S.; Watanabe, M. Polycationic biocides with pendant active groups: Molecular weight dependence of antibacterial activity. *Antimicrob. Agents Chemother.* **1986**, *30*, 132–136. [CrossRef]

52. Ikeda, T.; Yamaguchi, H.; Tazuke, S. Molecular weight dependence of antibacterial activity in cationic disinfectants. *J. Bioact. Compat. Polym.* **1990**, *5*, 31–41. [CrossRef]
53. Kapralos, V.; Koutroulis, A.; Ørstavik, D.; Sunde, P.T.; Rukke, H.V. Antibacterial Activity of Endodontic Sealers against Planktonic Bacteria and Bacteria in Biofilms. *J. Endod.* **2018**, *44*, 149–154. [CrossRef] [PubMed]
54. Harrison, J.J.; Ceri, H.; Stremick, C.; Turner, R.J. Differences in biofilm and planktonic cell mediated reduction of metalloid oxyanions. *FEMS Microbiol. Lett.* **2004**, *235*, 357–362. [CrossRef] [PubMed]
55. Bienek, D.R.; Frukhtbeyn, S.A.; Giuseppetti, A.A.; Okeke, U.C.; Pires, R.M.; Antonucci, J.M.; Skrtic, D. Ionic dimethacrylates for antimicrobial and remineralizing dental composites. *Ann. Dent. Oral Disord.* **2018**, *1*, 108.
56. Bienek, D.R.; Frukhtbeyn, S.A.; Giuseppetti, A.A.; Okeke, U.C.; Skrtic, D. Antimicrobial monomers for polymeric dental restoratives: Cytotoxicity and physicochemical properties. *J. Funct. Biomat.* **2018**, *9*, 20. [CrossRef] [PubMed]
57. Skrtic, D.; Antonucci, J.M. Bioactive polymeric composites for tooth mineral regeneration: Physicochemical and cellular aspects. *J. Funct. Biomat.* **2011**, *2*, 271–307. [CrossRef]
58. Bienek, D.R.; Giuseppetti, A.A.; Okeke, U.C.; Frukhtbeyn, S.A.; Dupree, P.J.; Khajotia, S.S.; Esteban Florez, F.L.; Hiers, R.D.; Skrtic, D. Antimicrobial, biocompatibility, and physicochemical properties of novel adhesive methacrylate dental monomers. *J. Bioact. Compat. Polym.* **2019**, in press.
59. Merritt, J.; Kreth, J.; Qi, F.; Sullivan, R.; Shi, W. Non-disruptive, real-time analyses of the metabolic status and viability of Streptococcus mutans cells in response to antimicrobial treatments. *J. Microbiol. Methods* **2005**, *61*, 161–170. [CrossRef]

13

Novel CaF_2 Nanocomposites with Antibacterial Function and Fluoride and Calcium Ion Release to Inhibit Oral Biofilm and Protect Teeth

Heba Mitwalli [1,2], Abdulrahman A. Balhaddad [1,3], Rashed AlSahafi [1,4], Thomas W. Oates [5], Mary Anne S. Melo [5,6], Hockin H. K. Xu [5,7,8] and Michael D. Weir [5,*]

1 Program in Dental Biomedical Sciences, University of Maryland School of Dentistry, Baltimore, MD 21201, USA; hmitwalli@umaryland.edu (H.M.); aabalhaddad@umaryland.edu (A.A.B.); rashed.alsahafi@umaryland.edu (R.A.)
2 Department of Restorative Dental Science, College of Dentistry, King Saud University, Riyadh 11451, Saudi Arabia
3 Department of Restorative Dental Sciences, College of Dentistry, Imam Abdulrahman bin Faisal University, Dammam 31441, Saudi Arabia
4 Department of Restorative Dental Sciences, College of Dentistry, Umm Al-Qura University, Makkah 24211, Saudi Arabia
5 Department of Advanced Oral Sciences and Therapeutics, School of Dentistry, University of Maryland, Baltimore, MD 21201, USA; TOates@umaryland.edu (T.W.O.); MMelo@umaryland.edu (M.A.S.M.); HXu2@umaryland.edu (H.H.K.X.)
6 Division of Operative Dentistry, Department of General Dentistry, University of Maryland School of Dentistry, Baltimore, MD 21201, USA
7 Center for Stem Cell Biology & Regenerative Medicine, University of Maryland School of Medicine, Baltimore, MD 21201, USA
8 Marlene and Stewart Greenebaum Cancer Center, University of Maryland School of Medicine, Baltimore, MD 21201, USA
* Correspondence: michael.weir@umaryland.edu

Abstract: (1) Background: The objective of this study was to develop a novel dental nanocomposite containing dimethylaminohexadecyl methacrylate (DMAHDM), 2-methacryloyloxyethyl phosphorylcholine (MPC), and nanoparticles of calcium fluoride ($nCaF_2$) for preventing recurrent caries via antibacterial, protein repellent and fluoride releasing capabilities. (2) Methods: Composites were made by adding 3% MPC, 3% DMAHDM and 15% $nCaF_2$ into bisphenol A glycidyl dimethacrylate (Bis-GMA) and triethylene glycol dimethacrylate (TEGDMA) (denoted BT). Calcium and fluoride ion releases were evaluated. Biofilms of human saliva were assessed. (3) Results: $nCaF_2$+DMAHDM+MPC composite had the lowest biofilm colony forming units (CFU) and the greatest ion release; however, its mechanical properties were lower than commercial control composite ($p < 0.05$). $nCaF_2$+DMAHDM composite had similarly potent biofilm reduction, with mechanical properties matching commercial control composite ($p > 0.05$). Fluoride and calcium ion releases from $nCaF_2$+DMAHDM were much more than commercial composite. Biofilm CFU on composite was reduced by 4 logs ($n = 9$, $p < 0.05$). Biofilm metabolic activity and lactic acid were also substantially reduced by $nCaF_2$+DMAHDM, compared to commercial control composite ($p < 0.05$). (4) Conclusions: The novel nanocomposite $nCaF_2$+DMAHDM achieved strong antibacterial and ion release capabilities, without compromising the mechanical properties. This bioactive nanocomposite is promising to reduce biofilm acid production, inhibit recurrent caries, and increase restoration longevity.

Keywords: dental nanocomposite; calcium fluoride nanoparticles; remineralization; antibacterial; protein repellent; oral biofilm

1. Introduction

Dental resin composites are an excellent material for direct restorations of anterior teeth and in many cases posterior teeth due to their esthetics and ease of placement [1]. Nevertheless, composites are known to accumulate more oral bacterial plaque and biofilm than other direct restorative materials, which could expose the restored tooth to a higher risk for future recurrent caries [2]. Indeed, most failed restorations due to secondary caries are restored with composites [3,4]. The formation of plaque starts with the salivary-acquired pellicle formation. The glycoprotein found in the acquired pellicle promotes bacterial cell adherence. The microbes in the biofilm then produce acids which lowers the pH and lead to mineral loss over time resulting in dissolution of the tooth structure, the formation of caries, and failure of the restoration [5–7]. Unfortunately, currently available commercial composites lack antibacterial properties. Accordingly, efforts were made to overcome the presence of cariogenic bacteria, in an effort to prevent recurrent caries [8].

The incorporation of calcium fluoride nanoparticles ($nCaF_2$) into composites has the potential to reduce demineralization [9]. Fluoride (F) ions work by stimulating the remineralization and suppressing the oral microorganisms [10,11]. The presence of F ions in the event of demineralization enhances the precipitation of calcium and phosphate ions and forms fluorapatite [$Ca_5(PO_4)_3F$] to protect the tooth surface [12–14]. Fluoride was also shown to have the advantage of reducing bacterial acid production to reduce recurrent caries.

Designing a composite containing calcium fluoride nanoparticles would enhance the fluorapatite deposition in the affected tooth structure. When the tooth structure is subjected to acidic attack by the cariogenic pathogens, calcium and phosphate ions are lost from enamel. Using remineralization approaches to restore the lost minerals is required to enforce and strengthen the tooth structure. Therefore, the composite with calcium fluoride nanoparticles would enhance remineralization and form fluorapatite that is able to resist future acidic challenges. Several studies have demonstrated the ability of forming fluorapatite using nanotechnology [15,16]. In one study, they manufactured fluorapatite nanoparticles and examined its doping with silver ion nanoparticles and evaluated its physical and antimicrobial effects. The results showed 30% inhibition of bacterial growth after 4 h of incubation while maintaining the natural morphology of fluorapatite [15]. In another study, fluorapatite was incorporated into chitosan scaffolds. Fluorapatite maintained its structure, granted antimicrobial effects, and showed osteoconductive capability [16].

Furthermore, the incorporation of antibacterial agents into composites have also been investigated. Imazato et al. integrated 12-methacryloyloxydodecylpyridinium bromide (MDPB) into composites and showed successful antibacterial effects [17–20]. The incorporation of quaternary ammonium polyethylenimine (QPEI) into composites also produced a potent and wide-spectrum antimicrobial effect against salivary microorganisms [21]. Antimicrobial peptides (AMPs) were also demonstrated to have antimicrobial properties by bacterial membrane permeabilization and intracellular targeting [22]. Other studies developed antibacterial agents such as dimethylaminohexadecyl methacrylate (DMAHDM) [23,24] and showed a strong antibiofilm activity without compromising the mechanical properties [25].

Previous studies indicated that the salivary protein accumulation on composite surface could lower the efficiency of "contact-killing" mechanisms [26,27]. Accordingly, efforts were made to improve protein-repellent strategies including the addition of protein-repellent agents such as (2-methacryloyloxyethyl phosphorylcholine, or MPC) into resins [28–30]. This method provided resistance to protein adsorption and bacterial adhesion due to the hydrophilic characteristic of MPC [29,30]. However, to date, there has been no report on the development of a novel bioactive dental composite that contains $nCaF_2$, DMAHDM, and MPC in combination.

The objectives of this study were to develop a new composite consisting $nCaF_2$, DMAHDM, and MPC, and to investigate the mechanical, ion release and oral biofilm properties for the first time. The following hypotheses were tested: (1) Adding DMAHDM and MPC into the $nCaF_2$ composite would have mechanical properties similar to a commercial control composite; (2) Adding DMAHDM and MPC into the $nCaF_2$ composite would not compromise the F and Ca ion release; and (3) The new bioactive composite would have much less microorganisms, produce less biofilm acid, and have better remineralizing properties than the commercial control composite.

2. Materials and Methods

2.1. Fabrication of Composites

The experimental resin consisted of bisphenol A glycidyl dimethacrylate (BisGMA, Esstech, Essington, PA, USA), and triethylene glycol dimethacrylate (TEGDMA, Esstech) at 50:50 mass ratio. Camphorquinone at 0.2% (Millipore Sigma, Burlington, MA, USA) and 0.8% ethyl 4-N, N-diethylaminobenzoate (Millipore Sigma) were incorporated for photoactivation. The resin is referred to as BT resin. MPC (Millipore Sigma) was added at a mass fraction of 3% and incorporated into the BT resin with magnetic stirring bar at 150 rpm to be dissolved completely into the resin.

The synthesis of DMAHDM was performed using a modified Menschutkin reaction [31]. Briefly, 10 mmol of 2-(dimethylamino) ethyl methacrylate (Millipore Sigma), 10 mmol of 1-bromohexadecane (TCI America, Portland, OR, USA), and 3 g of ethanol were combined in a reaction vessel and then stirred for 24 h at 70 °C. After the evaporation of the solvent and removal of impurities, the DMADHM was collected. DMAHDM was added into the BT resin at a mass fraction of 3% and was stirred using a magnetic stirring bar at 150 rpm until it was completely dissolved into the resin.

The $nCaF_2$ was manufactured using a spray-dry method as described in previous studies, yielding a mean particle size of 32 nm [9,32–34]. The mass fraction of $nCaF_2$ incorporated into BT resin was 15%, based on our preliminary study. A previous study tested different concentrations of $nCaF_2$ in composite and, after long-term water-aging, the composite with 20% $nCaF_2$ had a flexural strength of 60 MPa [33]. In the present study, 15% $nCaF_2$ was integrated into the resin to achieve good mechanical strength. Silanized barium boroaluminosilicate glass particles with a mean size of 1.4 μm (Dentsply Sirona, Milford, DE, USA) were incorporated into the BT resin for mechanical enhancement. As a commercial control composite, Heliomolar (Ivoclar Vivadent, Mississauga, ON, Canada) was also tested. Heliomolar contains 66.7% filler mass fraction of ytterbium-trifluoride and nanofillers of 40–200 nm of silica. The following groups were tested (Table 1 summarizes the materials used in the study):

1. Heliomolar (referred to as commercial control (CC));
2. BT Resin + 70% glass (referred to as experimental control (EC));
3. Remineralizing composite: BT + 15% $nCaF_2$ + 55% glass (referred to as $nCaF_2$);
4. Antibacterial and remineralizing composite: BT + 15% $nCaF_2$ + 3% DMAHDM + 55% glass (referred to as $nCaF_2$+DMAHDM);
5. Protein-repellent and remineralizing composite: BT + 15% $nCaF_2$ + 3% MPC + 55% glass (referred to as $nCaF_2$+MPC);
6. Antibacterial, protein-repellent, and remineralizing composite: BT + 15% $nCaF_2$ + 3% DMAHDM + 3% MPC + 55% glass (referred to as $nCaF_2$+DMAHDM+MPC).

Table 1. Materials used in the study.

Formulation/Manufacturer	Abbreviation	Fluoride	DMAHDM	MPC
Heliomolar, Ivoclar Vivadent, Mississauga, ON, Canada (Commercial control)	CC	+	-	-
30% BT+70% Glass (Experimental Control)	EC	-	-	-
30% BT+15% $nCaF_2$+55% Glass	$nCaF_2$	+	-	-
27% BT+15% $nCaF_2$+3%DMAHDM +55% Glass	$nCaF_2$+ DMAHDM	+	+	-
27% BT+15% $nCaF_2$+3% MPC +55% Glass	$nCaF_2$+MPC	+	-	+
24% BT+15% $nCaF_2$+3% DMAHDM +3% MPC+55% Glass	$nCaF_2$+DMAHDM+MPC	+	+	+

2.2. *Characterization of $nCaF_2$*

Transmission electron microscopy (TEM, Tecnai T12, FEI, Hillsboro, OR, USA) was used to assess the nanoparticles. Samples were prepared through placing nanoparticles on a perforated copper grid coated by a carbon film. To avoid particle agglomeration, the sample was ultrasonicated for 5 min in acetone prior to deposition. Particle size distribution was measured using a laser diffraction particle size analyzer (SALD-2300, Shimadzu North America, Columbia, MD, USA).

2.3. *Mechanical Properties Testing*

Each composite paste was mixed in a disposable plastic container using a speed mixer (DAC 150.1 FVZ-K SpeedMixer™, FlackTec Inc., Landrum, SC, USA) at a speed of 2800 rpm for 1 min, and then thoroughly mixed by hand on a plastic slab for 5 min. The paste was then placed in a rectangular mold of $2 \times 2 \times 25$ mm^3. Mylar strips were placed on both sides, followed by two glass slides. The specimen was light-cured using a curing unit at 1200 mW/cm^2 (Labolight DUO, GC America, Alsip, IL, USA) on each side for 1 min [35]. After demolding, the samples were stored in a 100% humidity chamber for 24 h at 37 °C. Flexural strength and elastic modulus were tested at a crosshead-speed of 1 mm/min with a 10 mm span with a three-point flexural test using a computer-controlled universal testing system (Insight 1, MTS, Eden Prairie, MN, USA) [36,37]. Flexural strength and elastic modulus were measured after 24 h of specimen immersion in distilled water at 37 °C. Flexural strength: $S = 3P_{max}/L(2bh^2)$, where P_{max} is the fracture load, L is span, b is sample width and h is thickness. Elastic modulus: $E = (P/d)\ (L^3/[4bh^3])$, where load P was divided by displacement d which is the slope in the linear elastic region. Six specimens were tested for each group ($n = 6$).

2.4. *Ca and F Ion Release*

The ion releases for all groups containing $nCaF_2$ were tested. A solution of sodium chloride (NaCl) (133 mmol/L) was buffered with 50 mmol/L HEPES to pH 7 [36,38]. Three specimens of $2 \times 2 \times 12$ mm^3 were placed into 50 mL of solution, accommodating a specimen volume/solution ratio of 3.0 mm^3/mL, similar to those in previous studies [36,38,39]. The specimen's F and Ca ions release were measured at 1, 2, 4, 7, 14, 21, 28, 35, 42, 49, 56, 63, and 70 days. At every time point, aliquots of 2 mL were collected and substituted by a fresh 2 mL solution of NaCl. The aliquots were investigated for Ca ions by a colorimetric assay using a microplate reader (SpectraMax M5, Molecular Probes, San Jose, CA, USA) as previously described, using known standard and calibration curves [36,38,39]. The F ion release was tested with a F ion selective electrode (Orion, Cambridge, MA, USA). Fluoride standard solutions were measured to form a standard curve. The standard curve was used to establish the F concentration. The F ion concentration measurement was performed by combining 0.5 mL of sample and 0.5 mL of undiluted TISAB solution (Fisher Scientific, Pittsburgh, PA, USA).

2.5. *Sample Preparation for Biofilm Tests*

The cover of a 96 well plate was used to fabricate composite discs for microbiological experiments yielding samples 0.5 mm in thickness and 8 mm in diameter [31]. Composite paste was placed at each indent in the in 96-well plate cover then covered with Mylar strips and glass slides to form a smooth surface. It was then light cured as described previously and then stored for 24 h at 37 °C. The following day discs were magnetically stirred for 1 h at 100 rpm in distilled water to remove uncured monomers [18,40,41]. The specimens were sterilized using ethylene oxide (Anprolene AN 74i, Andersen Products, Haw River, NC, USA) for 24 and allowed to de-gas for 7 days, following the instructions of the manufacturer.

2.6. *Saliva Collection and Dental Plaque Microcosm Biofilm Model*

Saliva collection was conducted in accordance with the Declaration of Helsinki, and the protocol was approved by the Institutional Review Board at the University of Maryland Baltimore (IRB #: HP-00050407). The advantage of the dental plaque microcosm biofilm model is the use of an inoculum of human saliva to mimic the heterogeneity and complexity of the bacteria that are present in human dental plaque [18]. An equal amount of saliva was simultaneously gathered from ten healthy contributors with normal dentition, free of active caries, and no antibiotic use within the prior 3 months. Contributors were instructed not to brush their teeth 24 h preceding collection and not to eat or drink 2 h preceding the collection. Subsequently, the collected saliva from all participants was mixed and diluted to 70% in sterile glycerol. Then the saliva–glycerol solution was stored at −80 °C until use [42].

For all biofilm experiments, McBain artificial saliva growth medium was used. McBain medium contained 2.5 g/L Type II mucin (porcine, gastric, Millipore Sigma), 2.0 g/L bacteriological peptone (Becton Dickinson, Sparks, MD, USA), 2.0 g/L tryptone (Becton Dickinson), 0.35 g/L NaCl, 1.0 g/L yeast extract (Fisher Scientific), 0.2 g/L potassium chloride (Millipore Sigma), 0.1 g/L cysteine hydrochloride (Millipore Sigma), 0.2 g/L calcium chloride (Millipore Sigma). The pH of the medium was adjusted to 7 and autoclaved. After cooling the medium, 0.0002 g/L vitamin K_1, 0.001 g/L hemin were added. During biofilm experiments, 2% sucrose solution and the saliva–glycerol solution were used as an inoculum at a ratio of 1:50. The sucrose and inoculum were added to the medium and 1.5 mL of the medium was placed in each well of a 24-well plate containing a composite specimen from each groups. Specimen were incubated in 5% CO_2 at 37 °C for 8 h to permit biofilm growth on the samples. The same procedure was repeated after 8 h without the addition of saliva and incubation occurred again for 16 h. After 16 h the samples were moved to a new 24-well plate which contained fresh medium and sucrose, and was further incubated for 24 h. Composites were exposed to bacterial culture for a total of 48 h, which resulted in reasonably mature dental plaque microcosm biofilms on composites [25,43].

2.7. *Biofilm Colony Forming Units (CFU) Counts*

Nine discs were prepared for each group. Following the 48 h incubation, the disc samples containing biofilm were transported into a vial filled with 1 mL of cysteine peptone water (CPW). This was vortexed for 5 s then sonicated for 5 min and vortexed again to harvest the biofilm [29]. Serial dilutions of the suspensions of bacteria were prepared and transported to agar plates to grow. The CFU were counted on three different agar plates. To determine total streptococci count, mitis salivarius agar (MSA, Becton Dickinson, Sparks, MD, USA) were used. To determine the growth of mutans streptococci, 0.2 units per mL bacitracin (Millipore Sigma) was added to the mitis salivarius agar (MSB). To evaluate the growth of the total microorganisms, tryptic soy blood agar (TSBA) agar plates were used by adding defibrinated sheep blood to tryptic soy agar (TSA, Becton Dickinson). The agar plates were kept at 37 °C in a 5% CO_2 incubator for 48 h. CFU calculation was based on the colony number and multiplied by the dilution factor [29].

2.8. *Biofilms Metabolic Activity Evaluation (MTT)*

The MTT (3-[4,5-dimethylthiazol-2-yl]-2,5- diphenyltetrazolium bromide) assay was performed to investigate the biofilm metabolic activity. Following 48 h of incubation, the discs (n = 9) were transferred into a clean 24-well plate, then 1 mL of tetrazolium dye was placed to every disc. The discs were then incubated in an incubator of 5% CO_2 at 37 °C. Discs were then transported to another 24-well plate, and 1 mL of dimethyl sulfoxide (DMSO) was added to every disc and incubated for 20 min in a dark room [29,44]. After incubation, 200 µL of the DMSO solution was collected and the absorbance at 540 nm was measured [29,44] using a microplate reader (SpectraMax® M5, Molecular Devices, San Jose, CA, USA).

2.9. *Biofilms Lactic Acid Production*

Following 48 h incubation, discs (n = 9) were moved to a different 24-well plate comprising 1.5 mL buffered-peptone water (BPW) with 0.2% sucrose then incubated for 3 h in a 5% CO_2 incubator at 37 °C to release acids. After 3 h, the BPW solution lactic acid concentrations were measured by recording the absorbance at 340 nm [29,44] using a microplate reader (SpectraMax® M5, Molecular Devices). Standard curves were produced by means of lactic acid standards.

2.10. *Scanning Electron Microscopy (SEM) of Biofilms*

For biofilm visualization and confirmation of bacterial attachments on composite discs, biofilms formed at 24 h, 48 h, and 96 h were sputter-coated with platinum. Scanning electron microscopy (SEM, Quanta 200, FEI Company, Hillsboro, OR, USA) was used to examine the bacterial accumulation (Figure 7).

3. Statistical Analysis

All data were evaluated with one-way analysis of variance (ANOVA), and post hoc multiple comparison using Tukey's honestly significant difference test was performed. All statistical analysis was completed using the GraphPad Prism 8 software package (GraphPad Software, San Diego, CA, USA) at 0.05 level of significance.

4. Results

A representative TEM image of calcium fluoride ($nCaF_2$) nanoparticles is shown in Figure 1A. The nanoparticle size distribution ranged from 22 nm to 57 nm, with a mean particle size of 32 nm and is illustrated in Figure 1B.

Flexural strength and elastic modulus of the six composite groups (mean ± sd; n = 6) are shown in Figure 2A,B, respectively. The flexural strength was measured after one day of immersion in water at 37 °C. The flexural strength was significantly higher in EC and $nCaF_2$ composites, when compared to the commercial Heliomolar control ($p < 0.05$). Flexural strength in groups with $nCaF_2$+DMAHDM and $nCaF_2$+MPC matched those of Heliomolar control composite ($p > 0.05$). However, flexural strength in $nCaF_2$+DMAHDM+MPC was significantly lower than commercial Heliomolar control ($p < 0.05$).

The elastic modulus values of EC and $nCaF_2$ were significantly greater than all other groups ($p < 0.05$). Other groups had comparable elastic modulus values to Heliomolar control ($p < 0.05$).

The accumulative F ion release is shown in Figure 3. At 70 days, the composite $nCaF_2$+MPC had the highest F release of (0.40 ± 0.02) mmol/L ($p < 0.05$). Meanwhile, $nCaF_2$+DMAHDM+MPC had F release of (0.25 ± 0.03) mmol/L, $nCaF_2$+DMAHDM had (0.20 ± 0.03) mmol/L, and $nCaF_2$ had (0.04 ± 0.01) mmol/L of fluoride ion release. Heliomolar control had the lowest F release of (0.004 ± 0.0003) mmol/L.

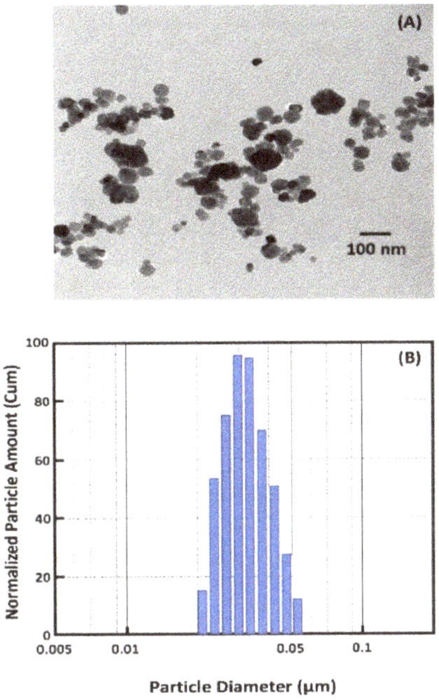

Figure 1. (**A**) TEM of nanoparticles of CaF_2 ($nCaF_2$) synthesized in this study. (**B**) Particle size distribution of $nCaF_2$. The $nCaF_2$ were synthesized via a spray-drying technique and collected using an electrostatic precipitator.

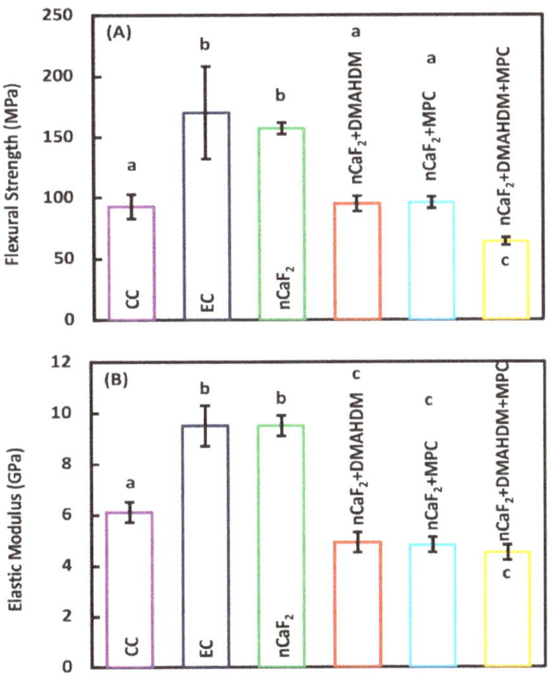

Figure 2. Mechanical properties of composites: (**A**) Flexural strength, and (**B**) Elastic modulus (mean ± sd; $n = 6$). The flexural strength was higher in experimental control (EC) and $nCaF_2$ than commercial Heliomolar control ($p < 0.05$). Flexural strength in $nCaF_2$+DMAHDM and $nCaF_2$+MPC matched Heliomolar control ($p > 0.05$). However, the flexural strength in $nCaF_2$+DMAHDM+MPC was reduced ($p < 0.05$). The elastic modulus of the EC and $nCaF_2$ were higher than Heliomolar control ($p < 0.05$). All other groups had comparable elastic moduli to Heliomolar control after 1 day of immersion ($p > 0.05$). In each plot, different letters (a, b, c) indicate values that are significantly different from each other ($p < 0.05$).

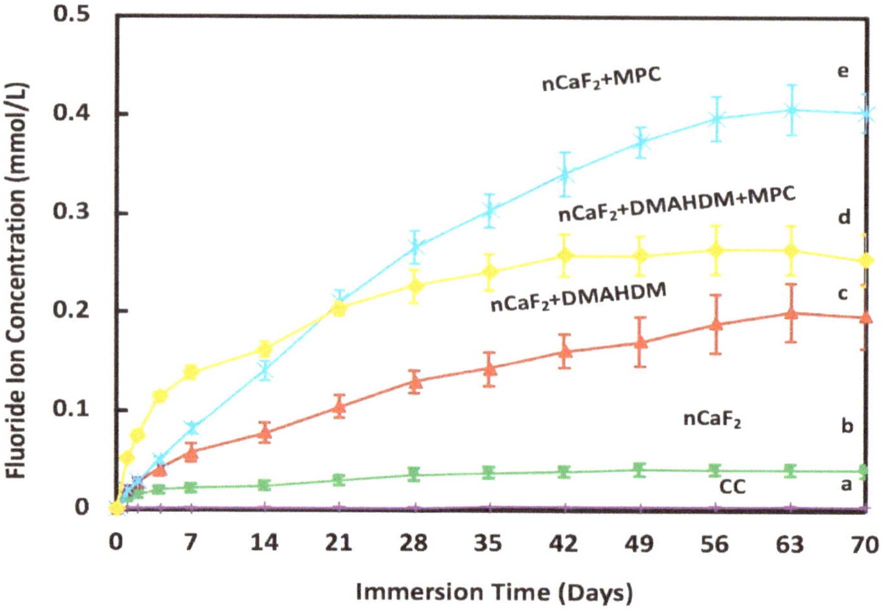

Figure 3. Fluoride (F) ion release from composites (mean ± sd; $n = 6$) at pH 7.0. The incorporation of $nCaF_2$, DMAHDM, and MPC increased the release of F ions with time ($p < 0.05$). Different letters (a, b, c, d, e) indicate significant differences between groups at day 70 ($p < 0.05$).

The calcium ion release is plotted in Figure 4. At 70 days, $nCaF_2$+MPC had a Ca ion release of (0.32 ± 0.005) mmol/L, and $nCaF_2$+DMAHDM+MPC had a similar ion release at (0.35 ± 0.006) mmol/L. Groups containing MPC had ion releases that were significantly higher when compared to other groups ($p < 0.05$). $nCaF_2$ had a Ca ion release of (0.11 ± 0.004) mmol/L. $nCaF_2$+DMAHDM had (0.18 ± 0.005) mmol/L, and Heliomolar control had close to zero Ca ion release.

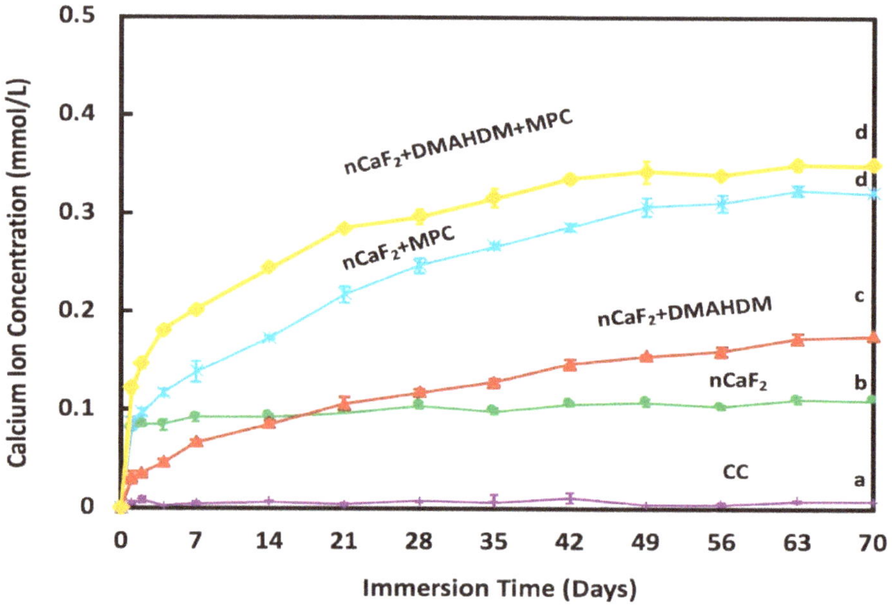

Figure 4. Calcium (Ca) ion release from composite resins (mean ± sd; $n = 6$) at pH 7.0. The incorporation of $nCaF_2$, DMAHDM, and MPC increased the release of Ca ions with time ($p < 0.05$). Different letters (a, b, c, d) indicate significant differences between groups at day 70 ($p < 0.05$).

Two-day biofilm colony forming units CFU on composites are shown in Figure 5: (A) Total microorganisms, (B) total streptococci and (C) mutans streptococci (mean ± SD; $n = 9$). CFU was reduced by 6 logs from a mean of 2.51×10^8 counts for Heliomolar control to 1.00×10^2 counts for the new $nCaF_2$+DMAHDM+MPC composite ($p < 0.05$). $nCaF_2$+DMAHDM reduced the CFU by 4 logs ($p < 0.05$). The combination of $nCaF_2$+DMAHDM+MPC yielded the smallest CFU counts.

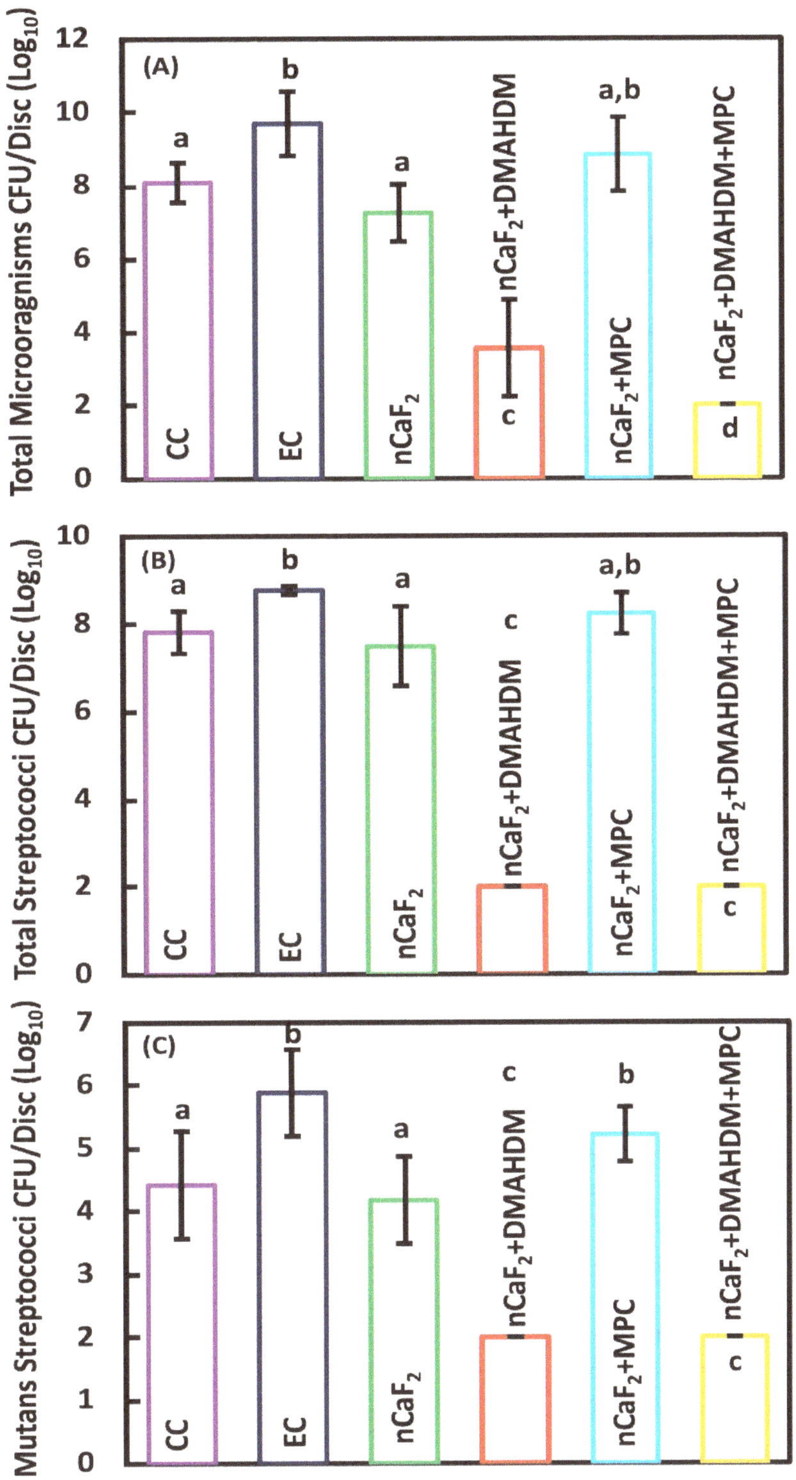

Figure 5. Colony-forming unit (CFU) counts of 2-day biofilm on composite discs (mean ± sd; $n = 9$): (**A**) Total microorganisms, (**B**) total streptococci, and (**C**) mutans streptococci (mean ± sd; $n = 9$).The incorporation of $nCaF_2$+DMAHDM+MPC had the lowest CFU, followed by $nCaF_2$+DMAHDM in the total microorganisms. The reduction of CFU in $nCaF_2$+DMAHDM+MPC and $nCaF_2$+DMAHDM was similar in total streptococci and mutans streptococci ($p < 0.05$). In each plot, different letters (a, b, c, d) indicate significant differences between groups ($p < 0.05$).

The bacterial metabolic activity of 2 days biofilm on composites is shown in Figure 6A. Metabolic activity was decreased from 0.18 (OD_{540}/cm^2) for commercial Heliomolar composite control, to 0.02 for the $nCaF_2$+DMAHDM+MPC composite ($p < 0.05$). Biofilm lactic acid production results can be seen in Figure 6B. The lactic acid production was reduced from 0.72 mmol/L on commercial Heliomolar control composite to 0.29 mmol/L in the $nCaF_2$+DMAHDM+MPC composite.

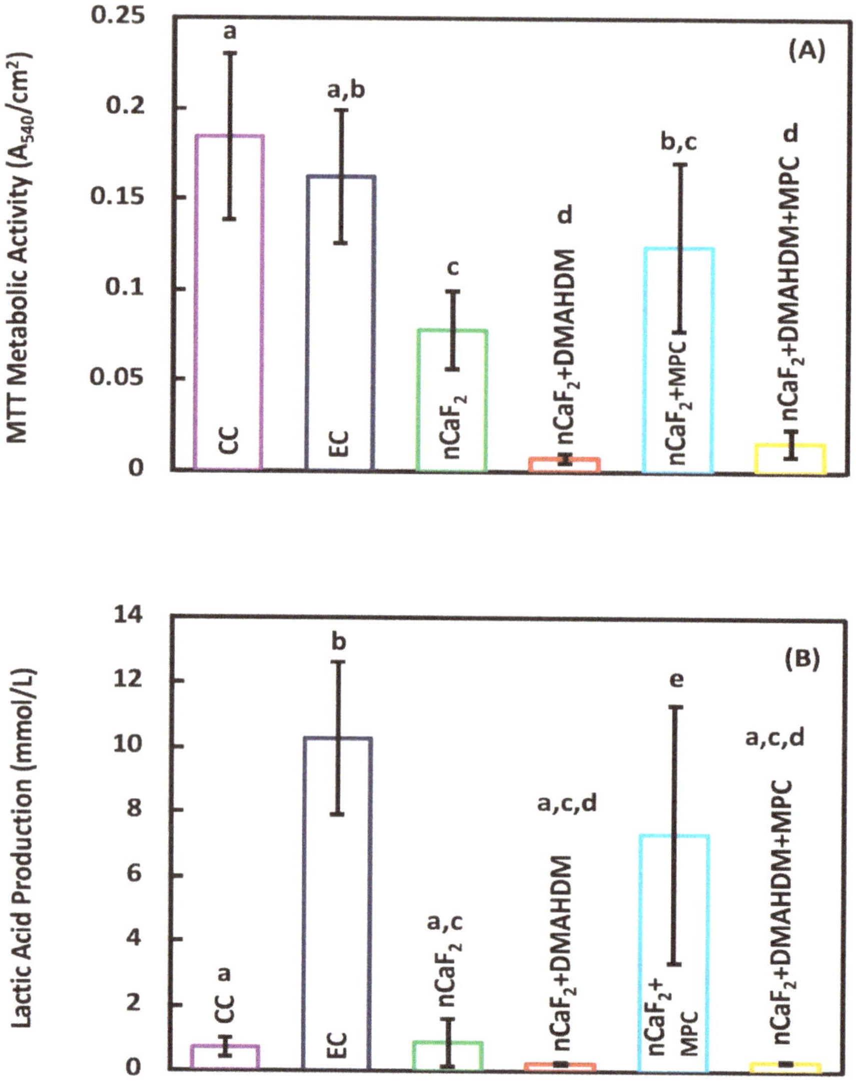

Figure 6. (**A**) The total metabolic activity, and (**B**) Lactic acid production (mean ± sd; $n = 9$) of composite specimens exposed to salivary biofilm. The incorporation of $nCaF_2$+ DMAHDM had the best reduction in the metabolic activity and lactic acid production ($p < 0.05$). In each plot, different letters (a, b, c, d) indicate significant differences between groups ($p < 0.05$).

SEM results in Figure 7 indicate an extensive biofilm formation at 24 h, 48 h, and 96 h in all groups except those containing the antimicrobial DMAHDM. Heliomolar (CC), experimental control (EC), and $nCaF_2$+MPC groups had the most biofilm formation at all time points, followed by the $nCaF_2$ group. Biofilm formation increased with time. However, in DMAHDM-containing groups there was minimal attachment of biofilm observed. At 96 h, the DMAHDM-containing groups showed a reduction in biofilm attachment compared with earlier time points.

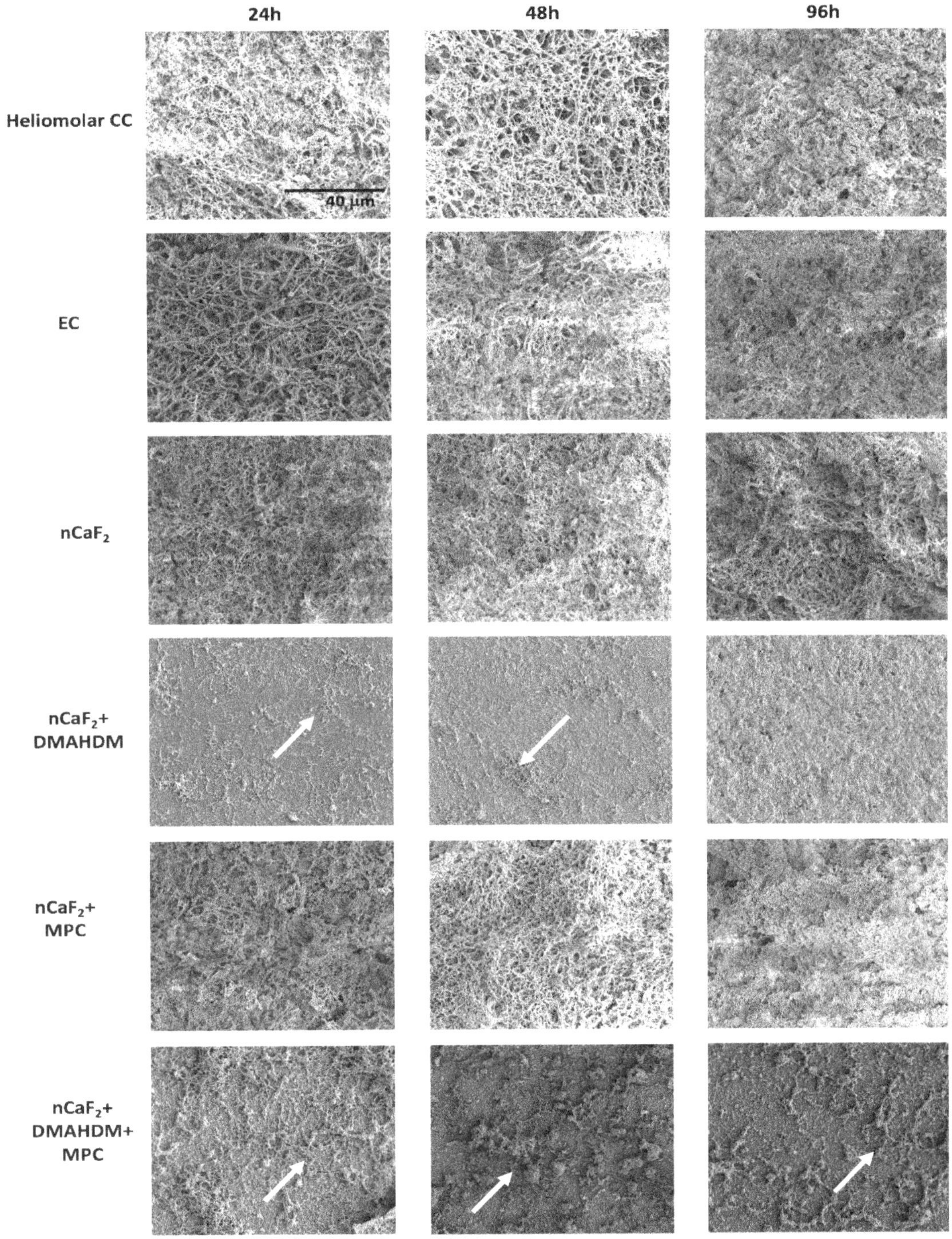

Figure 7. Scanning Electron Microscopy (SEM) images of biofilm formed on composite disc surfaces at 24 h, 48 h, and 96 h. All images are at 3000× magnification. Arrows indicate presence of minimal biofilm on DMAHDM-containing specimens. All other groups had full coverage of a substantial and mature biofilm.

5. Discussion

The present study developed a new composite consisting of $nCaF_2$, DMAHDM and MPC, and investigated the mechanical, ion release and oral biofilm properties. The protein-repellant $nCaF_2$+DMAHDM+MPC had slightly lower mechanical properties when compared to all other groups. However, $nCaF_2$+DMAHDM had good mechanical properties matching those of a commercial composite, while possessing high levels of F and Ca ion release and a strong antibacterial effect.

The new bioactive composite $nCaF_2$+DMAHDM decreased biofilm CFU by four orders of magnitude over that of commercial control composite, and substantially reduced acid production to inhibit caries.

Critical to the development of any new composite restorative material are its mechanical properties. The flexural strength of EC was around (170 ± 38) MPa. With the addition of 15% $nCaF_2$, the strength was reduced slightly to (157 ± 5) MPa. Those values are consistent with the results in a previous study [32]. The composite in that study had 65% total fillers and 20% CaF_2, similar to the 70% total fillers and 15% $nCaF_2$ composition in the present study. The flexural strength for the control group containing no $nCaF_2$ in the previous study was (145 ± 9) MPa, while the group which had 20% $nCaF_2$ had a flexural strength of 121 MPa. The $nCaF_2$+DMAHDM and $nCaF_2$+MPC had similar strengths of (95 ± 6), and (96 ± 5) MPa, respectively. Meanwhile, for $nCaF_2$+DMAHDM+MPC, the flexural strength was around (64 ±3) MPa. Those are similar to the results of a previous study using the same filler mass fraction where the flexural strength was around 90 MPa when 3% MPC and 3% DMAHDM were added to the BT resin [43]. The decreased strength in $nCaF_2$+DMAHDM+MPC could be due to two reasons. First, the BT base resin is composed of BisGMA and TEGDMA, which contain two reactive groups each. However, both DMAHDM and MPC are monomethacrylates and contain one reactive group. The addition of these monomethacrylates may substantially change the reaction kinetics and resulting crosslinked network, which can result in inferior mechanical properties. Another possible explanation for the decrease in mechanical properties is due to the hydrophilic nature of MPC. The specimens for flexural strength were stored for 24 h in water at 37 °C. The hydrophilicity of MPC makes it more likely that the composite would absorb water during the 24 h immersion prior to testing. This would likely lead to the reduction in flexural strength compared with the non-MPC groups.

Fluoride releasing materials have been known to render teeth more resistant to decay [45]. However, many available materials with fluoride-releasing properties, such as glass ionomer and resin modified glass ionomers, have inferior mechanical properties that do not serve the high load requirements for restorations in stress-bearing areas. Therefore, the incorporation of F ions into composite restorations would have the dual benefit of fluoride release and improved mechanical properties [46–48]. The current study synthesized $nCaF_2$ through a spray-drying method, which produced nanoparticles of CaF_2 with a median particle size of about 32 nm. The use of small amounts of $nCaF_2$ fillers prevented the mechanical properties to be compromised. As seen in previous studies, the use of fluoride fillers with larger particle sizes require higher mass fractions of fillers to achieve significant fluoride ion release. This would lead to a decrease in the composite mechanical properties [49].

The incorporation of nanoparticles with a high surface area resulted in the release of high levels of F and Ca ions using a low $nCaF_2$ filler level [33]. F ions foster remineralization by forming fluoroapatite [$Ca_5(PO_4)_3F$] [50]. Furthermore, it was shown that the lower the pH, the higher the release of ions. In this study, the release of F ions was significantly increased with the integration of 15% $nCaF_2$ at a pH of 7, measuring (0.04 ± 0.01) mmol/L. This was comparable to the 0.03 mmol/L F release level in a study that had a pH of 6, yet with an increased percentage of CaF_2 (23%) [51]. Groups containing MPC had the highest F ion release over time. The levels of release in $nCaF_2$+MPC and $nCaF_2$+DMAHDM+MPC were (0.40 ± 0.02) mmol/L and (0.25 ± 0.03) mmol/L, respectively. This could be due to the hydrophilic nature of MPC, resulting in a higher level of water uptake. As more water was absorbed by the composite, the Ca and F ions were solubilized, leading to an increase in the initial ion release. However, $nCaF_2$+DMAHDM F ion release was (0.20 ± 0.03) mmol/L, which was superior to the control. While the amount of $nCaF_2$ was the same in the two groups, the lower level of initial release in $nCaF_2$+DMAHDM, when compared to MPC containing groups, could result in a more sustained level of F ion release over a longer period. The releasing trend of F and Ca ions were the same for all groups. The groups containing $nCaF_2$ had a high F release initially, and subsequently were followed by a steady state release. The higher release of Ca and F ions in all $nCaF_2$ composites revealed that CaF_2 nanoparticles were fast released from the $nCaF_2$ composites because of the hydrolytic breakdown of the interface between the resin matrix and the CaF_2 nanoparticles. A likely explanation for such a trend is that the ions were released from the near-surface Ca and F reservoir of the $nCaF_2$ composite, and the reservoir near the surface diminished with the increase in immersion time. However, in clinical situations, the superficial layer of $nCaF_2$ would experience repeated chewing forces and tooth-brushing, hence the CaF_2-depleted surface would be removed by wear. As a result, a fresh surface would be exposed with the ability to further continue the calcium and fluoride release. Further studies are needed to investigate the outcome of wear on Ca and F ion release, as well as whether these materials can be made rechargeable to extend the lifetime of ion release.

Recurrent caries is considered a major drawback of composite restorations [1,52,53]. Studies proposed that the greater vulnerability to recurrent caries may be associated with the absence of composites' antibacterial capability when compared to other commonly used restorative materials such as glass ionomers and amalgams [2,54]. Therefore, the improvement of composites by incorporating antibacterial, protein repellent, and remineralizing properties is essential to lengthen the service life of composite restorations. DMAHDM has demonstrated strong antibacterial effects on an extensive antimicrobial spectrum through its contact-killing properties [26,55]. Since DMAHDM contains a reactive methacrylate group, it is copolymerized within the resin matrix, rendering it immobilized and preventing its release or loss over time [26,56]. Hence, its antibacterial capability is long-lasting. However, the antibacterial ability of DMAHDM is limited to biofilms that contact the composite surface [26], as biofilms that are not in contact with DMAHDM cannot be killed via DMAHDM's mechanism of action. Even with this limitation, the composite containing $nCaF_2$+DMAHDM substantially lowered the biofilm development and production of lactic acid, reducing the CFU of biofilm by 4 logs.

It can be seen in Figure 6B that the experimental control group and the group containing $nCaF_2$ and MPC exhibited a greater lactic acid production when compared with the other groups. DMAHDM has been shown in previous work to have a strong antibacterial effect, as illustrated by the CFU data in Figure 5. This antibacterial activity is reflected indirectly by the lactic acid production. When an *S mutans* biofilm accumulates, the secretion of lactic acid occurs. In the absence of a viable biofilm, the concentration of lactic acid is expected to be very low, as is the case in the DMAHDM-containing groups. Interestingly, the $nCaF_2$ and $nCaF_2$+MPC groups did not have a significant reduction in CFU (Figure 5), but the $nCaF_2$ group showed a significant reduction in lactic acid production in contrast to the $nCaF_2$+MPC group. Previously, it has been shown that the inclusion of CaF_2 in a composite formulation has a moderating effect on the lactic acid production [57]. It has been speculated that the F ion release helped reduce the acid production of the bacteria via the inhibition of metabolic pathways such as the fermentation pathway for lactic acid production, biofilm plaque, and hydrodynamic effects on mass transfer, fluoride delivery, and caries [58]. However, when MPC was added to the composite containing $nCaF_2$, there was no decrease in lactic acid production. This response may be related to the interactions between the calcium and fluoride ions and the phosphorylcholine fragment of MPC. The protein-repellent nature of MPC from the hydrogen bond network of water molecules surrounding the phosphorylcholine fragment limited the ability of the protein to adsorb on the surface. It was found, however, that the presence of halide ions (Cl^-, Br^-, I^-) influenced the hydrogen bond network and the diffusion through it [59]. It is possible that the presence of F^- ions would have a similar result, which may affect F ion diffusion and disrupt the creation of a protein-repellant coating, leading to biofilm formation.

SEM images in Figure 7 confirm the presence of substantial biofilm on all groups except those containing DMAHDM. At 24 h and 48 h, Heliomolar (CC), experimental control (EC), $nCaF_2$, and $nCaF_2$+MPC groups exhibited the formation of microcolonies and early biofilm multilayers. The biofilms on these groups at 96 h were fully mature, substantial, and dense. However, in DMAHDM-containing groups there was minimal attachment of biofilm observed. At 96 h the DMAHDM-containing groups showed a reduction in biofilm attachment compared to earlier time points. It is possible that the antimicrobial effect of DMAHDM as a contact-killing agent had eliminated the bacteria left on the samples over time. These results correlate very well with the CFU results.

It is possible that the salivary proteins adsorption on composite resin surfaces might reduce the effectiveness of this "contact-killing" mechanism. Therefore, a protein repellent agent was added. MPC is a methacrylate that contains phospholipid polar groups. MPC is highly hydrophilic and has been shown to decrease the adsorption of protein and reduce bacterial attachments [60]. Previous work indicated that integrating MPC into the resin decreased the adsorption of proteins by approximately one order of magnitude [43,61]. Additionally, it was shown that surfaces containing MPC were resistant to brushing mechanical stresses [62]. In this study, MPC was incorporated into the resin, and copolymerized into the composite resin. This is analogous to the process of incorporating DMAHDM, with a similar result of a stable, covalently bonded, and non-releasing functionality.

In the current study, the antibacterial capability of the experimental composite was improved with $nCaF_2$ and was further substantially improved with the use of both $nCaF_2$ and DMAHDM. However, the $nCaF_2$+MPC group showed no reduction in the CFU counts. The composite that had $nCaF_2$+DMAHDM+MPC displayed the most potent antibacterial effect with CFU 6 log biofilm reduction. Therefore, these results confirmed that the addition of DMAHDM is vital to improving the antibacterial effect. It is thought that DMAHDM serves to reduce the accumulation of biofilm and, as a result, improves the efficacy of MPC in resisting protein adsorption. However, in the absence of DMAHDM, the bacterial biofilm will accumulate and render MPC less effective.

The combination of $nCaF_2$+DMAHDM promoted remineralization and had a significant antibacterial effect. Another potential benefit of using $nCaF_2$ is that the release of F ions could act as a transmembrane proton carrier and an inhibitor to the glycolytic enzyme, thus preventing oral microorganisms by stimulating acidification of the cytoplasm and providing antibacterial effect at a long-distance to inhibit caries [10,63]. These properties would be highly valuable to inhibit recurrent caries around the margins of the restoration, since this is the location that most dental plaque tends to accumulate. In addition to its superior antibacterial and remineralization properties, the $nCaF_2$+DMAHDM composite exhibits excellent mechanical properties which make it suitable in a variety of restoration applications. In comparison, the composite consisting of $nCaF_2$+DMAHDM+MPC exhibited lower mechanical properties. However, the strength and modulus achieved by this group was still high enough to be used for restorations in low load areas such as class V restorations [37]. This is a critical area of utilization, since older patients tend to have exposed root surfaces that are more prone to caries. Further studies are needed to investigate the $nCaF_2$+DMAHDM combination in dental cements, bonding agents, fissure sealants, and composites to remineralize tooth lesions and suppress biofilm and plaque buildup, especially in patients with a high caries risk.

6. Conclusions

A novel composite with remineralization and antibacterial properties was established by combining $nCaF_2$+DMAHDM for the first time. Release of F and Ca ions from the composite was significantly achieved through the incorporation of $nCaF_2$. The new composite exhibited strong antibacterial and ion release capabilities, prevented biofilm production of lactic acid, and decreased biofilm CFU by 4 log. This bioactive nanocomposite is promising to protect tooth structures, inhibit demineralization, and provide a reservoir for the release of calcium and fluoride ions. The combined effect of $nCaF_2$+DMAHDM shows promise in a variety of dental applications where remineralization and prevention of recurrent caries is a priority.

Author Contributions: H.M. contributed to design, data acquisition, and analysis, and drafted the manuscript; A.A.B. contributed to data acquisition, and analysis; R.A. contributed to data acquisition and analysis; T.W.O. contributed to data interpretation and funding acquisition; M.A.S.M. contributed to data acquisition, analysis, and interpretation; H.H.K.X. contributed to conception, design, data interpretation and critically revised the manuscript; M.D.W. contributed to design, data acquisition, analysis, and interpretation, and critically revised the manuscript. All authors have read and agreed to the published version of the manuscript.

Acknowledgments: We thank Quan Dai, Jianghong Gao, Maria Ibrahim, Bashayer Baras, Pei Feng, Nancy J. Lin, Jirun Sun, and Laurence C. Chow for discussions and assistance. We thank the technical support of the Core Imaging Facility of the University of Maryland Baltimore. We are grateful to Dentsply Sirona (Milford, DE) for the donation of the glass fillers. This work was supported by The University of Maryland School of Dentistry bridge fund (HX) and University of Maryland seed grant (HX).

References

1. Ferracane, J.L. Resin composite—State of the art. *Dent. Mater.* **2011**, *27*, 29–38. [CrossRef]
2. Beyth, N.; Domb, A.J.; Weiss, E.I. An in vitro quantitative antibacterial analysis of amalgam and composite resins. *J. Dent.* **2007**, *35*, 201–206. [CrossRef] [PubMed]
3. Deligeorgi, V.; Mjör, I.A.; Wilson, N.H. An overview of reasons for the placement and replacement of restorations. *Prim. Dent. Care* **2001**, *8*, 5–11. [CrossRef] [PubMed]
4. Jokstad, A.; Bayne, S.; Blunck, U.; Tyas, M.; Wilson, N. Quality of dental restorations. FDI Commission Project 2-95. *Int. Dent. J.* **2001**, *51*, 117–158. [CrossRef]
5. Takahashi, N.; Nyvad, B. Ecological Hypothesis of Dentin and Root Caries. *Caries Res.* **2016**, *50*, 422–431. [CrossRef]
6. Kidd, E.A.M.; Fejerskov, O. What constitutes dental caries? Histopathology of carious enamel and dentin related to the action of cariogenic biofilms. *J. Dent. Res.* **2004**, *83*, C35–C38. [CrossRef]
7. Kidd, E. *Essentials of Dental Caries: The Disease and Its Management*, 3rd ed.; OUP Oxford: Oxford, UK, 2005; ISBN 978-0-19-852978-1.
8. Xu, X.; Ling, L.; Wang, R.; Burgess, J.O. Formulation and characterization of a novel fluoride-releasing dental composite. *Dent. Mater.* **2006**, *22*, 1014–1023. [CrossRef]
9. Xu, H.H.K.; Moreau, J.L.; Sun, L.; Chow, L.C. Novel CaF2 Nanocomposite with High Strength and Fluoride Ion Release. *J. Dent. Res.* **2010**, *89*, 739–745. [CrossRef]
10. Zheng, X.; Cheng, X.; Wang, L.; Qiu, W.; Wang, S.; Zhou, Y.; Li, M.; Li, Y.; Cheng, L.; Li, J.; et al. Combinatorial effects of arginine and fluoride on oral bacteria. *J. Dent. Res.* **2015**, *94*, 344–353. [CrossRef]
11. Koo, H. Strategies to enhance the biological effects of fluoride on dental biofilms. *Adv. Dent. Res.* **2008**, *20*, 17–21. [CrossRef]
12. Rošin-Grget, K. The cariostatic mechanisms of fluoride. *Acta Med. Acad.* **2013**, *42*, 179–188. [CrossRef]
13. ten Cate, J.M. Current concepts on the theories of the mechanism of action of fluoride. *Acta Odontol. Scand.* **1999**, *57*, 325–329. [CrossRef]
14. ten Cate, J.M. Contemporary perspective on the use of fluoride products in caries prevention. *Br. Dent. J.* **2013**, *214*, 161–167. [CrossRef]
15. Wojnarowska-Nowak, R.; Rzeszutko, J.; Barylyak, A.; Nechyporenko, G.; Zinchenko, V.; Leszczyńska, D.; Bobitski, Y.; Kus-Liśkiewicz, M. Structural, physical and antibacterial properties of pristine and Ag+ doped fluoroapatite nanomaterials. *Adv. Appl. Ceram.* **2017**, *116*, 108–117. [CrossRef]
16. Anastasiou, A.D.; Nerantzaki, M.; Gounari, E.; Duggal, M.S.; Giannoudis, P.V.; Jha, A.; Bikiaris, D. Antibacterial properties and regenerative potential of Sr2+ and Ce3+ doped fluorapatites; a potential solution for peri-implantitis. *Sci. Rep.* **2019**, *9*. [CrossRef]
17. Imazato, S.; Russell, R.R.; McCabe, J.F. Antibacterial activity of MDPB polymer incorporated in dental resin. *J. Dent.* **1995**, *23*, 177–181. [CrossRef]
18. Imazato, S.; Ehara, A.; Torii, M.; Ebisu, S. Antibacterial activity of dentine primer containing MDPB after curing. *J. Dent.* **1998**, *26*, 267–271. [CrossRef]
19. Imazato, S. Bio-active restorative materials with antibacterial effects: New dimension of innovation in restorative dentistry. *Dent. Mater. J.* **2009**, *28*, 11–19. [CrossRef]
20. Imazato, S.; Torii, M.; Tsuchitani, Y.; McCabe, J.F.; Russell, R.R. Incorporation of bacterial inhibitor into resin composite. *J. Dent. Res.* **1994**, *73*, 1437–1443. [CrossRef]
21. Beyth, N.; Yudovin-Farber, I.; Perez-Davidi, M.; Domb, A.J.; Weiss, E.I. Polyethyleneimine nanoparticles incorporated into resin composite cause cell death and trigger biofilm stress in vivo. *Proc. Natl. Acad. Sci. USA* **2010**, *107*, 22038–22043. [CrossRef]
22. Jiao, Y.; Tay, F.R.; Niu, L.-N.; Chen, J.-H. Advancing antimicrobial strategies for managing oral biofilm infections. *Int. J. Oral Sci.* **2019**, *11*, 28. [CrossRef] [PubMed]

23. Imazato, S. Antibacterial properties of resin composites and dentin bonding systems. *Dent. Mater.* **2003**, *19*, 449–457. [CrossRef]
24. Faust, D.; Dolado, I.; Cuadrado, A.; Oesch, F.; Weiss, C.; Nebreda, A.R.; Dietrich, C. p38alpha MAPK is required for contact inhibition. *Oncogene* **2005**, *24*, 7941–7945. [CrossRef] [PubMed]
25. Li, F.; Weir, M.D.; Xu, H.H.K. Effects of quaternary ammonium chain length on antibacterial bonding agents. *J. Dent. Res.* **2013**, *92*, 932–938. [CrossRef]
26. Beyth, N.; Yudovin-Farber, I.; Bahir, R.; Domb, A.J.; Weiss, E.I. Antibacterial activity of dental composites containing quaternary ammonium polyethylenimine nanoparticles against Streptococcus mutans. *Biomaterials* **2006**, *27*, 3995–4002. [CrossRef]
27. Namba, N.; Yoshida, Y.; Nagaoka, N.; Takashima, S.; Matsuura-Yoshimoto, K.; Maeda, H.; Van Meerbeek, B.; Suzuki, K.; Takashiba, S. Antibacterial effect of bactericide immobilized in resin matrix. *Dent. Mater.* **2009**, *25*, 424–430. [CrossRef]
28. Müller, R.; Eidt, A.; Hiller, K.-A.; Katzur, V.; Subat, M.; Schweikl, H.; Imazato, S.; Ruhl, S.; Schmalz, G. Influences of protein films on antibacterial or bacteria-repellent surface coatings in a model system using silicon wafers. *Biomaterials* **2009**, *30*, 4921–4929. [CrossRef]
29. Xie, X.; Wang, L.; Xing, D.; Zhang, K.; Weir, M.D.; Liu, H.; Bai, Y.; Xu, H.H.K. Novel dental adhesive with triple benefits of calcium phosphate recharge, protein-repellent and antibacterial functions. *Dent. Mater.* **2017**, *33*, 553–563. [CrossRef]
30. Zhang, N.; Weir, M.D.; Romberg, E.; Bai, Y.; Xu, H.H.K. Development of novel dental adhesive with double benefits of protein-repellent and antibacterial capabilities. *Dent. Mater.* **2015**, *31*, 845–854. [CrossRef]
31. Zhou, H.; Li, F.; Weir, M.D.; Xu, H.H.K. Dental plaque microcosm response to bonding agents containing quaternary ammonium methacrylates with different chain lengths and charge densities. *J. Dent.* **2013**, *41*, 1122–1131. [CrossRef]
32. Xu, H.H.K.; Moreau, J.L.; Sun, L.; Chow, L.C. Strength and fluoride release characteristics of a calcium fluoride based dental nanocomposite. *Biomaterials* **2008**, *29*, 4261–4267. [CrossRef] [PubMed]
33. Weir, M.D.; Moreau, J.L.; Levine, E.D.; Strassler, H.D.; Chow, L.C.; Xu, H.H.K. Nanocomposite containing CaF2 nanoparticles: Thermal cycling, wear and long-term water-aging. *Dent. Mater.* **2012**, *28*, 642–652. [CrossRef] [PubMed]
34. Sun, L.; Chow, L.C. Preparation and properties of nano-sized calcium fluoride for dental applications. *Dent. Mater.* **2008**, *24*, 111–116. [CrossRef]
35. Trujillo-Lemon, M.; Ge, J.; Lu, H.; Tanaka, J.; Stansbury, J.W. Dimethacrylate derivatives of dimer acid. *J. Polym. Sci. Part A Polym. Chem.* **2006**, *44*, 3921–3929. [CrossRef]
36. Xu, H.H.K.; Moreau, J.L.; Sun, L.; Chow, L.C. Nanocomposite containing amorphous calcium phosphate nanoparticles for caries inhibition. *Dent. Mater.* **2011**, *27*, 762–769. [CrossRef]
37. ISO 4049:200.9. *Dentistry—Polymer-Based Restorative Materials*; International Organization for Standardization: Geneva, Switzerland, 2009.
38. Xu, H.H.K.; Weir, M.D.; Sun, L.; Takagi, S.; Chow, L.C. Effects of calcium phosphate nanoparticles on Ca-PO4 composite. *J. Dent. Res.* **2007**, *86*, 378–383. [CrossRef]
39. Skrtic, D.; Antonucci, J.M.; Eanes, E.D. Improved properties of amorphous calcium phosphate fillers in remineralizing resin composites. *Dent. Mater.* **1996**, *12*, 295–301. [CrossRef]
40. Wang, L.; Xie, X.; Li, C.; Liu, H.; Zhang, K.; Zhou, Y.; Chang, X.; Xu, H.H.K. Novel bioactive root canal sealer to inhibit endodontic multispecies biofilms with remineralizing calcium phosphate ions. *J. Dent.* **2017**, *60*, 25–35. [CrossRef]
41. Xie, X.; Wang, L.; Xing, D.; Arola, D.D.; Weir, M.D.; Bai, Y.; Xu, H.H.K. Protein-repellent and antibacterial functions of a calcium phosphate rechargeable nanocomposite. *J. Dent.* **2016**, *52*, 15–22. [CrossRef]
42. McBain, A.J. In Vitro Biofilm Models: An Overview. In *Advances in Applied Microbiology*; Elsevier: Cambridge, MA, USA, 2009; Volume 69, pp. 99–132.
43. Zhang, N.; Ma, J.; Melo, M.A.S.; Weir, M.D.; Bai, Y.; Xu, H.H.K. Protein-repellent and antibacterial dental composite to inhibit biofilms and caries. *J. Dent.* **2015**, *43*, 225–234. [CrossRef]
44. Al-Dulaijan, Y.A.; Cheng, L.; Weir, M.D.; Melo, M.A.S.; Liu, H.; Oates, T.W.; Wang, L.; Xu, H.H.K. Novel rechargeable calcium phosphate nanocomposite with antibacterial activity to suppress biofilm acids and dental caries. *J. Dent.* **2018**, *72*, 44–52. [CrossRef] [PubMed]

45. Deng, D.M.; van Loveren, C.; ten Cate, J.M. Caries-preventive agents induce remineralization of dentin in a biofilm model. *Caries Res.* **2005**, *39*, 216–223. [CrossRef] [PubMed]
46. Kus-Liśkiewicz, M.; Rzeszutko, J.; Bobitski, Y.; Barylyak, A.; Nechyporenko, G.; Zinchenko, V.; Zebrowski, J. Alternative Approach for Fighting Bacteria and Fungi: Use of Modified Fluorapatite. *J. Biomed. Nanotechnol.* **2019**, *15*, 848–855. [CrossRef] [PubMed]
47. Montazeri, N.; Jahandideh, R.; Biazar, E. Synthesis of fluorapatite–hydroxyapatite nanoparticles and toxicity investigations. *Int. J. Nanomed.* **2011**, *6*, 197–201. [CrossRef]
48. Wiegand, A.; Buchalla, W.; Attin, T. Review on fluoride-releasing restorative materials—Fluoride release and uptake characteristics, antibacterial activity and influence on caries formation. *Dent. Mater.* **2007**, *23*, 343–362. [CrossRef]
49. Balhaddad, A.A.; Kansara, A.A.; Hidan, D.; Weir, M.D.; Xu, H.H.K.; Melo, M.A.S. Toward dental caries: Exploring nanoparticle-based platforms and calcium phosphate compounds for dental restorative materials. *Bioact. Mater.* **2019**, *4*, 43–55. [CrossRef]
50. Lata, S.; Varghese, N.O.; Varughese, J.M. Remineralization potential of fluoride and amorphous calcium phosphate-casein phospho peptide on enamel lesions: An in vitro comparative evaluation. *J. Conserv. Dent.* **2010**, *13*, 42–46. [CrossRef]
51. Anusavice, K.J.; Zhang, N.-Z.; Shen, C. Effect of CaF2 content on rate of fluoride release from filled resins. *J. Dent. Res.* **2005**, *84*, 440–444. [CrossRef]
52. Sakaguchi, R.L. Review of the current status and challenges for dental posterior restorative composites: Clinical, chemistry, and physical behavior considerations. Summary of discussion from the Portland Composites Symposium (POCOS) June 17–19, 2004, Oregon Health and Science University, Portland, Oregon. *Dent. Mater.* **2005**, *21*, 3–6. [CrossRef]
53. Demarco, F.F.; Corrêa, M.B.; Cenci, M.S.; Moraes, R.R.; Opdam, N.J.M. Longevity of posterior composite restorations: Not only a matter of materials. *Dent. Mater.* **2012**, *28*, 87–101. [CrossRef]
54. Nedeljkovic, I.; Teughels, W.; De Munck, J.; Van Meerbeek, B.; Van Landuyt, K.L. Is secondary caries with composites a material-based problem? *Dent. Mater.* **2015**, *31*, e247–e277. [CrossRef] [PubMed]
55. Imazato, S.; Ebi, N.; Takahashi, Y.; Kaneko, T.; Ebisu, S.; Russell, R.R.B. Antibacterial activity of bactericide-immobilized filler for resin-based restoratives. *Biomaterials* **2003**, *24*, 3605–3609. [CrossRef]
56. Xu, X.; Wang, Y.; Liao, S.; Wen, Z.T.; Fan, Y. Synthesis and characterization of antibacterial dental monomers and composites. *J. Biomed. Mater. Res. Part B Appl. Biomater.* **2012**, *100B*, 1151–1162. [CrossRef]
57. Cheng, L.; Weir, M.D.; Xu, H.H.K.; Kraigsley, A.M.; Lin, N.J.; Lin-Gibson, S.; Zhou, X. Antibacterial and physical properties of calcium-phosphate and calcium-fluoride nanocomposites with chlorhexidine. *Dent. Mater.* **2012**, *28*, 573–583. [CrossRef]
58. Stoodley, P.; Wefel, J.; Gieseke, A.; Debeer, D.; von Ohle, C. Biofilm plaque and hydrodynamic effects on mass transfer, fluoride delivery and caries. *J. Am. Dent. Assoc.* **2008**, *139*, 1182–1190. [CrossRef]
59. Zhang, Z.J.; Madsen, J.; Warren, N.J.; Mears, M.; Leggett, G.J.; Lewis, A.L.; Geoghegan, M. Influence of salt on the solution dynamics of a phosphorylcholine-based polyzwitterion. *Eur. Polym. J.* **2017**, *87*, 449–457. [CrossRef]
60. Sibarani, J.; Takai, M.; Ishihara, K. Surface modification on microfluidic devices with 2-methacryloyloxyethyl phosphorylcholine polymers for reducing unfavorable protein adsorption. *Colloids Surf. B Biointerfaces* **2007**, *54*, 88–93. [CrossRef]
61. Zhang, N.; Chen, C.; Melo, M.A.; Bai, Y.-X.; Cheng, L.; Xu, H.H. A novel protein-repellent dental composite containing 2-methacryloyloxyethyl phosphorylcholine. *Int. J. Oral Sci.* **2015**, *7*, 103–109. [CrossRef]
62. Tateishi, T.; Kyomoto, M.; Kakinoki, S.; Yamaoka, T.; Ishihara, K. Reduced platelets and bacteria adhesion on poly(ether ether ketone) by photoinduced and self-initiated graft polymerization of 2-methacryloyloxyethyl phosphorylcholine. *J. Biomed. Mater. Res. A* **2014**, *102*, 1342–1349. [CrossRef]
63. Van Loveren, C. Antimicrobial activity of fluoride and its in vivo importance: Identification of research questions. *Caries Res.* **2001**, *35* (Suppl. S1), 65–70. [CrossRef]

14

Use of Protein Repellents to Enhance the Antimicrobial Functionality of Quaternary Ammonium Containing Dental Materials

Leopoldo Torres Jr and Diane R. Bienek *

ADA Science & Research Institute, LLC, Innovative & Technology Research, Frederick, MD 21704, USA; torresl@ada.org

* Correspondence: bienekd@ada.org

Abstract: An advancement in preventing secondary caries has been the incorporation of quaternary ammonium containing (QAC) compounds into a composite resin mixture. The permanent positive charge on the monomers allows for electrostatic-based killing of bacteria. Spontaneous adsorption of salivary proteins onto restorations dampens the antimicrobial capabilities of QAC compounds. Protein-repellent monomers can work with QAC restorations to achieve the technology's full potential. We discuss the theory behind macromolecular adsorption, direct and indirect characterization methods, and advances of protein repellent dental materials. The translation of protein adsorption to microbial colonization is covered, and the concerns and fallbacks of the state-of-the-art protein-resistant monomers are addressed. Last, we present new and exciting avenues for protein repellent monomer design that have yet to be explored in dental materials.

Keywords: protein repellent; restorations; zwitterionic polymers; dental materials; antimicrobial; antifouling

---

1. Introduction

Tooth decay, also known as dental caries, is one of the most prevalent infections globally that afflicts both the developed and developing world. It affects young and old at large percentages, while being a preventable disease. Due to the high incidence of patient affliction, the economic toll is large in the US, approximately $442 billion [1]. To combat caries, clinicians remove the decayed tissue and replace with restorative materials. These composite materials consist of a stiff polymeric matrix (e.g., bisphenol A-glycidyl methacrylate (BisGMA) [2], urethane dimethacrylate [3], or methacryl polyhedral oligomeric silsesquioxane [4,5]) and inorganic filler components (i.e., amorphous calcium phosphate nanoparticles [6], borosilicate microparticles [7], and hydroxyapatite [8]). Additional problems arise from secondary caries, subsequent infections beneath or in the micro-cracks of the composite [9]. This occurs up to 44% for all adult patients and could be mitigated by antimicrobial technologies [10].

Integration of polymerizable antimicrobial methacrylates in dental resin offers the benefit of providing lasting antimicrobial activity, while being chemically stable. Specifically, quaternary ammonium containing (QAC) monomers have been incorporated into dental resins, to enable contact-killing of microorganisms. This concept was first introduced in 1993 by Imazato et al. [11]. Briefly, a quaternary ammonium compound, 12-methacryloyloxydodecylpyridinium bromide (MDPB), was incorporated into a resin, to formulate an antimicrobial composite [12]. Reports have indicated that QAC compounds destroy bacterial cell membrane integrity and eventually lead to cell death [13–15].

The design of these monomers has been heavily studied to optimize antimicrobial capabilities and elucidate the mechanism of bacterial killing [16]. For example, Li and coworkers synthesized QAC monomers with varying carbon lengths, following the positive quaternary amine, to enhance the insertion of the dangling monomer into the *Streptococcus mutans* membrane [17]. Another strategy has been to investigate monomers with varying degrees of flexibility, for improved incorporation into the bacterial membrane. The effect of alkyl chain length on antimicrobial properties of monomethacrylate monomers suggested a rise in antibacterial activity with the increasing alkyl chain [18,19]. However, the antimicrobial efficacy–structure relationships are not strictly linear. For instance, the longer chain length of novel adhesive methacrylate dental monomers had a less marked effect on reducing *S. mutans* biofilms [20]. Furthermore, when drawing conclusions about chain length, it is important to consider that antimicrobial functionality is also affected by molecular mass, spacer rigidity, hydrophobicity, charge density, and charge distribution [21,22]. Since the first Imazato and coworkers' QAC resin manuscript, advances have been made in synthesizing QAC monomers with dual functionality, such as increased shear bond strength [20,23,24] and silane-coupling capabilities [25–27]. Similarly, other antimicrobial approaches have been studied in dentistry, including metallic nanoparticles with inherent bactericidal properties [28] and are not discussed in this review.

While previous studies on QAC dental materials are significant, their impact has been dampened by the reduction in antimicrobial efficacy due to protein adsorption [29]. Salivary proteins form a thin coating onto the enamel surface, called the pellicle [30]. The pellicle allows for the attachment of early colonizing bacteria [31]. Many bacterial species possess surface structures (i.e., fimbriae and fibrils), which facilitate their attachment [32]. In the early stages of biofilm formation, planktonic bacteria directly attach to surfaces or indirectly bind to other bacteria that have already colonized [33]. Acidic and high-molecular-weight mucin fractions, acidic proline-rich proteins, and a multidomain glycosylated protein of the salivary pellicle are reported to bind bacteria and adhere to the non-native surface, to support biofilm attachment at the composite–adhesive–tooth interfaces [34]. The proteins and pathogens (and their interactions) attributing to failure at the composite–tooth interfaces have been presented in an elegant review [35]. After attachment, the bacterial cells proliferate, form microcolonies, and mature. Generally, biofilms can be morphologically heterogeneous 3D structures with the shape affected by spatiotemporal stress [36]. The 3D biofilm structures can be interspersed with bacteria-free channels used as diffusion pathways [32]. Dental caries and periodontal disease are a net result of the cross-talk between pathogenic dental-plaque biofilm and the host-tissue response [36]. While clinical examination and X-rays are commonly used to diagnose oral disease, advancement of salivary biomarkers and metaproteomic analyses of the oral microbiota may be exploited for future diagnosis of opportunistic and infectious disease [37].

To improve the antimicrobial properties of QAC monomers, protein-repellent functionality should be incorporated to prevent the extent of adsorption that current restorations experience (Figure 1). To accomplish this, the dental-material community has implemented approaches from the surface-science and blood-contacting material literature. Much of the recent literature has focused on 2-methacryloyloxyethyl phosphorylcholine (MPC), a commercially available and U.S. Food and Drug Administration-cleared zwitterionic polymer with well-studied protein-repellent capability.

The objective of this review is to focus on (1) the theoretical and practical considerations of protein adsorption; (2) methods to quantify protein adsorption; and (3) protein repelling functionality in dental restoratives and mouthwash technologies. Moreover, we also identify challenges with commonly used protein repellants and consider the potential of developing novel monomers.

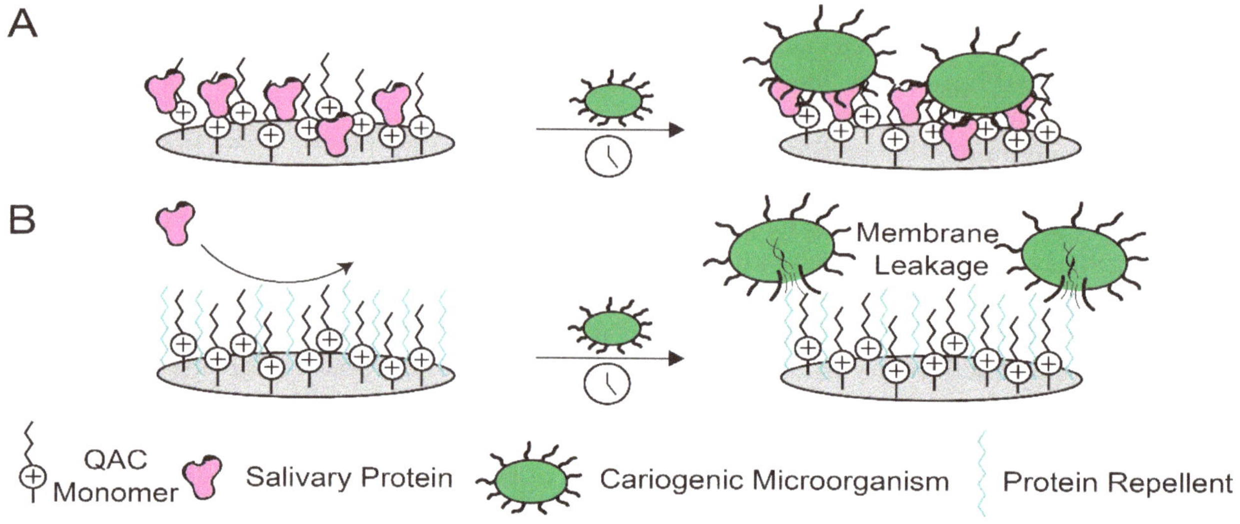

Figure 1. Dual functional dental materials enable contact-killing of cariogenic microorganisms by repelling proteins and disrupting bacterial membranes via charged interactions. (**A**) Salivary proteins adsorb to quaternary ammonium-containing (QAC) monomers, inhibiting their long-term antimicrobial properties. (**B**) Protein-repellent molecules work with QAC monomers to disrupt the formation of biofilms.

2. Theoretical and Practical Considerations for Protein Adsorption

Protein adsorption is a spontaneous process arising from a contribution of electrostatic and hydrophobic interactions, or hydrogen bonding [38]. Net charges on proteins can electrostatically bond with surfaces that are oppositely charged. This process can be reversed as the pH is altered, owing to the proteins pKa [39]. Additionally, hydrophobic regions of proteins can unravel (face outward) to bond with hydrophobic surfaces, minimizing the interactions between water and salivary proteins and between the surface and salivary proteins [40]. Lastly, both proteins and dental materials can participate in hydrogen bonding with each other if that is more favorable than surface solvation interactions [41].

Understanding the mechanisms of adsorption has led to the development of design principles for protein-repellent materials. The Whitesides group in 1993 reported a method for fabricating self-assembled monolayers (SAMs) as a tool to study protein adsorption [42]. These SAMs consisted of densely packed alkylthiol molecules that aligned parallel with one another on the surface of gold substrates. The tail end of the alkylthiol molecules were terminated with a functional group that could be covalently bonded to a chemical group of interest. Surface Plasmon Resonance (SPR) was coupled with a SAMs device to quantify the adsorption, observed as a change in frequency of the plasmon resonance. Their group subsequently followed their initial article with a survey of chemical structure relationship on adsorption, for which they reported four distinct rules for effective protein-repellent surfaces: The surface exposed monomers should be (1) hydrophilic; (2) contain hydrogen bond acceptors; (3) have no hydrogen bond donors; and (4) be electrically neutral [43–45]. Poly(ethylene glycol) (PEG)-based polymers [46] and many zwitterions [47] fall into this set of criteria and have been widely used for coatings in blood-contacting materials and implants.

In practice, additional considerations need to be taken into account to ensure effective protein repelling. The findings of the Whitesides' group can only translate if a critical density of antifouling monomers is on the surface of the material. Surface-coating treatment of protein-repellent monomers will not be as effective in dentistry, due to the formation of micro-cracks in composite materials produced during polymerization shrinkage [3]. These cracks are susceptible to bacterial colonization and consequently secondary caries, which are largely responsible for the failure of composite fillings [10]. It is imperative that dental materials contain protein-repellent molecules on their surface and in the bulk without (or minor) effect on the mechanical properties. In the same vein, researchers have developed hydrogels with protein-repellent monomers incorporated in the bulk and surface [48–50]. Last, the QAC monomers have functional groups that inherently adsorb proteins more readily. Specifically, the charged quaternary amine will participate in electrostatic interactions with proteins, leading toward adsorption. The long alkyl chain in many QAC monomers will also aid in hydrophobic–hydrophobic interactions, causing unfavorable adsorption. Therefore, dental materials require sufficient coverage of protein-repellent monomers to minimize attractive forces between proteins and QAC monomers.

3. Characterization Methods for Quantifying Protein Adsorption

Several techniques and assays have been developed to study the degree of protein coating on material surfaces (Figure 2). These methods range in sensitivity and each have trade-offs and should be considered for studying the adsorption of protein on dental materials. A comprehensive guide to characterization techniques for protein adsorption can be found in a previous article [51].

The most sensitive techniques (able to detect 1 ng to 1 μg of protein) commonly utilized are SPR or quartz crystal microbalance (QCM). Both analyze the surface of a small (<5 × 5 mm) substrate that is functionalized with a protein repellent of interest. Samples are prepared by coating or chemically functionalizing the surface with the protein repellent of interest. By preparing a thin sample, the interactions between a protein solution and protein-repellent monomer can be probed. In a typical SPR detection apparatus, a thin gold-coated slide is coated with the monomer of interest [42,52]. The slide is mounted, glass side down, onto a prism, and the functionalized side is used as part of a microfluidic channel. A light source with narrow range emission is projected through the prism and glass slide and reflected off the thin gold layer. A detector collects the angle of the reflected light, which corresponds to the index of refraction of the functionalized gold layer. When a protein solution flows onto the functionalized surface, the index of refraction increases, causing the angle of the reflected light to change. This change can then be used to calculate the mass of protein on the surface of the substrate.

QCM devices implement a piezoelectric functionalized substrate [53–55]. When a current is applied to the substrate, the material vibrates at a frequency proportional to its mass. The piezoelectric material surface is coated or chemically bonded with a material of interest, to probe how much protein adsorbs to the material surface. These substrates are incorporated into microfluidic devices that flow protein solutions onto the substrate surface and are coupled with real-time sensing. When proteins adsorb onto the substrate, the frequency at which it vibrates changes. This change in frequency is converted to the mass of protein adsorbed to the substrate. QCM can be used to yield dynamic properties of adsorbed proteins, such as revealing changes to the salivary pellicle on hydroxyapatite surfaces when various detergents are flowed over the substrates [56]. In addition to monitoring protein adsorption, QCM has been used to probe the formation of biofilms and bacterial death in a clinically relevant microorganism model [57]. SPR and QCM techniques are useful for protein interactions with high-density surfaces and are best for studying low adsorption, as they saturate with milligram quantities of protein.

Dental composite materials exhibit polymerization stress, causing the composite to crack when curing [3]. These cracks expose the bulk, leaving sites for adsorption without a surface-modified layer. A more practical method for detection of protein adsorption is through colorimetric analysis of protein solution surrounding a dental material. Biochemical assays such as the bicinchoninic acid (BCA), Lowry protein, or Bradford assay utilize reagents that alter their visible-light absorbance upon reacting with a protein in solution. In this regard, three protocol variations have been widely used by the dental materials community. A material sample is submerged in a protein solution for a predetermined time. (1) The material is rinsed with saline solution, to remove non-adsorbed proteins, and the adsorbed protein is removed by rinsing the material with a sodium dodecyl sulfate (SDS) solution. This SDS solution is then used in a colorimetric assay [58]. While this method is the most used in the dental material literature, a comprehensive investigation determined that SDS rinsing does not adequately remove adsorbed proteins [59]. This may lead researchers to conclude a protein-repelling capacity that is inaccurate. (2) In lieu of rinsing the material with SDS to remove the adsorbed protein, the protein solution and material can be vortexed to remove non-adsorbed proteins, and the protein solution surrounding the material is analyzed. This method yields quantification of the remaining solution compared to the initial starting concentration. (3) A small sample of protein solution is placed on a flat, clear, and polymerized dental resin. After the desired time, the non-adherent protein is removed by rinsing with saline. The material is then submerged in the reagents of a colorimetric assay, allowing the adsorbed proteins to react with the assay reagents. The optical density at the assays absorbance wavelength is then performed to quantify the adsorbed proteins [60,61].

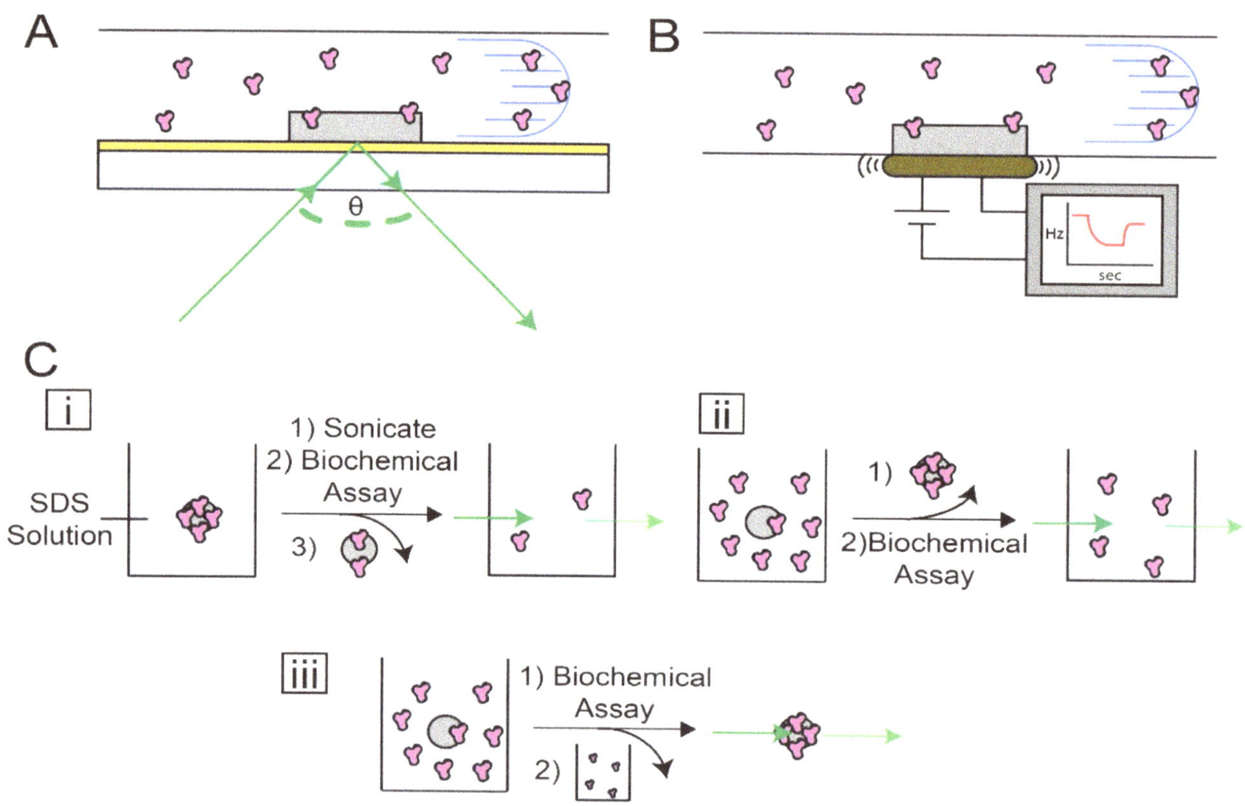

Figure 2. Characterization methods for quantifying protein adsorption on dental materials. (**A**) A general Surface Plasmon Resonance (SPR) device setup. Protein solution is flowed through a microfluidic channel and onto the material of interest bonded to a thin gold layer. Light is projected through a prism and onto the gold layer to discern protein–material interactions. (**B**) A general quartz crystal microbalance (QCM) device setup. The material of interest is fabricated onto a piezoelectric sensor. As protein accumulates onto the material, the vibration frequency changes. (**C**) Colorimetric methods for quantifying protein adsorption. (**i**) A disk with protein adsorbed to the surface is placed into a sodium dodecyl sulfate (SDS) buffer, to remove the protein. This solution is then analyzed by using an amino acid colorimetric reactive dye. (**ii**) A material of interest is placed in a protein solution of known concentration. After some time, the material is removed, and the remaining solution is analyzed. (**iii**) A material is placed in protein solution and is removed from the solution after a desired time point. The material with adsorbed protein is placed in a solution with colorimetric reagents, and the optical density is measured.

Topographical features and visualization of adsorption are important in understanding the growth of biofilm formation on dental materials. Looking toward the future, dental materials researchers should explore atomic force microscopy as a characterization tool. This technique probes the surface of materials, using a cantilever tip (100 nm–100 μm) and a laser to gauge the position of the tip, producing geometric information of a material [62]. Few dental material groups have explored the use of atomic force microscopy. to visualize protein adsorption on the surface [63]. Information that could be useful to researchers include the homogeneity of the adsorption layer, thickness of the adsorption layer, and force required to break bonds between the material surface and adsorbed proteins.

4. Dental Materials with Protein-Repellent Functionality

MPC is a methacrylate zwitterionic polymer that contains a negatively charged phosphorylcholine and a positively charged quaternary ammonium head. It is the most investigated molecule for protein-repelling dental materials [47,64,65]. It blends well into BisGMA/triethylene glycol methacrylate (TEGMA) and other hydrophilic resins. It was first introduced in the dental material literature by the Xu group in 2015 as an additive to a 50:50 BisGMA and TEGMA (BT) resin with dimethylaminohexyadecyl methacrylate (DMAHDM) and barium boroaluminosilicate filler [58]. The authors found that, out of various compositions investigated, a 3% (wt/wt) MPC and 1.5% (wt/wt) DMAHDM composite demonstrated nine times less bovine serum albumin (BSA) adsorption (~1 $\mu g/cm^2$), compared to the commercial control. For this composition, the flexural strength decreased from 100 to 80 MPa and elastic modulus from 6.7 to 6.5 MPa, compared to the resin without MPC. Oral biofilms, derived from the saliva of human donors, were cultured on the composites, to assess the antimicrobial capabilities of the MPC composites, with and without DMAHDM. Compared to the commercial control, a 3% MPC composite exhibited an order of magnitude lower total microorganisms, while the 3% MPC + 1.5% DMAHDM exhibited a three order of magnitude decrease of total microorganisms. This result demonstrated that the full potential of QAC resins could be realized with the addition of MPC.

The Xu lab continued their efforts into investigating the capability of MPC in many facets of materials in dentistry. A subsequent article optimized the addition of MPC into BT resins to identify a formulation with high protein repellency, without compromising the mechanical properties of the material [66]. They demonstrated that the flexural strength and elastic modulus suffer with materials containing 4.5% MPC and above. Specifically, the 4.5% MPC composite exhibited a flexural strength decrease to ~60 MPa compared to ~85 MPa in the case of the control. Moreover, the elastic modulus decreased to 5 MPa, compared to 6 MPa, as it was with the control. In a BSA adsorption assay, the researchers reported that a 3% MPC sample decreased the amount adsorbed by 85%, as compared to a polymerized BT sample. This same formulation also exhibited eight times fewer total microorganisms compared to the BT control.

MPC was then incorporated into a dental primer, to establish whether it could be useful as a restoration [67]. In conjunction with DMAHDM, MPC mixed into a commercial dental bond primer (3M Scotchbond Multi-Purpose Adhesive and Primer). A 7.5% MPC composite demonstrated less than 1 $\mu g/cm^2$ of protein adsorption, nearly 10 times less than the control. The same formulation had a comparable dentin shear bond strength, at ~27 MPa, compared to the control, at ~33 MPa. The degree of conversion was minimally impacted in all the formulations tested, indicating that MPC blends well with conventional dental resins. Last, the 7.5% MPC formulation was the most effective at reducing the total microbial count, by four orders of magnitude lower than the primer control. A follow-up investigation with amorphous calcium phosphate nanoparticles as the filler revealed that the shear bond strength decreased from 30 to 22 MPa [68]. The addition of the particles did decrease the shear bond strength to 25 from 30 MPa for a filler content of 30%, but did not alter the protein-repelling effects or antimicrobial efficacy. Even in long-term water aging of 180 days, MPC composites demonstrated closely similar protein-repelling and antimicrobial efficacy, likely due to the high degree of conversion [69].

To probe whether MPC inhibited or enhanced the release of calcium and phosphate ions from ACP particles, a 1:1 mixture of ethoxylated bisphenol A dimethacrylate (EBPADMA) and pyromellitic dianhydride glycerol dimetrocralte (PMGDM) was used as the resin matrix, abbreviated to EBPM [70]. This resin formulation was found to allow for the release of calcium and phosphorous ions when used with a ACP particle filler [71]. The combination of resin, MPC, and DMAHDM did not alter the protein-repelling properties of a 3% MPC formulation. In a four-organism biofilm challenge, a 3% MPC

+ 3% DMAHDM composite inhibited the colony count of *Porphyromonas gingivalis* and *Aggregatibacter actinomycetemcomitans* by four orders of magnitude and *Prevotella intermedia* and *Fusobacterium nucleatum* by three orders of magnitude, as compared to the resin alone [70]. The hydrophilicity of MPC caused more swelling in the composites, leading to a higher release of calcium and phosphorous ions, compared to the formulation without MPC [72]. By altering the amount of MPC, the amount of ions released could be tuned [73].

Poly(methyl methacrylate) (PMMA) is a common biomaterial routinely used in dentures and can be a breeding ground for oral microbes due to the heavy coating of salivary proteins it endures. MPC was incorporated into a methyl methacrylate monomer mixture and thermally cured. A 3% MPC formulation was enough to substantially decrease the amount of BSA adsorbed to ~2.0 $\mu g/cm^2$ compared to bare PMMA (~12 $\mu g/cm^2$) [74]. Computational modeling of surface interactions of MPC grafted onto PMMA revealed that MPC forms a tight hydration layer and a network of hydrogen bonding between adjacent MPC chains (in high-density grafting), which inhibits the adsorption of proteins and the anchoring of bacteria to the material surface [75].

More recently, there has been an effort to understand how QAC composites affect the microbial composition in biofilm models. MPC in QAC composites were shown to be more effective at decreasing the microbial growth of a single species biofilm of *P. gingivalis* [76]. As the microbial diversity increased, the composite was less effective at decreasing growth. Ultimately, the composite decreased the total microbe count by three orders of magnitude, compared to the resin control. It is well-documented that genetic information is shared between microbes in biofilm communities that act as a defense against chemical agents [77]. These composites also have shown to decrease the *S. mutans* composition in biofilms, leaving non-cariogenic species to thrive [78]. A summary of the protein repellent dental material capabilities discussed can be found in Table 1.

5. Mouthwash Coating Technology

A potential solution to repetitive cariogenic bacterial attachment to dental tissue is through the use of oral rinses with safe protein-repellent molecules that bind to enamel, root, or dentin surfaces. Recently, this concept was tested in a small clinical study by evaluating the number of microbes in dental plaque before and after rinsing with a solution of 5% MPC in saline [79]. Twenty patients had oral samples collected via gargle immediately after and 5 h after brushing their teeth. Half of the subjects were given a saline rinse as a control and the other half the MPC treatment. The patients treated with MPC saw a microbial decrease of 45%, compared to the control, through electric counting of the patients' gargle, indicating that protein adsorption was lessened. The number of fusobacteria, a mediator of bacterial aggregation and plague formation, was inhibited by this treatment. While no chemical modification of the oral environment was mentioned, a more biologically compatible material may be necessary for frequent rinses. In a separate study, a self-assembly approach was used to coat the oral cavity with lysozyme aggregated particles tethered to PEG to repel proteins [53]. Lysozyme was reduced with tris(2-carboxyethyl)phosphine (TCEP) to induce aggregation. These particles have a high tendency to physically bond to many material surfaces, including dentin and enamel surfaces. The particles densely pack at the surface, allowing for the formation of a tight hydration shell around the outward facing PEG molecules, yielding an effective protein repellent monolayer. The authors successfully tested their coatings against BSA, concanavalin A, fibronectin, saliva, fetal bovine serum, milk, egg whites, and various polysaccharides. Importantly, the authors found they can overcome the potential of esterase degradation by incorporating both positive and negative charges into the PEG molecules to induce a zwitterion effect and increase protein repellency of esterases. These approaches are novel and justify further investigations to determine feasibility and effect on the biofilm formation.

Table 1. Summary of bovine serum albumin (BSA) adsorption values for references in this review.

Protein Repellent Compound	Bulk Material	Filler	Adsorption Value (ng/cm^2)	Quantification Method	Reference
3% MPC (w/w)	25.5% 1:1 BisGMA/TEGDMA	70% Barium boroaluminosilicate	1240	SDS removal + BCA Assay	[58]
3% MPC	27% 1:1 BisGMA/TEGDMA	70% Barium boroaluminosilicate	960	SDS removal + BCA Assay	[66]
7.5% MPC	75% 1:1 Scotchbond Multi-Purpose Primer and Adhesive	15% Amorphous calcium phosphate	321	SDS removal + BCA Assay	[68]
3% MPC	25.5% 50:50 BisGMA/TEGDMA	70% Barium boroaluminosilicate	972 (with 180 days water aging)	SDS removal + BCA Assay	[69]
3% MPC	24% 1:1 EBPM	20% Amorphous calcium phosphate; 50% barium boroaluminosilicate	1200	SDS removal + BCA Assay	[70]
3% MPC	44.5% PMGDM, 39.5% EBPADMA, 10% 2-hydroxyethyl methacrylate, 5% BisGMA	30% Amorphous calcium phosphate	416	SDS removal + BCA Assay	[72]
3% MPC	47.75% Nature Cryl^{TM} liquid	47.75% Nature Cryl^{TM} powder	2150	SDS removal + BCA Assay	[74]
3% MPC	24% 1:1 EBPM	20% NACP, 50% barium boroaluminosilicate	1000	SDS removal + BCA Assay	[76]
PEG	Self-assembled PEG lysozyme	N/A	8	QCM	[53]
33% trimethylamine *N*-oxide Zwitterionic Hydrogel	N/A	N/A	3 *	SPR	[80]
9% Poly(carboxybetaine acrylamide) Zwitterionic Hydrogel	N/A	N/A	4.3 *	SPR	[49]

* Adsorption values for human serum, not BSA.

6. Limitations of Existing Technologies

While MPC has gained attention in the dental material literature, it has several shortcomings: (1) MPC contains an ester group connecting the zwitterionic component and the polymerizable methacrylate group. It is well-documented that ester bonds can be cleaved by esterases in saliva via hydrolysis [81]. (2) To achieve low levels of protein adsorption (ng/cm^2), MPC concentrations $\geq$ 5% need to be included into the bulk, which has a detrimental effect on the flexural strength, elastic modulus, and hardness. (3) Currently, there is a paucity of information regarding the long-term protein adsorption of dental resins containing MPC [82]. (4) Although, in theory, MPC meets many design criteria for being the superior protein-repellent candidate, many groups have shown that other conventional polymers outperform MPC in various experimental models [83–86]. New zwitterionic polymers are needed to overcome some of the long-term concerns with MPC. In addition, the potential clinical benefit needs to be confirmed, as MPC may have a deleterious effect on the remineralization capacity of restoratives (i.e., possible binding of the re-mineralizing calcium ions by MPC).

Recently, a zwitterionic polymer was synthesized by oxidizing an acrylamide monomer with 50% hydrogen peroxide, resulting in a permanently positive quaternary amine bonded to a permanently negative oxygen atom [80]. The proximity of the two charged atoms forms a tight hydration layer in an aqueous environment, leading to high repellent efficacy (5 ng/cm^2 by SPR). The polymer also exhibited satisfactory cytotoxicity and immunogenicity in a mouse model and should be studied as a candidate for protein repellency in dental materials. A separate group also synthesized amide-based mono- and bi-functional monomers to create hydrogels, which also demonstrated excellent compatibility in vivo and high protein repellency (4.3 ng/cm^2 by SPR) [49,87]. Further investigations are warranted to determine if these types of molecules can produce dental materials with satisfactory mixing with resin monomers, mechanical properties, and degree of conversion.

7. Conclusions

Protein-repellent technology has the potential to decrease the global burden of dental caries. When incorporated into composites alone or with QAC monomers, protein-repellent technology can inhibit the adsorption of proteins onto dental materials and thus slow the formation of biofilm and associated oral diseases. Many research groups have contributed to the understanding of protein adsorption and material design, and it is now time for dental material researchers to make an impact in the clinical setting. A concerted effort should be placed on understanding the long-term effect on the oral microflora with protein-repellent restorations, as it is not ideal to remove "good" bacteria from the oral cavity. New, more design-driven monomers should be explored to enhance the stability and protein repellency of QAC restorations, to allow for prolonged antimicrobial properties. Last, the dental material field should unify in using reliable protein-adsorption protocols, to ensure consistent comparisons across different material platforms.

Author Contributions: L.T.J. and D.R.B. contributed to the preparation/review of this manuscript. All authors have read and agreed to the published version of the manuscript.

Disclaimer: The sole purpose of identifying certain commercial materials and equipment in this article was to adequately define the experimental protocols. Such identification, in no instance, implies recommendation or endorsement by the ADA or ADA Science & Research Institute, LLC, or means that the material/equipment specified is the best available for the purpose.

References

1. Sugars and Dental Caries. Available online: https://www.who.int/news-room/fact-sheets/detail/sugars-and-dental-caries (accessed on 15 June 2020).
2. Venhoven, B.A.M.; de Gee, A.J.; Davidson, C.L. Polymerization contraction and conversion of light-curing BisGMA-based methacrylate resins. *Biomaterials* **1993**, *14*, 871–875. [CrossRef]
3. O'Donnell, J.N.R.; Skrtic, D. Degree of Vinyl Conversion, Polymerization Shrinkage and Stress Development in Experimental Endodontic Composite. *J. Biomim. Biomater. Tissue Eng.* **2009**, *4*, 1–12. [CrossRef] [PubMed]
4. Wang, J.; Liu, Y.; Yu, J.; Sun, Y.; Xie, W. Study of POSS on the Properties of Novel Inorganic Dental Composite Resin. *Polymers* **2020**, *12*, 478. [CrossRef] [PubMed]
5. Liu, Y.; Wu, X.; Sun, Y.; Xie, W. POSS Dental Nanocomposite Resin: Synthesis, Shrinkage, Double Bond Conversion, Hardness, and Resistance Properties. *Polymers* **2018**, *10*, 369. [CrossRef]
6. Skrtic, D.; Antonucci, J.M.; Eanes, E.D. Amorphous calcium phosphate-based bioactive polymeric composites for mineralized tissue regeneration. *J. Res. Natl. Inst. Stand. Technol.* **2003**, *108*, 167. [CrossRef]
7. Tanaka, J.; Inoue, K.; Masamura, H.; Matsumura, K.; Najai, H.; Inoue, K. The Application of Fluorinated Aromatic Dimethacrylates to Experimental Light-cured Radiopaque Composite Resin, Containing Barium-Borosilicate Glass Filler—A Progress in Nonwaterdegradable Properties. *Dent. Mater. J.* **1993**, *12*, 1–11. [CrossRef]
8. Arcís, R.W.; López-Macipe, A.; Toledano, M.; Osorio, E.; Rodríguez-Clemente, R.; Murtra, J.; Fanovich, M.A.; Pascual, C.D. Mechanical properties of visible light-cured resins reinforced with hydroxyapatite for dental restoration. *Dent. Mater.* **2002**, *18*, 49–57. [CrossRef]

9. Kuper, N.K.; van de Sande, F.H.; Opdam, N.J.M.; Bronkhorst, E.M.; de Soet, J.J.; Cenci, M.S.; Huysmans, M.C.D.J.N.M. Restoration Materials and Secondary Caries Using an In Vitro Biofilm Model. *J. Dent. Res.* **2015**, *94*, 62–68. [CrossRef]
10. Nedeljkovic, I.; Teughels, W.; De Munck, J.; Van Meerbeek, B.; Van Landuyt, K.L. Is secondary caries with composites a material-based problem? *Dent. Mater.* **2015**, *31*, e247–e277. [CrossRef]
11. Imazato, S.; Torri, M.; Tsuchitani, Y. Immobilization of an antibacterial component in composite resin. *Dent. Jpn.* **1993**, *30*, 63–68.
12. Imazato, S.; Torii, M.; Tsuchitani, Y.; McCabe, J.F.; Russell, R.R.B. Incorporation of Bacterial Inhibitor into Resin Composite. *J. Dent. Res.* **1994**. [CrossRef]
13. Gottenbos, B.; van der Mei, H.C.; Klatter, F.; Nieuwenhuis, P.; Busscher, H.J. In vitro and in vivo antimicrobial activity of covalently coupled quaternary ammonium silane coatings on silicone rubber. *Biomaterials* **2002**, *23*, 1417–1423. [CrossRef]
14. Murata, H.; Koepsel, R.R.; Matyjaszewski, K.; Russell, A.J. Permanent, non-leaching antibacterial surfaces—2: How high density cationic surfaces kill bacterial cells. *Biomaterials* **2007**, *28*, 4870–4879. [CrossRef] [PubMed]
15. Lu, G.; Wu, D.; Fu, R. Studies on the synthesis and antibacterial activities of polymeric quaternary ammonium salts from dimethylaminoethyl methacrylate. *React. Funct. Polym.* **2007**, *67*, 355–366. [CrossRef]
16. Jain, A.; Duvvuri, L.S.; Farah, S.; Beyth, N.; Domb, A.J.; Khan, W. Antimicrobial Polymers. *Adv. Healthc. Mater.* **2014**, *3*, 1969–1985. [CrossRef]
17. Li, F.; Weir, M.D.; Xu, H.H.K. Effects of Quaternary Ammonium Chain Length on Antibacterial Bonding Agents. *J. Dent. Res.* **2013**, *92*, 932–938. [CrossRef]
18. Gozzelino, G.; Lisanti, C.; Beneventi, S. Quaternary ammonium monomers for UV crosslinked antibacterial surfaces. *Colloids Surf. A Physicochem. Eng. Asp.* **2013**, *430*, 21–28. [CrossRef]
19. He, J.; Söderling, E.; Österblad, M.; Vallittu, P.K.; Lassila, L.V.J. Synthesis of Methacrylate Monomers with Antibacterial Effects Against S. Mutans. *Molecules* **2011**, *16*, 9755–9763. [CrossRef]
20. Bienek, D.R.; Giuseppetti, A.A.; Okeke, U.C.; Frukhtbeyn, S.A.; Dupree, P.J.; Khajotia, S.S.; Florez, F.L.E.; Hiers, R.D.; Skrtic, D. Antimicrobial, biocompatibility, and physicochemical properties of novel adhesive methacrylate dental monomers. *J. Bioact. Compat. Polym.* **2020**. [CrossRef]
21. Xue, Y.; Xiao, H.; Zhang, Y. Antimicrobial Polymeric Materials with Quaternary Ammonium and Phosphonium Salts. *Int. J. Mol. Sci.* **2015**, *16*, 3626–3655. [CrossRef]
22. Makvandi, P.; Jamaledin, R.; Jabbari, M.; Nikfarjam, N.; Borzacchiello, A. Antibacterial quaternary ammonium compounds in dental materials: A systematic review. *Dent. Mater.* **2018**, *34*, 851–867. [CrossRef] [PubMed]
23. Antonucci, J.M.; Zeiger, D.N.; Tang, K.; Lin-Gibson, S.; Fowler, B.O.; Lin, N.J. Synthesis and characterization of dimethacrylates containing quaternary ammonium functionalities for dental applications. *Dent. Mater.* **2012**, *28*, 219–228. [CrossRef] [PubMed]
24. Bienek, D.; Frukhtbeyn, S.; Giuseppetti, A.; Okeke, U.; Skrtic, D. Antimicrobial Monomers for Polymeric Dental Restoratives: Cytotoxicity and Physicochemical Properties. *JFB* **2018**, *9*, 20. [CrossRef] [PubMed]
25. Daood, U.; Parolia, A.; Elkezza, A.; Yiu, C.K.; Abbott, P.; Matinlinna, J.P.; Fawzy, A.S. An in vitro study of a novel quaternary ammonium silane endodontic irrigant. *Dent. Mater.* **2019**, *35*, 1264–1278. [CrossRef] [PubMed]
26. Bienek, D.R.; Giuseppetti, A.A.; Frukhtbeyn, S.A.; Hiers, R.D.; Esteban Florez, F.L.; Khajotia, S.S.; Skrtic, D. Physicochemical, Mechanical, and Antimicrobial Properties of Novel Dental Polymers Containing Quaternary Ammonium and Trimethoxysilyl Functionalities. *JFB* **2019**, *11*, 1. [CrossRef] [PubMed]
27. Daood, U.; Matinlinna, J.P.; Pichika, M.R.; Mak, K.-K.; Nagendrababu, V.; Fawzy, A.S. A quaternary ammonium silane antimicrobial triggers bacterial membrane and biofilm destruction. *Sci. Rep.* **2020**, *10*, 10970. [CrossRef] [PubMed]
28. Makvandi, P.; Wang, C.; Zare, E.N.; Borzacchiello, A.; Niu, L.; Tay, F.R. Metal-Based Nanomaterials in Biomedical Applications: Antimicrobial Activity and Cytotoxicity Aspects. *Adv. Funct. Mater.* **2020**, *30*, 1910021. [CrossRef]
29. Imazato, S. Bio-active restorative materials with antibacterial effects: New dimension of innovation in restorative dentistry. *Dent. Mater. J.* **2009**, *28*, 11–19. [CrossRef]
30. Li, F.; Weir, M.D.; Fouad, A.F.; Xu, H.H.K. Effect of salivary pellicle on antibacterial activity of novel antibacterial dental adhesives using a dental plaque microcosm biofilm model. *Dent. Mater.* **2014**, *30*, 182–191. [CrossRef]

31. Ten Cate, J.M. Biofilms, a new approach to the microbiology of dental plaque. *Odontology* **2006**, *94*, 1–9. [CrossRef]
32. Saini, R.; Saini, S.; Sharma, S. Biofilm: A dental microbial infection. *J. Nat. Sci. Biol. Med.* **2011**, *2*, 71. [CrossRef]
33. Hojo, K.; Nagaoka, S.; Ohshima, T.; Maeda, N. Bacterial Interactions in Dental Biofilm Development. *J. Dent. Res.* **2009**, *88*, 982–990. [CrossRef] [PubMed]
34. Gibbons, R.J.; Hay, D.I. Adsorbed Salivary Acidic Proline-rich Proteins Contribute to the Adhesion of Streptococcus mutans JBP to Apatitic Surfaces. *J. Dent. Res.* **1989**, *68*, 1303–1307. [CrossRef] [PubMed]
35. Spencer, P.; Ye, Q.; Misra, A.; Goncalves, S.E.P.; Laurence, J.S. Proteins, Pathogens, and Failure at the Composite-Tooth Interface. *J. Dent. Res.* **2014**, *93*, 1243–1249. [CrossRef]
36. Seneviratne, C.J.; Zhang, C.F.; Samaranayake, L.P. Dental plaque biofim in oral health and disease. *Chin. J. Dent. Res.* **2011**, *14*, 87–94.
37. Castagnola, M.; Scarano, E.; Passali, G.C.; Messana, I.; Cabras, T.; Iavarone, F.; Cintio, G.D.; Fiorita, A.; Corso, E.D.; Paludetti, G. Salivary biomarkers and proteomics: Future diagnostic and clinical utilities. *Acta Otorhinolaryngolog. Italica* **2017**, *37*, 94.
38. McPherson, T.B.; Lee, S.J.; Park, K. Analysis of the Prevention of Protein Adsorption by Steric Repulsion Theory. In *Proteins at Interfaces II*; Horbett, T.A., Brash, J.L., Eds.; ACS Symposium Series; American Chemical Society: Washington, DC, USA, 1995; Volume 602, pp. 395–404. ISBN 978-0-8412-3304-1.
39. Müller, C.; Wald, J.; Hoth-Hannig, W.; Umanskaya, N.; Scholz, D.; Hannig, M.; Ziegler, C. Protein adhesion on dental surfaces—A combined surface analytical approach. *Anal. Bioanal. Chem.* **2011**, *400*, 679–689. [CrossRef]
40. Tilton, R.D.; Robertson, C.R.; Gast, A.P. Manipulation of hydrophobic interactions in protein adsorption. *Langmuir* **1991**, *7*, 2710–2718. [CrossRef]
41. Chen, S.; Li, L.; Zhao, C.; Zheng, J. Surface hydration: Principles and applications toward low-fouling/nonfouling biomaterials. *Polymer* **2010**, *51*, 5283–5293. [CrossRef]
42. KL Prime; G Whitesides Self-assembled organic monolayers: Model systems for studying adsorption of proteins at surfaces. *Science* **1991**, *252*, 1164–1167. [CrossRef]
43. Ostuni, E.; Chapman, R.G.; Holmlin, R.E.; Takayama, S.; Whitesides, G.M. A Survey of Structure−Property Relationships of Surfaces that Resist the Adsorption of Protein. *Langmuir* **2001**, *17*, 5605–5620. [CrossRef]
44. Chapman, R.G.; Ostuni, E.; Takayama, S.; Holmlin, R.E.; Yan, L.; Whitesides, G.M. Surveying for Surfaces that Resist the Adsorption of Proteins. *J. Am. Chem. Soc.* **2000**, *122*, 8303–8304. [CrossRef]
45. Holmlin, R.E.; Chen, X.; Chapman, R.G.; Takayama, S.; Whitesides, G.M. Zwitterionic SAMs that Resist Nonspecific Adsorption of Protein from Aqueous Buffer. *Langmuir* **2001**, *17*, 2841–2850. [CrossRef]
46. Bernhard, C.; Roeters, S.J.; Franz, J.; Weidner, T.; Bonn, M.; Gonella, G. Repelling and ordering: The influence of poly(ethylene glycol) on protein adsorption. *Phys. Chem. Chem. Phys.* **2017**, *19*, 28182–28188. [CrossRef]
47. Baggerman, J.; Smulders, M.M.J.; Zuilhof, H. Romantic Surfaces: A Systematic Overview of Stable, Biospecific, and Antifouling Zwitterionic Surfaces. *Langmuir* **2019**, *35*, 1072–1084. [CrossRef] [PubMed]
48. Jain, P.; Hung, H.-C.; Lin, X.; Ma, J.; Zhang, P.; Sun, F.; Wu, K.; Jiang, S. Poly(ectoine) Hydrogels Resist Nonspecific Protein Adsorption. *Langmuir* **2017**, *33*, 11264–11269. [CrossRef] [PubMed]
49. Chou, Y.-N.; Sun, F.; Hung, H.-C.; Jain, P.; Sinclair, A.; Zhang, P.; Bai, T.; Chang, Y.; Wen, T.-C.; Yu, Q.; et al. Ultra-low fouling and high antibody loading zwitterionic hydrogel coatings for sensing and detection in complex media. *Acta Biomater.* **2016**, *40*, 31–37. [CrossRef] [PubMed]
50. Sabaté del Río, J.; Henry, O.Y.F.; Jolly, P.; Ingber, D.E. An antifouling coating that enables affinity-based electrochemical biosensing in complex biological fluids. *Nat. Nanotechnol.* **2019**, *14*, 1143–1149. [CrossRef]
51. Migliorini, E.; Weidenhaupt, M.; Picart, C. Practical guide to characterize biomolecule adsorption on solid surfaces (Review). *Biointerphases* **2018**, *13*, 06D303. [CrossRef]
52. Prabowo, B.; Purwidyantri, A.; Liu, K.-C. Surface Plasmon Resonance Optical Sensor: A Review on Light Source Technology. *Biosensors* **2018**, *8*, 80. [CrossRef]
53. Li, C.; Lu, D.; Deng, J.; Zhang, X.; Yang, P. Amyloid-Like Rapid Surface Modification for Antifouling and In-Depth Remineralization of Dentine Tubules to Treat Dental Hypersensitivity. *Adv. Mater.* **2019**, *31*, 1903973. [CrossRef] [PubMed]

54. Bhakta, S.A.; Evans, E.; Benavidez, T.E.; Garcia, C.D. Protein adsorption onto nanomaterials for the development of biosensors and analytical devices: A review. *Anal. Chim. Acta* **2015**, *872*, 7–25. [CrossRef] [PubMed]
55. Höök, F.; Vörös, J.; Rodahl, M.; Kurrat, R.; Böni, P.; Ramsden, J.J.; Textor, M.; Spencer, N.D.; Tengvall, P.; Gold, J.; et al. A comparative study of protein adsorption on titanium oxide surfaces using in situ ellipsometry, optical waveguide lightmode spectroscopy, and quartz crystal microbalance/dissipation. *Colloids Surf. B Biointerfaces* **2002**, *24*, 155–170. [CrossRef]
56. Ash, A.; Mulholland, F.; Burnett, G.R.; Wilde, P.J. Structural and compositional changes in the salivary pellicle induced upon exposure to SDS and STP. *Biofouling* **2014**, *30*, 1183–1197. [CrossRef]
57. Xu, Z.; Coriand, L.; Loeffler, R.; Geis-Gerstorfer, J.; Zhou, Y.; Scheideler, L.; Fleischer, M.; Gehring, F.K.; Rupp, F. Saliva-coated titanium biosensor detects specific bacterial adhesion and bactericide caused mass loading upon cell death. *Biosens. Bioelectron.* **2019**, *129*, 198–207. [CrossRef] [PubMed]
58. Zhang, N.; Ma, J.; Melo, M.A.S.; Weir, M.D.; Bai, Y.; Xu, H.H.K. Protein-repellent and antibacterial dental composite to inhibit biofilms and caries. *J. Dent.* **2015**, *43*, 225–234. [CrossRef] [PubMed]
59. Kratz, F.; Grass, S.; Umanskaya, N.; Scheibe, C.; Müller-Renno, C.; Davoudi, N.; Hannig, M.; Ziegler, C. Cleaning of biomaterial surfaces: Protein removal by different solvents. *Colloids Surf. B Biointerfaces* **2015**, *128*, 28–35. [CrossRef]
60. Kwon, J.-S.; Lee, M.-J.; Kim, J.-Y.; Kim, D.; Ryu, J.-H.; Jang, S.; Kim, K.-M.; Hwang, C.-J.; Choi, S.-H. Novel anti-biofouling light-curable fluoride varnish containing 2-methacryloyloxyethyl phosphorylcholine to prevent enamel demineralization. *Sci. Rep.* **2019**, *9*. [CrossRef]
61. Lee, M.-J.; Kwon, J.-S.; Kim, J.-Y.; Ryu, J.-H.; Seo, J.-Y.; Jang, S.; Kim, K.-M.; Hwang, C.-J.; Choi, S.-H. Bioactive resin-based composite with surface pre-reacted glass-ionomer filler and zwitterionic material to prevent the formation of multi-species biofilm. *Dent. Mater.* **2019**, *35*, 1331–1341. [CrossRef]
62. Binnig, G.; Quate, C.F.; Gerber, C. Atomic Force Microscope. *Phys. Rev. Lett.* **1986**, *56*, 930–933. [CrossRef]
63. Chen, X.; Davies, M.C.; Roberts, C.J.; Tendler, S.J.B.; Williams, P.M.; Davies, J.; Dawkes, A.C.; Edwards, J.C. Recognition of Protein Adsorption onto Polymer Surfaces by Scanning Force Microscopy and Probe–Surface Adhesion Measurements with Protein-Coated Probes. *Langmuir* **1997**, *13*, 4106–4111. [CrossRef]
64. Cao, L.; Wu, J.; Zhang, Q.; Baras, B.; Bhadila, G.; Li, Y.; Melo, M.A.S.; Weir, M.D.; Bai, Y.; Zhang, N.; et al. Novel Protein-Repellent and Antibacterial Resins and Cements to Inhibit Lesions and Protect Teeth. *Int. J. Polym. Sci.* **2019**, *2019*, 1–11. [CrossRef]
65. Zhang, N.; Zhang, K.; Xie, X.; Dai, Z.; Zhao, Z.; Imazato, S.; Al-Dulaijan, Y.; Al-Qarni, F.; Weir, M.; Reynolds, M.; et al. Nanostructured Polymeric Materials with Protein-Repellent and Anti-Caries Properties for Dental Applications. *Nanomaterials* **2018**, *8*, 393. [CrossRef] [PubMed]
66. Zhang, N.; Chen, C.; Melo, M.A.; Bai, Y.-X.; Cheng, L.; Xu, H.H. A novel protein-repellent dental composite containing 2-methacryloyloxyethyl phosphorylcholine. *Int. J. Oral Sci.* **2015**, *7*, 103–109. [CrossRef]
67. Zhang, N.; Weir, M.D.; Romberg, E.; Bai, Y.; Xu, H.H.K. Development of novel dental adhesive with double benefits of protein-repellent and antibacterial capabilities. *Dent. Mater.* **2015**, *31*, 845–854. [CrossRef]
68. Zhang, N.; Melo, M.A.S.; Chen, C.; Liu, J.; Weir, M.D.; Bai, Y.; Xu, H.H.K. Development of a multifunctional adhesive system for prevention of root caries and secondary caries. *Dent. Mater.* **2015**, *31*, 1119–1131. [CrossRef]
69. Zhang, N.; Zhang, K.; Melo, M.; Weir, M.; Xu, D.; Bai, Y.; Xu, H. Effects of Long-Term Water-Aging on Novel Anti-Biofilm and Protein-Repellent Dental Composite. *IJMS* **2017**, *18*, 186. [CrossRef]
70. Wang, L.; Xie, X.; Imazato, S.; Weir, M.D.; Reynolds, M.A.; Xu, H.H.K. A protein-repellent and antibacterial nanocomposite for Class-V restorations to inhibit periodontitis-related pathogens. *Mater. Sci. Eng. C* **2016**, *67*, 702–710. [CrossRef]
71. Zhang, L.; Weir, M.D.; Chow, L.C.; Antonucci, J.M.; Chen, J.; Xu, H.H.K. Novel rechargeable calcium phosphate dental nanocomposite. *Dent. Mater.* **2016**, *32*, 285–293. [CrossRef]
72. Al-Qarni, F.D.; Tay, F.; Weir, M.D.; Melo, M.A.S.; Sun, J.; Oates, T.W.; Xie, X.; Xu, H.H.K. Protein-repelling adhesive resin containing calcium phosphate nanoparticles with repeated ion-recharge and re-releases. *J. Dent.* **2018**, *78*, 91–99. [CrossRef]
73. Al-Dulaijan, Y.A.; Weir, M.D.; Melo, M.A.S.; Sun, J.; Oates, T.W.; Zhang, K.; Xu, H.H.K. Protein-repellent nanocomposite with rechargeable calcium and phosphate for long-term ion release. *Dent. Mater.* **2018**, *34*, 1735–1747. [CrossRef] [PubMed]

74. Cao, L.; Xie, X.; Wang, B.; Weir, M.D.; Oates, T.W.; Xu, H.H.K.; Zhang, N.; Bai, Y. Protein-repellent and antibacterial effects of a novel polymethyl methacrylate resin. *J. Dent.* **2018**, *79*, 39–45. [CrossRef]
75. Choi, W.; Jin, J.; Park, S.; Kim, J.-Y.; Lee, M.-J.; Sun, H.; Kwon, J.-S.; Lee, H.; Choi, S.-H.; Hong, J. Quantitative Interpretation of Hydration Dynamics Enabled the Fabrication of a Zwitterionic Antifouling Surface. *ACS Appl. Mater. Interfaces* **2020**, *12*, 7951–7965. [CrossRef] [PubMed]
76. Wang, L.; Xie, X.; Qi, M.; Weir, M.D.; Reynolds, M.A.; Li, C.; Zhou, C.; Xu, H.H.K. Effects of single species versus multispecies periodontal biofilms on the antibacterial efficacy of a novel bioactive Class-V nanocomposite. *Dent. Mater.* **2019**, *35*, 847–861. [CrossRef] [PubMed]
77. Chen, H.; Tang, Y.; Weir, M.D.; Lei, L.; Masri, R.; Lynch, C.D.; Oates, T.W.; Zhang, K.; Hu, T.; Xu, H.H.K. Effects of *S. mutans* gene-modification and antibacterial calcium phosphate nanocomposite on secondary caries and marginal enamel hardness. *RSC Adv.* **2019**, *9*, 41672–41683. [CrossRef]
78. Wang, H.; Wang, S.; Cheng, L.; Jiang, Y.; Melo, M.A.S.; Weir, M.D.; Oates, T.W.; Zhou, X.; Xu, H.H.K. Novel dental composite with capability to suppress cariogenic species and promote non-cariogenic species in oral biofilms. *Mater. Sci. Eng. C* **2019**, *94*, 587–596. [CrossRef]
79. Fujiwara, N.; Yumoto, H.; Miyamoto, K.; Hirota, K.; Nakae, H.; Tanaka, S.; Murakami, K.; Kudo, Y.; Ozaki, K.; Miyake, Y. 2-Methacryloyloxyethyl phosphorylcholine (MPC)-polymer suppresses an increase of oral bacteria: A single-blind, crossover clinical trial. *Clin. Oral Investig.* **2019**, *23*, 739–746. [CrossRef]
80. Li, B.; Jain, P.; Ma, J.; Smith, J.K.; Yuan, Z.; Hung, H.-C.; He, Y.; Lin, X.; Wu, K.; Pfaendtner, J.; et al. Trimethylamine N-oxide–derived zwitterionic polymers: A new class of ultralow fouling bioinspired materials. *Sci. Adv.* **2019**, *5*. [CrossRef]
81. Gonzalez-Bonet, A.; Kaufman, G.; Yang, Y.; Wong, C.; Jackson, A.; Huyang, G.; Bowen, R.; Sun, J. Preparation of Dental Resins Resistant to Enzymatic and Hydrolytic Degradation in Oral Environments. *Biomacromolecules* **2015**, *16*, 3381–3388. [CrossRef]
82. Tone, S.; Hasegawa, M.; Puppulin, L.; Pezzotti, G.; Sudo, A. Surface modifications and oxidative degradation in MPC-grafted highly cross-linked polyethylene liners retrieved from short-term total hip arthroplasty. *Acta Biomater.* **2018**, *66*, 157–165. [CrossRef] [PubMed]
83. Van Andel, E.; Lange, S.C.; Pujari, S.P.; Tijhaar, E.J.; Smulders, M.M.J.; Savelkoul, H.F.J.; Zuilhof, H. Systematic Comparison of Zwitterionic and Non-Zwitterionic Antifouling Polymer Brushes on a Bead-Based Platform. *Langmuir* **2019**, *35*, 1181–1191. [CrossRef] [PubMed]
84. Gu, M.; Vegas, A.J.; Anderson, D.G.; Langer, R.S.; Kilduff, J.E.; Belfort, G. Combinatorial synthesis with high throughput discovery of protein-resistant membrane surfaces. *Biomaterials* **2013**, *34*, 6133–6138. [CrossRef] [PubMed]
85. Imbrogno, J.; Williams, M.D.; Belfort, G. A New Combinatorial Method for Synthesizing, Screening, and Discovering Antifouling Surface Chemistries. *ACS Appl. Mater. Interfaces* **2015**, *7*, 2385–2392. [CrossRef] [PubMed]
86. Li, Q.; Imbrogno, J.; Belfort, G.; Wang, X.-L. Making polymeric membranes antifouling via "grafting from" polymerization of zwitterions. *J. Appl. Polym. Sci.* **2015**, *132*. [CrossRef]
87. Zhang, P.; Sun, F.; Tsao, C.; Liu, S.; Jain, P.; Sinclair, A.; Hung, H.-C.; Bai, T.; Wu, K.; Jiang, S. Zwitterionic gel encapsulation promotes protein stability, enhances pharmacokinetics, and reduces immunogenicity. *Proc. Natl. Acad. Sci. USA* **2015**, *112*, 12046–12051. [CrossRef] [PubMed]

15

Substituted Nano-Hydroxyapatite Toothpastes Reduce Biofilm Formation on Enamel and Resin-Based Composite Surfaces

Andrei C. Ionescu [1,*], Gloria Cazzaniga [1], Marco Ottobelli [1], Franklin Garcia-Godoy [2] and Eugenio Brambilla [1]

1 Oral Microbiology and Biomaterials Laboratory, Department of Biomedical, Surgical and Dental Sciences, University of Milan, via Pascal 36, 20133 Milan, Italy; gloria.cazzaniga@yahoo.it (G.C.); marco.ottobelli@unimi.it (M.O.); eugenio.brambilla@unimi.it (E.B.)

2 Bioscience Research Center and Clinical Research, College of Dentistry, University of Tennessee Health Science Center, 875 Union Avenue, Memphis, TN 38163, USA; fgarciagodoy@gmail.com

* Correspondence: andrei.ionescu@unimi.it

Abstract: *Background*: Toothpastes containing nano-hydroxyapatite (n-HAp) substituted with metal ions provide calcium and phosphate ions to dental hard tissues, reducing demineralization, and promoting remineralization. Few data are available about the effect of these bioactive compounds on oral microbiota. *Methods*: This in vitro study evaluated the influence of two commercially-available substituted n-HAp-based toothpastes (α: Zn-carbonate substituted n-HAp; β: F, Mg, Sr-carbonate substituted n-HAp) on early colonization (EC, 12 h) and biofilm formation (BF, 24 h) by oral microbiota. Controls were brushed with distilled water. Artificial oral microcosm and *Streptococcus mutans* biofilms were developed using human enamel and a resin-based composite (RBC) as adherence surfaces. Two test setups, a shaking multiwell plate and a modified drip-flow reactor (MDFR), were used to simulate clinical conditions during the night (low salivary flow and clearance) and daytime, respectively. Energy-dispersive X-ray spectrometry (EDS) was used to evaluate specimens' surfaces after toothpaste treatment. Fluoride release from β toothpaste was evaluated. Viable adherent biomass was quantified by MTT assay, and biofilms' morphology was highlighted using confocal microscopy. *Results*: EDS showed the presence of remnants from the tested toothpastes on both adherence surfaces. β toothpaste showed significantly lower EC and BF compared to control using the artificial oral microcosm model, while α toothpaste showed lower EC and BF compared to control, but higher EC and BF compared to β toothpaste. The effect shown by β toothpaste was, to a minimal extent, due to fluoride release. Interestingly, this result was seen on both adherence surfaces, meaning that the tested toothpastes significantly influenced EC and BF even on RBC surfaces. Furthermore, the effect of toothpaste treatments was higher after 12 h than 24 h, suggesting that toothbrushing twice a day is more effective than brushing once. *Conclusions*: The efficacy of these treatments in reducing microbial colonization of RBC surfaces may represent a promising possibility in the prevention of secondary caries.

Keywords: fluoride(s); biofilm(s); *Streptococcus mutans*; bioreactor(s); enamel; composite materials; biomaterials; hydroxyapatite; nanostructured materials; dental

---

1. Introduction

Biofilms colonizing dental surfaces represent the habitat of a wide range of microorganisms. In healthy conditions, this microbial community provides fundamental benefits to host surfaces, including homeostasis of critical environmental parameters such as pH, as well as protection against colonization by exogenous species. However, loss of this equilibrium can result in dysbiosis, leading to the onset of oral diseases, including dental caries [1,2].

Mechanical biofilm control can be beneficially associated with the use of active compounds to reduce biofilm formation, positively affecting the biological equilibrium of the ecosystem [3]. The search for new bioactive compounds to prevent dental caries development and progression has led researchers to focus their attention on the use of nanotechnologies, especially hydroxyapatite (HAp), metals, and metal oxide nanoparticles [4–6]. Nanotechnology applications offer the opportunity to modulate the formation of dental biofilms using nanoparticles with bioactive effects. Indeed, their possible use in biofilm control is related to some peculiar characteristics that materials acquire when nano-sized: shape, surface-to-volume ratio, chemical reactivity, and ability to interact with the bacterial cell wall directly [6–8]. Considerable efforts have been made to clarify the transfer mechanisms of such nanoparticles through biofilms, indicating that nanoparticles can diffuse through water channels inside biofilms, interacting both with the microbial cells and with the hard tissue surface.

Toothpastes containing nano-hydroxyapatite (n-HAp) and its precursors can provide calcium and phosphate ions to dental hard tissues, reducing demineralization, and promoting remineralization. N-HAp may also form a protective layer on dental hard tissues with chemical characteristics very close to natural tissues, showing biomimetic properties [9,10]. Biomimetic n-HAp or other calcium phosphate-based nanosystems have been shown to actively shift the ionic balance toward remineralization [11,12]. Recently, n-HAp-based toothpastes containing metal ions such as Zn, F, Mg, and Sr have been introduced to improve the remineralization processes. The small quantity of metal ions with which nHAp is doped modulates the properties of the compound already from its deposition, influencing crystal growth and length, and influencing its solubility and strength. They are firmly embedded inside the lattice and are not supposed to be released. Most studies, therefore, provide data about the remineralization potential of these compounds on surface lesions, with few reporting their influence on early microbial colonization (EC) and biofilm formation (BF) [13–16].

Resin-based composites (RBCs) provide an example of artificial surfaces intensely colonized by cariogenic biofilms due to their lack of buffering effect [17]. This characteristic has been put into relation with the high occurrence of secondary caries in the sound dental tissues surrounding an RBC restoration [17]. The possibility of influencing microbial colonization of RBCs, therefore, can be seen as a means to prevent the occurrence of such lesions. For this reason, RBCs are a potential target of preventive measures exploiting the potential of nanotechnologies in order to reduce secondary caries occurrence.

The aim of this study was to evaluate the in vitro effect of two n-Hap-based toothpastes on early colonization (EC) (12 h) and biofilm formation (BF) (24 h) of human enamel and RBC surfaces. The study was performed by aerobically culturing the monospecies *Streptococcus mutans* and an artificial oral microcosm using both a static and a continuous flow setup. The aim of the two models was to assess the effect of the tested toothpastes under environments simulating clinical conditions during the night (low salivary flow and clearance) and day (high salivary flow and clearance). The null hypothesis was that toothpaste treatment would not influence EC and BF on sound enamel surfaces in the tested models. An additional null hypothesis was that toothpaste treatment would not influence EC and BF on RBC surfaces in the tested models.

2. Materials and Methods

2.1. Preparation of Specimens

Reagents, culture media, and disposables used in this study were obtained from E. Merck AG (Darmstadt, Germany). A total of 110 human teeth extracted for clinical reasons were obtained and stored at −20 °C until use. The Institutional Review Board of the University of Milan approved the protocol (codename: SALTiBO-2017). Enamel disks 6.0 mm in diameter and 1.5 mm thick were cut from the teeth surfaces by means of custom-made water-cooled diamond trephine burs (Indiam, Carrara,

Italy). A total of 213 enamel disks were prepared for the study, using this procedure to obtain more than one disk from each tooth.

A total of 213 disks (6.0 mm diameter and 1.5 mm thickness) of a nanohybrid resin-based composite (RBC, Clearfil Majesty ES-2, shade A2, Kuraray Europe GmbH, Hattersheim am Main, Germany) were obtained by packing an excess of uncured material into a custom-made PTFE mold. The top and bottom surfaces of the RBC were covered with a cellulose acetate strip (Mylar) and condensed against a glass plate by applying a load of 1 kg for 20 s. The specimens were then irradiated for 40 s by placing the tip of a light-curing unit (MiniLED, Satelec, Acteon Group, Merignac, France, 420–480 nm emission, 1250 mW/cm^2 irradiance) into direct contact with the acetate strip. To remove most of leachates, RBC specimens were then stored under light-proof conditions in phosphate-buffered saline (PBS) for 6 days at 37 °C, with the buffer replaced twice a day.

Both enamel and RBC disks were polished using grinding paper (1000, 2000, and 4000 grit) to obtain a surface roughness with Ra < 0.2 µm. They were then randomly divided into three groups (α, β, and control, n = 71/group, Figure 1).

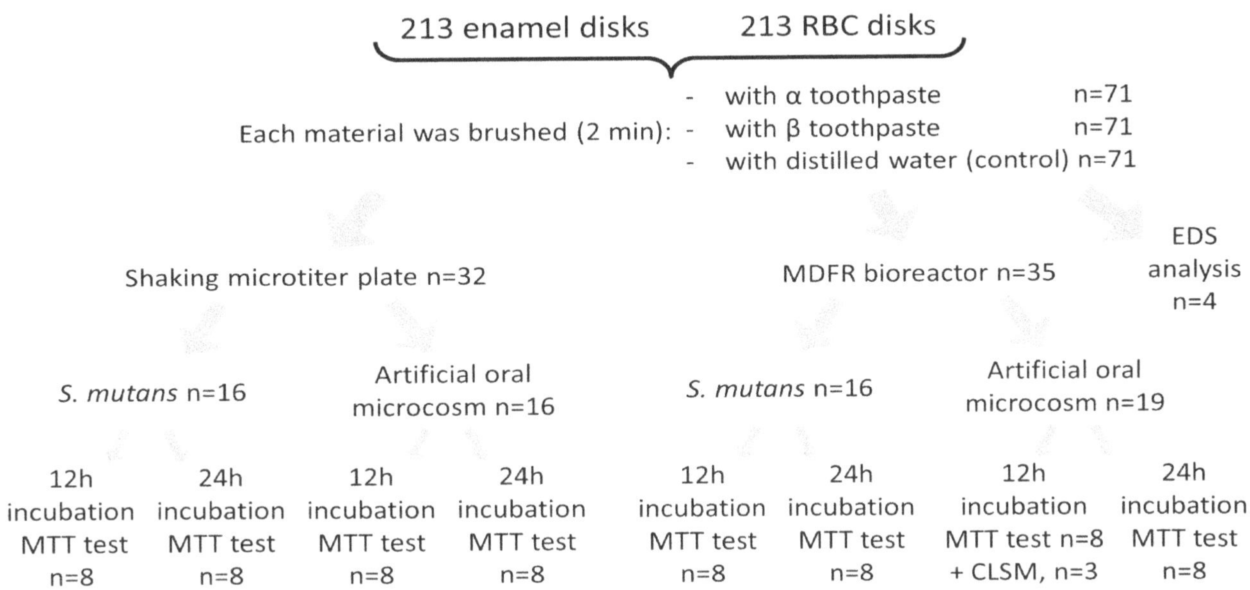

Figure 1. Diagram of specimens processing for the present study. After brushing with the tested toothpastes or with distilled water, enamel and RBC specimens were rinsed, sterilized, then subjected to microbiological analysis and surface imaging (SEM, CLSM) and analysis (EDS). The microbiological analysis included two test setups, two microbiological models, and two incubation times.

2.2. Toothpastes

Two toothpastes containing n-HAp were tested (Table 1). The toothpastes were inserted into test tubes coded by the Greek letter corresponding to the first two groups (α, β). In this way, the experimenters performing microbiological procedures were blinded regarding their composition. Each toothpaste was mixed to a slurry using one part of toothpaste and two parts of distilled water. Then, enamel and RBC disks of groups α and β were manually brushed by a single operator with the corresponding toothpaste for 2 min and rinsed with distilled water for 1 min. Disks belonging to the control group were brushed with distilled water for 2 min, then rinsed for 1 min with distilled water. All disks were then sterilized using a chemical peroxide-ion plasma sterilizer (STERRAD, ASP, Irvine, CA, USA).

Table 1. Label, manufacturer and composition of the tested substituted n-Hap-containing toothpastes.

Label	Name	Company	Composition
Toothpaste α	Biorepair Total Protection Plus	Coswell Funo (BO), Italy	Purified water, zinc carbonate hydroxyapatite, glycerin, sorbitol, hydrated silica, silica, aroma, cellulose gum, tetrapotassium pyrophosphate, sodium myristoyl sarcosinate, sodium methyl cocoyl taurate, sodium saccharin, citric acid, phenoxyethanol, benzyl alcohol, sodium benzoate.
Toothpaste β	Biosmalto Caries, Abrasion and Erosion	Curasept Healthcare S.p.A. Saronno (VA), Italy	Purified water, glycerin, hydrated silica, fluoride-hydroxyapatite, Mg-Sr-carbonate hydroxyapatite conjugated with chitosan, cellulose gum, xylitol, cocamidopropyl betaine, xantham gum, aroma, acesulfame K, ethylhexylglycerin, phenoxyethanol, sodium benzoate, citric acid.

2.3. Surface Imaging and Analysis

Scanning electron microscopy (SEM) and energy-dispersive X-ray spectroscopy (EDS) analysis were performed (n = 4/group, Figure 1) using a TM4000Plus Tabletop scanning electron microscope (Hitachi, Schaumburg, IL, USA) equipped with an EDS probe (Q75, Bruker, Berlin, Germany) to investigate the presence of toothpaste residues on the specimen surface. Dry specimens were observed in surface-charge reduction mode without sputter-coating, using an accelerating voltage of 15 KV. Three randomly selected fields were acquired for each specimen at 500× magnification and were analyzed using the EDS probe in full-frame mode using an acquisition time of 150 s. SEM micrographs (backscattered electrons mode) and EDS elemental maps of the surfaces at 5000× magnification were also obtained. The acquired data represent the elemental composition of the ≈1 μm superficial layer.

2.4. Saliva Collection

Whole saliva was collected from five healthy volunteers, according to a previously described protocol [18]. They refrained from oral hygiene for 24 h, did not have any active dental disease, and did not have antibiotic therapy for at least three months prior to the experiment. Chilled test tubes were used for saliva collection. Saliva was then pooled, heated to 60 °C for 30 min and centrifuged (27,000× *g*, 4 °C, 30 min). The sterile supernatant was collected into sterile tubes and stored at −20 °C. Saliva was thawed at 37 °C for 1 h before use. The Institutional Review Board of the University of Milan approved the use of saliva (codename: SALTiBO-2017), and written, informed consent was obtained from all volunteers.

2.5. Microbiological Procedures

Two microbiological models were used in this study: a monospecific *S. mutans* culture and an artificial oral microcosm based on mixed oral flora (Figure 1).

A pure suspension of *S. mutans* strain ATCC 35668 was obtained as described elsewhere [19]. Briefly, Mitis Salivarius Bacitracin agar (MSB agar) plates were inoculated with the *S. mutans* strain and incubated aerobically in a 5% CO_2-supplemented atmosphere at 37 °C for 48 h. After transferring an inoculum in Brain Heart Infusion (BHI) broth and further incubating in a 5% CO_2-supplemented atmosphere at 37 °C for 12 h, a pure culture of the microorganism was obtained. Cells were harvested by centrifugation (2200× *g*, 19 °C, 5 min), washed twice with sterile phosphate-buffered saline (PBS), and resuspended in the same buffer., The suspension was sonicated using low-energy output (7W for 30 s, B-150 Sonifier, Branson, Danbury, CT, USA) to disperse bacterial chains. Finally, the suspension was adjusted to an optical density of 1.0 on the McFarland scale, corresponding to a concentration of approximately 6.0×10^8 cells/mL.

A mixed oral flora inoculum was obtained from fresh, pooled saliva expectorated from the same five donors previously described, filtered through sterile glass wool, vigorously stirred for 2 min, and immediately used. Two test setups were used in this study: a shaking multiwell plate and a modified drip-flow reactor (MDFR).

2.5.1. Shaking Multiwell Plate

Disks were placed in 48-well sterile plates and incubated at 37 °C for 24 h in sterile saliva; then, the saliva was removed by gentle aspiration. Each well was inoculated with 100 µl of either *S. mutans* suspension or mixed oral flora, and 900 µl of sterile modified artificial saliva medium. The medium composition was the following: 10.0 g/L sucrose, 2.5 g/L mucin (type II, porcine gastric), 2.0 g/L bacteriological peptone, 2.0 g/L tryptone, 1.0 g/L yeast extract, 0.35 g/L NaCl, 0.2 g/L KCl, 0.2 g/L $CaCl_2$, 0.1 g/L cysteine hydrochloride, 0.001 g/L hemin, and 0.0002 g/L vitamin K1 [20]. Plates were then incubated aerobically in an orbital shaker at 37 °C and 100 rpm. After either 12 h (colonization) or 24 h (biofilm formation), adherent viable biomass assessment was performed.

2.5.2. MDFR

The bioreactor used in the present study was a modification of a commercially available drip-flow reactor (DFR 110, BioSurface Technologies; Bozeman, MT, USA) according to previously described [21]. The modified design (MDFR) allowed the placement of customized PTFE trays on the bottom of the flow cells to submerge the specimen surfaces in the flowing medium. Specimens from each group were randomly divided into the eight flow cells of two identical MDFRs. After sterilization (STERRAD), the MDFR was assembled inside a sterile hood, and a salivary pellicle was obtained on the specimen surface after incubation with sterile saliva at 37 °C for 24 h. Saliva was then removed, each flow-cell was inoculated with 10 mL of either *S. mutans* suspension or mixed oral flora suspension to allow bacterial adherence. After 4 h, a peristaltic pump (RP-1k; Rainin, Emeryville, CA, USA) provided the constant flow of sterile modified artificial saliva medium through the flow cells (9.6 mL/h). For each microbiological inoculum, the amount of viable adherent biomass was evaluated after either 12 h or 24 h of further incubation in aerobic conditions (Figure 1).

2.6. Viable Biomass Assessment

Viable and metabolically active biomass adherent to the specimen surface was assessed using a tetrazolium-based assay as described previously [21]. In brief, a tetrazolium salt stock solution was prepared by dissolving 5 mg/mL 3-(4,5)-dimethylthiazol-2-yl-2,5-diphenyltetrazolium bromide (MTT) in sterile PBS; a phenazinium salt stock solution was prepared by dissolving 0.3 mg/mL of N-methylphenazinium methyl sulphate (PMS) in sterile PBS. The solutions were stored at 2 °C in light-proof vials until the day of the experiment when a fresh measurement solution (FMS) was prepared by diluting 1:10 v/v of MTT stock solution and 1:10 v/v of PMS stock solution in sterile PBS. A lysing solution (LS) was prepared by dissolving 10% v/v of sodium dodecyl sulphate (SDS) and 50% v/v dimethylformamide in distilled water and stored at 2 °C until the day of the experiment when it was warmed at 37 °C for 2 h before use. After the specified incubation times, the orbital shaker and the MDFR medium flow was halted, flow cells and plates were opened, the specimens were carefully removed and immediately placed into Petri plates containing sterile PBS at 37 °C. They were gently washed three times with sterile PBS to remove non-adherent cells and finally placed inside the wells of 48-well plates containing 300 µL of FMS each. The plates were incubated at 37 °C under light-proof conditions for 3 h. During incubation, electron transport across the microbial plasma membrane and, to a lesser extent, microbial redox systems, converted the yellow salt to insoluble purple formazan crystals. The conversion at the cell membrane level was facilitated by the intermediate electron acceptor (PMS). The unreacted FMS was gently removed by aspiration, and the formazan crystals were dissolved by adding 300 µL of LS to each well. The plates were stored for an additional 1 h under light-proof conditions at room temperature; 100 µL of the solution was then transferred into

96-well plates. The absorbance of the solution was measured using a spectrophotometer (Genesys 10-S, Thermo Spectronic, Rochester, NY, USA) at a wavelength of 550 nm; results were expressed as relative absorbance in optical density (OD) units corresponding to the amount of adherent, viable and metabolically active biomass.

2.7. Confocal Laser-Scanning Microscopy (CLSM)

A total of three specimens for each material and treatment group (Figure 1) were prepared for CLSM analysis. They were incubated using the MDFR test setup with the artificial oral microcosm model for 12 h. Then, they were gently removed from the flow cells, rinsed twice with sterile PBS, stained using the FilmTracer™ LIVE/DEAD® Biofilm Viability Kit (Invitrogen Ltd., Paisley, UK), and analyzed using confocal laser-scanning microscopy (CLSM; Eclipse Ti2 inverted CLSM, Nikon, Tokyo, Japan). Three randomly selected image stack sections were recorded for each specimen. Confocal images were obtained using a dry objective (20×; NA = 0.5) at a resolution of 2048 × 2048 pixels, with a zoom factor of 1.0 and a scan speed of 400 Hz, and digitalized using the Nikon Imaging Software (NIS)—Elements Viewer, v. 4.50. Three channels were acquired in parallel scanning; the first used an excitation at 405 nm and emission at 420–470 nm in order to subtract potential autofluorescence digitally. The other two channels had an excitation wavelength of 488 nm, and emission was acquired at 500–570 nm (green channel, live bacteria) and 610–760 nm (red channel, dead bacteria). For each image stack section, 3D-rendering reconstructions were obtained using Drishti (Ajay Limaye, Australian National University, CAN, AUS, http://sf.anu.edu.au/Vizlab/drishti/).

2.8. Fluoride Release Measurements

Measurements of fluoride release from the fluoride-hydroxyapatite-containing toothpaste (β) were performed to correlate it with the hypothesized antimicrobial activity of the toothpaste. A total of 48 enamel disks and 48 RBC disks were additionally prepared and brushed as previously specified (cf. Sections 2.1 and 2.2): one half (n = 24) was brushed with slurry from toothpaste β, and the other half was brushed with distilled water. Immediate fluoride release (t = 0) was evaluated from eight disks for each toothpaste. These disks were placed in 48-well plates containing 300 μL of sterile saliva in each well for 24 h. Disks were then discarded, 1:50 dilution of total ionic strength solution adjustment buffer, TISAB III (Orion Research Inc, Boston, MA, USA) was added, and the solution adjusted to pH = 5.5. The fluoride content of the solution was determined using the ion-selective electrode micro-method. The remaining disks were weighted with an analytical balance, then sterilized, and a monospecies *S. mutans* biofilm was allowed to develop on their surfaces after salivary pellicle formation using the MDFR as described in Section 2.5.2 for the same incubation times (12 h and 24 h). A total of eight disks for each toothpaste and time group were weighed again, and the weight of the adherent wet biomass was calculated. After that, each disk was inserted into one well of 48-well plates containing 300 μL of 10 vol% SDS in distilled water and 1:50 TISAB III (pH = 5.5), and the plates were sonicated for 5 min to allow dispersion of the biomass. Then, disks were discarded, and the fluoride content of the solution was determined.

The amount of released fluoride was calculated and displayed in parts per billion (ppb) after normalizing the fluoride readings by the disks' surfaces. The amount of fluoride incorporated in the biofilm structures was calculated and displayed in parts per million (ppm) after normalizing the fluoride readings by the amount of adherent biomass. All analyses were performed using the ion-selective electrode micro-method, as described previously [22]. In brief, a stock solution with a fluoride concentration of 1000 ppm was appropriately diluted with 10 vol% SDS in distilled water at pH = 5.5 to obtain fluoride standards with fluoride concentrations ranging from 0.0019 to 64 ppm. A calibration curve was obtained using a digital pH/mV meter (SA-720, Orion Research Inc, Boston, MA, USA). A 1:50 final dilution of TISAB III as an ionic strength adjustor was added to each standard before the analyses. A negative reference standard (0 ppm fluoride) was prepared by adding 1:50 TISAB III to the solution containing 10 vol% SDS in distilled water; this solution was also used to rinse the electrodes between measurements.

2.9. Statistical Analysis

All statistical analyses were performed using statistical software (JMP 12.0, SAS Institute, Inc., Cary, NC, USA). The OD and F data were reported as means and standard errors calculated from the natural values. The normality of distributions was preliminarily checked using Shapiro-Wilk test, and homogeneity of variances was preliminarily checked using Bartlett's test. A multi-way ANOVA model was used on OD dataset considering the factors: toothpaste (α, β, control), adherence surface (enamel, RBC), test setup (shaking multiwell plate, MDFR), microbiological model (*S. mutans*, oral microcosm), and incubation time (12 h, 24 h). A multi-way ANOVA model was used on fluoride dataset considering the factors: toothpaste (β, control), adherence surface (enamel, RBC), and incubation time (12 h, 24 h). Student-Newman-Keuls post-hoc test was used to highlight significant differences ($p < 0.05$).

3. Results

3.1. Surface Imaging and Analysis

To investigate the presence of toothpaste residues on enamel and RBC surfaces as well as the composition of the tested toothpastes, specimens were observed using SEM-EDS in surface-charge reduction mode without sputter-coating, using an accelerating voltage of 15 KV (Figure 2). EDS results showed that the elemental composition of both toothpastes was very similar, except that α toothpaste contained zinc, while β toothpaste contained strontium, magnesium, and fluoride (Figure 3). Enamel specimens showed a significant increase in surface zinc content after treatment with α toothpaste, and a significant increase in strontium and magnesium content after treatment with β toothpaste (Table 2). Very interestingly, EDS detected the presence of calcium and phosphate on the surfaces of RBC specimens treated with both toothpastes, as well as traces of zinc on specimens treated with α toothpaste and magnesium on specimens treated with β toothpaste (Figure 2, Table 2).

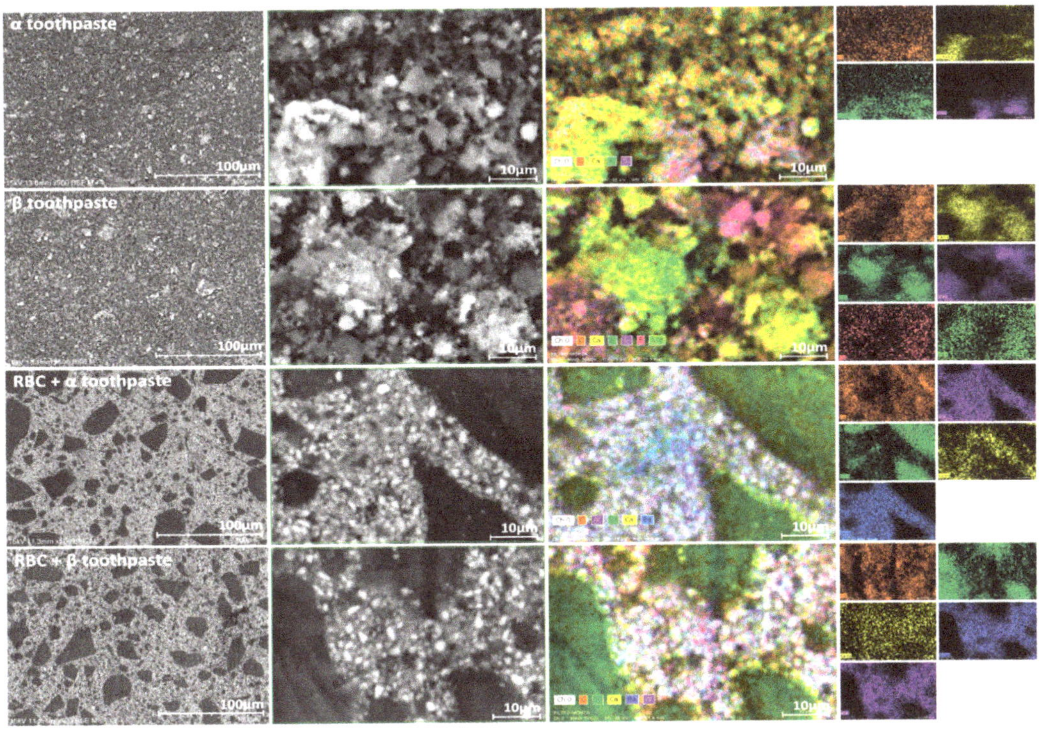

Figure 2. The panel, to be read horizontally, depicts the SEM backscattered electrons micrographs (500×

and 5000×, respectively) and EDS elemental maps (5000×) of the specimen surfaces. The EDS maps are additionally presented as single-channel maps to better identify the topographical presence of each element. The first two rows of the panel display the surfaces of the vacuum-dried toothpastes tested in this study: α toothpaste (containing Zn-carbonate substituted n-HAp) and β toothpaste (containing F, Mg, Sr-carbonate substituted n-HAp). Their aspect is very similar, showing silica microparticles (identified by Si signal) and clusters of n-HAp (identified by Ca and P signals). Zn and Sr signals were below the detection limits in mapping mode and were not displayed. The last two rows of the panel represent the surfaces of the tested restorative material after treatment with the toothpastes: RBC + α toothpaste and RBC + β toothpaste. The RBC composition included silica particles (identified by Si signal), and alumina and barium glass micro and nanoparticles (identified by Al and Ba signals). Ca signal was displayed as a marker of toothpaste remnants. It is noteworthy that toothpaste remnants could be associated with alumina and barium glass fillers rather than silica particles.

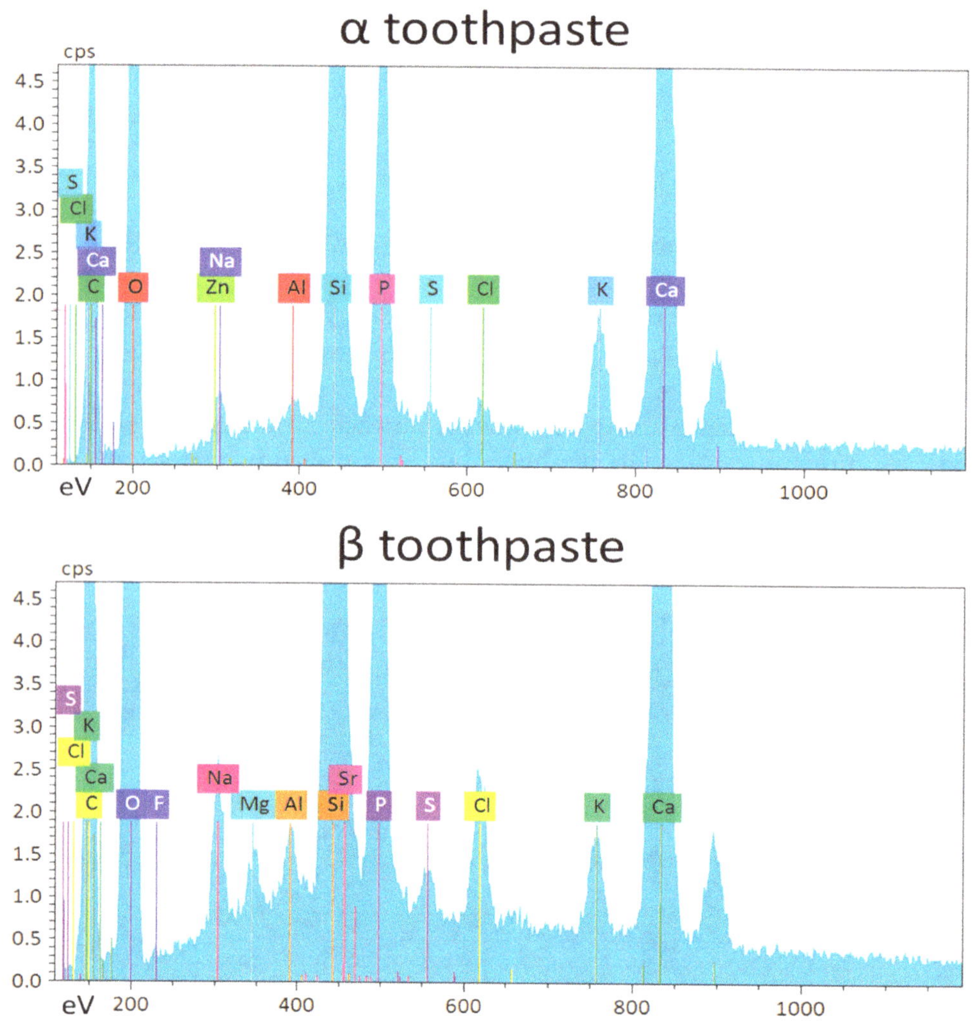

Figure 3. EDS spectra acquired from vacuum-dried tested toothpastes surfaces (α toothpaste containing Zn-carbonate substituted n-HAp, and β toothpaste containing F, Mg, Sr-carbonate substituted n-HAp). Strong Ca and P signals are identified belonging to the n-HAp, as well as the signals corresponding to the corresponding doping elements (Zn in α toothpaste and F, Mg, Sr, in β toothpaste). High counts of Si were also detected in both toothpastes, together with relatively low counts of Al and other elements. The relative amounts of n-HAp doping elements and other elements such as Al and S are below the conventionally considered detection limit of EDS (about 1 wt%). However, the presence of such elements is shown by peaks that were clearly identifiable on all acquired spectra. In this sense, the acquisition of several spectra over the surfaces of many specimens, and the use of statistical analysis on acquired data demonstrating low variability in signals among the different acquisitions (cf. Table 2) allows overcoming, to some extent, this detection limit, improving the performances of EDS analysis.

Table 2. Surface elemental composition of the experimental groups and vacuum-dried toothpastes (α toothpaste containing Zn-carbonate substituted n-HAp and β toothpaste containing F, Mg, Sr-carbonate substituted n-HAp), as assessed by EDS. Data are presented as mean (±1 SD); different letters indicate, for each element, significant differences between groups (Tukey test, $p < 0.05$).

Element	Control Enamel	Control RBC	α Toothpaste	β Toothpaste	Enamel+ α Toothpaste	Enamel+ β Toothpaste	RBC+ α Toothpaste	RBC+ β Toothpaste
C	6.19(0.32) c	33.36(0.49) a	26.08(2.01) b	25.53(1.10) b	5.49(0.75) c	6.12(0.20) c	32.77(1.86) a	33.96(0.34) a
O	38.21(1.38) a,b	33.04(0.33) c,d	43.75(3.23) a	42.69(0.38) a	40.12(2.93) a,b	36.06(1.78) b,c,d	32.89(2.21) d	32.63(0.60) c,d
Ca	38.71(0.90) a	0.00(0.00) c	12.12(2.22) b	9.80(0.40) b	36.97(2.30) a	39.13(0.74) a	1.26(0.12) c	0.30(0.13) c
P	16.31(0.45) a	0.00(0.00) c	4.95(0.95) b	4.93(0.42) b	15.78(1.39) a	16.59(1.20) a	0.76(0.17) c	0.12(0.06) c
Al	0.03(0.04) c	1.46(0.04) a,b	0.29(0.05) b,c	0.32(0.14) b,c	0.09(0.04) c	0.07(0.05) c	1.31(0.78) a,b	1.87(0.03) a
Si	0.08(0.02) d	20.50(0.32) a	9.36(1.81) c	12.12(0.59) b	0.49(0.15) d	0.39(0.04) d	20.23(0.69) a	20.24(0.64) a
Ba	0.00(0.00) c	11.37(0.56) a	0.00(0.00) c	0.00(0.00) c	0.00(0.00) c	0.00(0.00) c	10.52(0.39) b	10.74(0.09) a,b
F	0.00(0.00) b	0.00(0.00) b	0.00(0.00) b	0.18(0.08) a	0.00(0.00) b	0.04(0.02) b	0.00(0.00) b	0.00(0.00) b
Mg	0.18(0.01) b,c	0.00(0.00) d,e	0.00(0.00) d,e	0.35(0.01) a	0.13(0.03) c,d	0.28(0.11) a,b	0.00(0.00) e	0.03(0.01) c,d,e
Zn	0.05(0.06) c	0.00(0.00) c	0.27(0.05) a	0.00(0.00) c	0.17(0.04) a,b	0.05(0.06) c	0.09(0.03) b,c	0.00(0.00) c
Sr	0.00(0.00) c	0.00(0.00) c	0.00(0.00) c	0.93(0.09) a	0.00(0.00) c	0.38(0.10) b	0.00(0.00) c	0.00(0.00) c
Na	0.02(0.03) d	0.00(0.00) d	1.09(0.01) a	1.38(0.01) a	0.52(0.06) b,c	0.71(0.23) b	0.09(0.10) d	0.21(0.04) c,d
S	0.00(0.00) b	0.00(0.00) b	0.25(0.06) a	0.30(0.00) a	0.00(0.00) b	0.00(0.00) b	0.00(0.00) b	0.00(0.00) b
Cl	0.21(0.05) b,c	0.03(0.02) d	0.30(0.07) b	1.08(0.13) a	0.24(0.03) b	0.22(0.01) b,c	0.07(0.01) d	0.09(0.02) c,d
K	0.00(0.00) c	0.00(0.00) c	1.56(0.02) a	0.92(0.06) b	0.00(0.00) c	0.00(0.00) c	0.07(00.09) c	0.02(0.00) c

3.2. Microbiological Results

The effect of the tested toothpastes on EC and BF, expressed as mean OD values ± 1 standard error, according to test setup are shown in Figures 4 and 5. ANOVA results showed an overall significant influence of the tested toothpastes on both EC and BF, with a significant interaction between the factors, toothpaste, and microbiological model ($p = 0.017$). No significant interactions were found between toothpaste and incubation time, adherence surface, or test setup, meaning that the toothpastes had the same effect on microbial viability both in EC and BF, independently from the type of bioreactor used. Most importantly, the tested toothpastes had the same effect on microbial viability, both on enamel and RBC surfaces. On the contrary, ANOVA highlighted a significant interaction ($p < 0.0001$) among adherence surface, test setup, microbiological model, and incubation time.

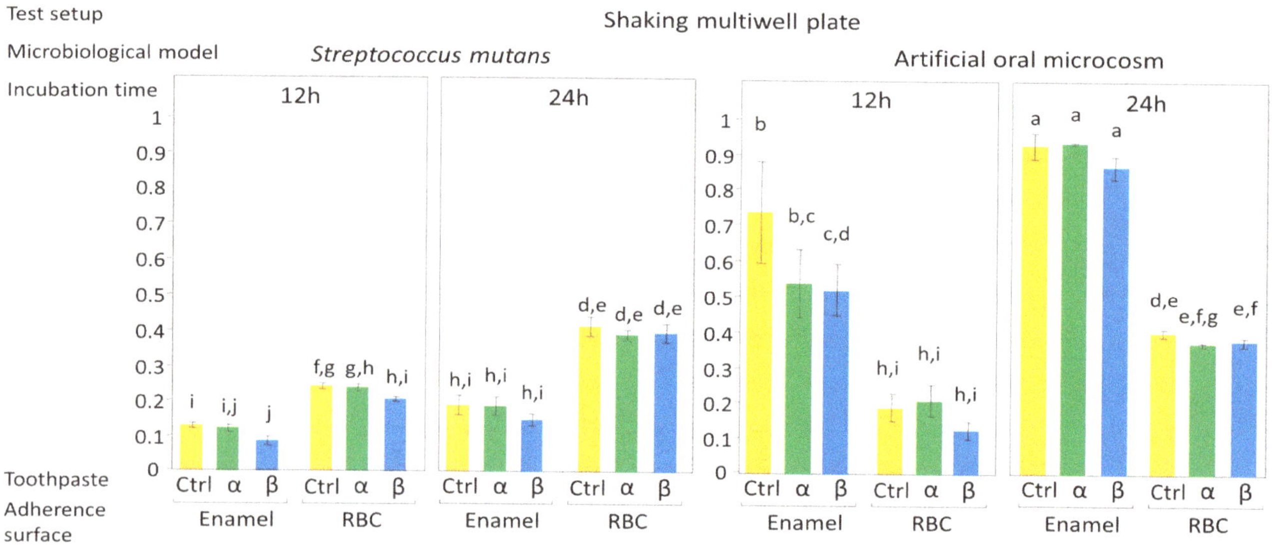

Figure 4. Biofilm formation on the surface of the tested specimens using the shaking multiwell plate test setup, according to the microbiological model (*S. mutans* monospecific biofilm or artificial oral microcosm, aerobically grown) and to the incubation time (12 h or 24 h). Sucrose-enriched sterile modified artificial saliva medium was used in all experiments. Low shear stress on specimens' surfaces was obtained by an orbital incubator, to simulate oral conditions during the night. Moreover, the closed system setup allows a progressive increase in microorganism catabolites and antimicrobial agents released from the surfaces. Results of viable biomass assay are expressed as mean OD ± SE. Different superscript letters indicate significant differences between groups (student's test, $p < 0.05$). α toothpaste contains Zn-carbonate substituted n-HAp; β toothpaste contains F, Mg, Sr-carbonate substituted n-HAp while Ctrl group was brushed with distilled water. β toothpaste significantly reduced the early colonization of the artificial oral microcosm on enamel surfaces when compared to the control.

Considering the results of the post-hoc test on the toothpaste factor, the artificial oral microcosm model showed significantly lower EC and BF on group β disks compared to the control, with group α disks showing lower EC and BF compared to control, but higher EC and BF compared to β toothpaste. Surprisingly, this pattern was found on both tested adherence surfaces, demonstrating an influence of toothpastes on EC and BF even over RBC surfaces. In the monospecific *S. mutans* model, the toothpastes did not significantly influence EC and BF.

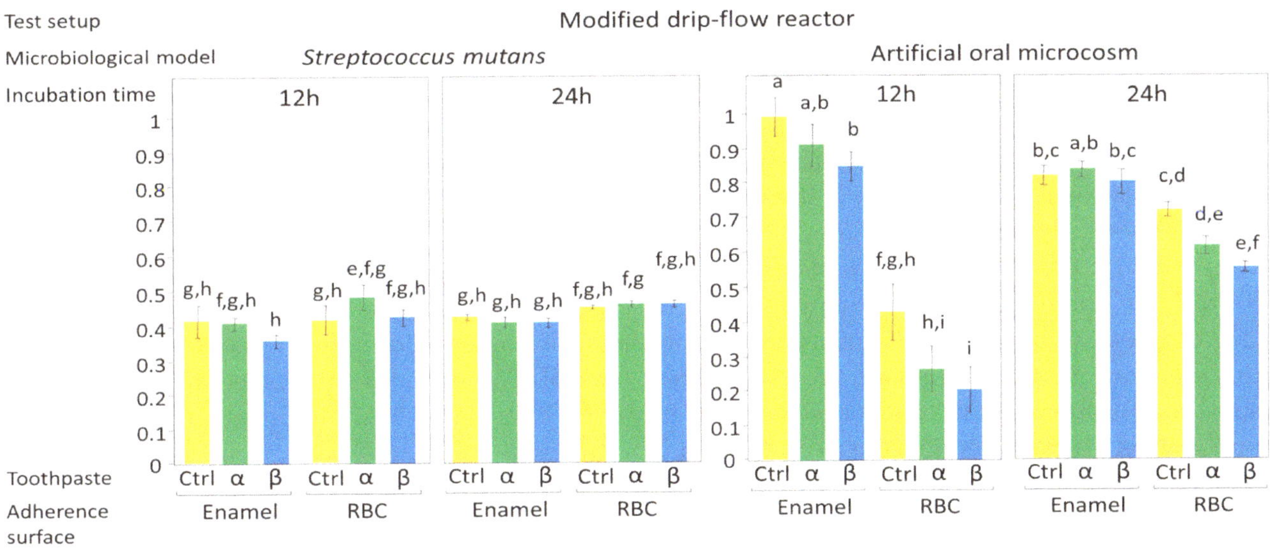

Figure 5. Biofilm formation on the surface of the tested specimens using the MDFR bioreactor test setup, according to the microbiological model (*S. mutans* monospecific biofilm or artificial oral microcosm, aerobically grown) and to the incubation time (12 h or 24 h). Sucrose-enriched sterile modified artificial saliva medium was used in all experiments, being pumped through the flow-cells of the bioreactor. High hydrodynamic stress conditions that occur during the daytime can thus be simulated. An elution of microorganism catabolites and antimicrobial agents released from the surfaces can also occur. Results of viable biomass assay are expressed as mean OD ± SE. Different superscript letters indicate significant differences between groups (student's test, $p < 0.05$). α toothpaste contains Zn-carbonate substituted n-HAp; β toothpaste contains F, Mg, Sr-carbonate substituted n-HAp while Ctrl group was brushed with distilled water. β toothpaste significantly reduced early colonization (enamel and RBC) and biofilm formation (RBC) of the artificial oral microcosm when compared to the control. Interestingly, the adherence surface showed a more considerable influence than toothpaste treatment on early colonization and biofilm formation, independent of the microbiological model or test setup applied. The effect of the toothpaste on RBC surfaces was not expected and opens the possibility to control microbial colonization on RBCs, and, ultimately, secondary caries prevention, by such treatments.

Considering the role of the adherence surface, the oral microcosm model showed significantly higher EC and BF on enamel than on the tested RBC in both test setups (shaking multiwell plate and MDFR). *S. mutans* showed significantly higher EC and BF on the tested RBC than on enamel in the shaking multiwell plate test setup and significantly higher BF on the tested RBC than on enamel in the MDFR.

Regarding incubation time, as expected, there was an overall significant increase in biomass over time. The artificial oral microcosm grown in the MDFR on enamel surfaces showed no significant difference in viable adherent biomass between 12 and 24 h incubation ($p = 0.0711$). Likewise, *S. mutans* grown in the MDFR on both adherence surfaces showed no significant difference in viable adherent biomass between 12 and 24 h incubation ($p = 0.5665$ and $p = 0.7691$ for enamel and RBC, respectively).

From the test setup point of view, MDFR showed an overall significantly higher EC and BF than the shaking multiwell plate, except for BF of artificial oral microcosm on enamel surfaces.

Considering the microbiological model, the artificial oral microcosm showed higher EC and BF than *S. mutans* on enamel surfaces in both test setups, whereas *S. mutans* showed higher EC and BF than the artificial oral microcosm in the shaking multiwell plate on RBC surfaces.

A set of additional enamel and RBC specimens were made and treated with the toothpastes or with the control, as described in the Methods section, to provide a morphological view of the microbial colonization. The most biologically meaningful result was found to be the one obtained using the MDFR test setup and the artificial oral microcosm model for 12 h (EC, Figure 5). Therefore, this particular situation was furtherly investigated using confocal laser-scanning microscopy and live/dead staining. The results are illustrated in Figure 6. Enamel specimens showed a uniform microbial layer colonizing all surfaces, with multilayered structures starting to develop. The aspect is in keeping with the viable biomass results, showing early colonization of β toothpaste < α toothpaste = control. On enamel specimens treated with β toothpaste, a slightly higher amount of dead cells and microcolonies can be seen. RBC specimens showed much lower colonization than enamel, showing early colonization of β toothpaste < α toothpaste < control. The surfaces of the specimens provided an intense red fluorescence that was not wholly subtracted by parallel scanning in the near-UV 405 nm channel. This artifact was not due to dead cells, but rather to autofluorescence coming from the RBC, and also to an affinity of the propidium iodide dye with RBC surfaces, as previously shown [22].

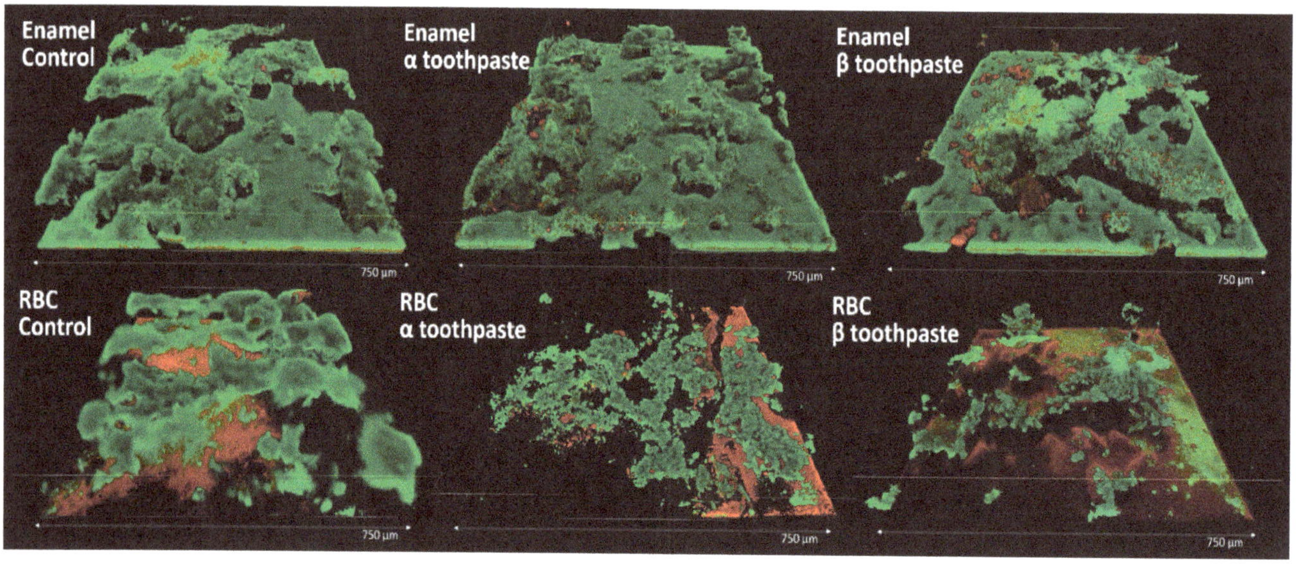

Figure 6. CLSM results of the adherence surfaces treated with the control and the tested toothpastes using the MDFR test setup and the artificial oral microcosm model for 12 h. Scans were analyzed 3D reconstructions obtained using Drishti software. Enamel surfaces provided a much higher early colonization than RBC surfaces. In the background of the enamel control specimen, a central microcolony shows a long tail detached from the surface and oriented horizontally downstream (to the right). This feature is typical of biofilms that develop on surfaces in the presence of relatively high shear stress and is also a means to colonize downstream surfaces rapidly. This feature demonstrates the good morphological resemblance of bioreactor-grown biofilms with in vivo ones. Enamel specimens treated with β toothpaste showed a higher amount of dead cells compared to the other groups. RBC specimens treated with β toothpaste showed the lowest early colonization overall, consistently with viable biomass results.

3.3. Fluoride Release Results

The fluoride release from the disks treated with the fluoride-hydroxyapatite containing toothpaste, and the fluoride content of the biofilms after 12 and 24 h are displayed in Figure 7. A significant albeit shallow release of fluoride was seen from enamel specimens treated with β toothpaste. Contrary to RBC specimens, enamel specimens showed biofilms containing significant amounts of fluoride at both incubation times. After 12 h, treatment with β toothpaste significantly decreased fluoride presence in the overlying biofilm compared to the control ($p < 0.001$).

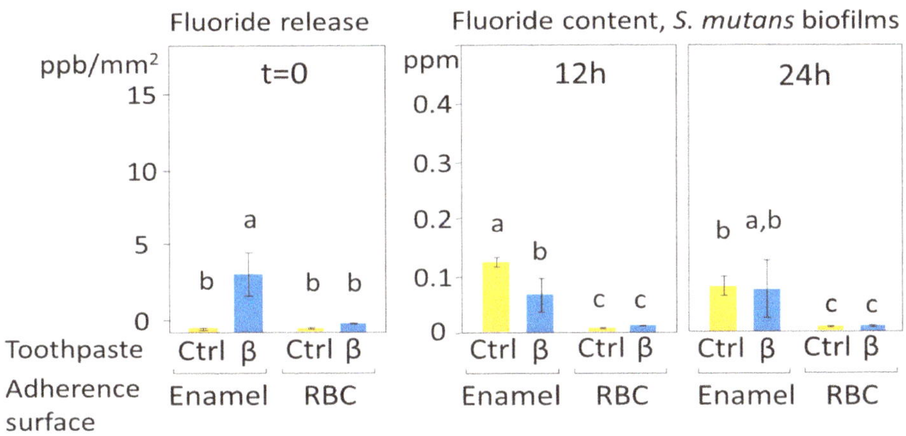

Figure 7. Immediate fluoride release (ppb/mm^2 ± SE) after disks' brushing and fluoride presence (ppm ± SE) in the biofilms grown over the disks' surfaces after 12 and 24 h. Different superscript letters indicate significant differences between groups (Student's test, $p < 0.05$). β toothpaste contains F, Mg, Sr-carbonate substituted n-HAp while Ctrl group was brushed with distilled water. β toothpaste did not increase the baseline fluoride presence in biofilms grown over enamel surfaces despite showing a low but significant immediate fluoride release. The reduction in fluoride presence seen in enamel specimens after 12 h of incubation when compared to the control may be due to an uptake of fluoride by the tested toothpaste.

4. Discussion

Nano-hydroxyapatite is considered one of the most promising bioactive materials with a broad spectrum of applications in preventive and restorative dentistry. N-HAp particles have been demonstrated to have a similar structure to natural enamel apatite crystals and can remineralize dental hard tissues [15,23–25]. Non-substituted n-HAp is also used for desensitizing and anti-erosion purposes [26,27]. The synthesis of nano-scaled zinc carbonate or magnesium-strontium carbonate hydroxyapatite ($ZnCO_3$/n-HAp, Mg-$SrCO_3$/n-HAp) represented significant progress in this field, allowing the introduction of n-HAp-based toothpastes with remineralization and antibacterial potential [28]. Different substituted n-Hap, coupled to other compounds with antibacterial activity, such as Zn PCA, chitosan, and fluoride, have been developed to achieve the goal of the remineralization of dental hard tissues [4,29–32]. Nevertheless, very few data are available in the literature about the antibacterial activity of these compounds, which is important in caries prevention because of the impact of oral biofilms in the dynamics of carious lesion formation.

Biofilms produce organic acids that cause the demineralization of the hard tissues. Moreover, biofilms can act as a reservoir of calcium and phosphate for remineralization, but also as a diffusion barrier for other compounds, such as fluoride, thus reducing the efficacy of some caries-preventive agents [16]. From a microbiological point of view, n-HAp-containing products might allow adsorbed nanoparticles to interact with bacterial cells, reducing adherence to hard tissue surfaces, thereby reducing biofilm formation.

The current in vitro study compared the effect of two substituted n-HAp-based toothpastes on early colonization and biofilm formation. Teeth specimens treated with the α toothpaste showed no significant differences in EC and BF compared to the control and β group, whereas specimens treated with β toothpaste showed a significantly lower EC and BF compared to the control (Figures 4 and 5). Both toothpaste formulations contained doping agents having antibacterial activity, namely zinc in α toothpaste and fluoride and strontium in β toothpaste, suggesting that n-HAp doping agents, rather than n-HAp itself, play a crucial role in determining the antibacterial properties of these compounds. Furthermore, fluoride and strontium have been shown to exhibit synergistic antibacterial performance [33,34]. EDS data (Table 2) showed that the zinc and fluoride concentrations were in the same range, while strontium in the β toothpaste was four times higher. A possible explanation of these results could be that the association of fluoride and strontium was more effective in reducing EC and BF than zinc alone at the tested concentrations. Nevertheless, fluoride release (Figure 7), which was only found on brushed enamel surfaces, did not help in explaining the reduced EC and BF by β toothpaste on RBC surfaces. Furthermore, despite a significant initial release of fluoride, the amount of this ion was not increased in biofilms grown over enamel and RBC surfaces treated with the β toothpaste, confirming the fact that biofilms do not tend to accumulate fluoride [16].

EDS data also showed the presence of calcium and phosphate on the surfaces of RBC specimens treated with both toothpastes, as well as traces of zinc on specimens treated with α toothpaste and magnesium on specimens treated with β toothpaste (Figure 2 and Table 1). It is noteworthy that toothpaste remnants could be associated with alumina and barium glass fillers rather than silica particles. This observation, needing further confirmation, opens the possibility for such compounds to actively interact with RBC surfaces with the effect of reducing or preventing secondary caries occurrence.

Regarding the influence of the adherence surface on the antibacterial activity of substituted n-HAp, as the surface features can deeply influence biological behavior, the roughness of all specimens was reduced below 0.2 μm Ra [35] to exclude the possible influence of this parameter on EC and BF. The two tested surfaces were selected considering their buffering capacity: a buffering surface (enamel) and a non-buffering one (RBC). The non-buffering surface was selected because it has been demonstrated to promote the growth of biofilms with a high concentration of cariogenic bacteria [17]. Our data showed that the adherence surfaces did not influence the effect of the tested toothpastes on EC and BF. This result was observed for both *S. mutans* and the oral microcosm, indicating that, unexpectedly, both substituted n-HAps had the same effect on buffering and non-buffering surfaces independent of their chemical composition, suggesting a similar interaction of the active components with the specimen surface. EDS results confirm the presence of active compounds from both toothpastes on both adherence surfaces. This presence was seen to a larger extent on enamel compared to RBC. However, the presence of such active compounds on the tested RBC surface, as seen in the present study, is very interesting from the perspective of controlling EC and BF on these surfaces, with the final aim of reducing secondary caries occurrence. Indeed, small but accumulative effects can prevent dysbiotic changes in dental biofilms and help maintain a beneficial oral microbiome [36]. In this sense, the use of this kind of active principles might be an efficient means of reducing secondary caries occurrence by actively promoting our natural microbiota and reducing the impact of the drivers of dysbiosis, such as, for instance, the presence of a non-buffering surface.

Two test setups were used, shaking multiwell plates and a drip-flow bioreactor to simulate clinical situations as close as possible, avoiding the variabilities that characterize in vivo studies. The first test setup was designed to evaluate EC and BF under low hydrodynamic stress conditions, for instance, during the night. Moreover, the first setup favors a progressive increase in microorganism catabolites and antimicrobial agents released from the surfaces. The second one simulated relatively high hydrodynamic stress conditions that occur during the daytime. *S. mutans* showed lower EC and BF in the first test setup compared to the second one, probably due to the limited amount of nutrients available and the accumulation of metabolic acids in the culture medium.

From the microbiological model point of view, the approach simulated as much as possible the clinical situation by testing an oral microcosm in addition to a monospecific *S. mutans* biofilm. The oral microcosm was used to evaluate the mixed oral flora developing on hard tissues, while the monospecific *S. mutans* model was used to assess the behavior of the cariogenic part of flora when treated with the tested compounds. In our study, *S. mutans* showed a higher affinity for RBC surfaces than for enamel, which is probably related to the buffering capacity of the tested surfaces being a crucial factor for both EC and BF.

Still, the microbiological models and incubation conditions may not be an accurate replica of all the complex interactions taking place in the oral environment. However, in vitro simulations are useful since they can push microenvironmental conditions to levels that might be difficult to control, or even unethical if replicated in vivo. The culture medium was made to have a high content in sucrose, therefore promoting the growth of fermentative Streptococcus as well as the acidogenic species in the mixed inoculum. The aim was to provide a shift in microbial composition towards a pathogenic biofilm, to test the activity of the toothpastes in a harsh environment. An active principle such as substituted n-HAp is especially useful if it can provide a controlled release of ions over time and, especially, in response to defined environmental conditions. A fermentative biofilm can reach pH values lower than 4.0, promoting the demineralization of enamel (critical pH $\approx$ 5.5). n-HAp is known to be very stable at neutral pH. Therefore, an acidogenic microbial challenge as the one produced in the present setups helped in understanding the effect of the toothpastes when challenged by pathogenic biofilms.

Considering incubation time, 12 h was selected as toothbrushing twice a day is the most frequently advised routine, while a 24 h incubation can provide a sufficient amount of time to evaluate BF. The results showed that the most relevant differences between the tested toothpaste groups were found on *S. mutans* EC, which means after 12 h of incubation. In a translational sense, this may suggest that the tested toothpastes provided the best effect when used twice a day, rather than a single time.

5. Conclusions

A toothpaste treatment based on substituted n-HAp showed an in vitro antibacterial effect both on natural and RBC surfaces, which was more pronounced after 12 h than after 24 h. On RBC surfaces, toothpaste remnants seemed to show selective affinity with some particles, such as alumina and barium glass fillers, rather than silica particles. This observation is worthy of future investigations aimed at clarifying the interactions between substituted n-HAp and RBC fillers from the perspective of secondary caries prevention. This phenomenon provides a basis to design clinical studies aimed to confirm in vivo the preventive efficacy of these active principles.

Author Contributions: Conceptualization, A.C.I. and E.B.; Data curation, A.C.I., G.C. and M.O.; Formal analysis, M.O., F.G.-G., and E.B.; Funding acquisition, E.B.; Investigation, A.C.I. and G.C.; Methodology, A.C.I., G.C. and M.O.; Project administration, E.B.; Resources, E.B.; Software, G.C. and M.O.; Supervision, A.C.I. and E.B.; Validation, A.C.I.; Visualization, E.B., F.G.-G.; Writing—original draft, A.C.I., G.C. and M.O.; Writing—review & editing, F.G.-G., and E.B. All authors have read and agreed to the published version of the manuscript.

Acknowledgments: The authors are grateful to Massimo Tagliaferro and to Nanovision S.R.L. for providing the SEM-EDS equipment.

References

1. Flemming, T.F.; Beikler, T. Control of oral biofilms. *Periodontology 2000* **2011**, *55*, 9–15. [CrossRef]
2. Rosier, B.T.; Marsh, P.D.; Mira, A. Resilience of the oral microbiota in health: Mechanisms that prevent dysbiosis. *J. Dent. Res.* **2018**, *97*, 371–380. [CrossRef] [PubMed]
3. Marsh, P.D. Plaque as a biofilm: Pharmacological principles of drug delivery and action in the sub-and supragingival environment. *Oral Dis.* **2003**, *9*, 16–22. [CrossRef] [PubMed]
4. Allaker, R.P. The use of nanoparticles to control oral biofilm formation. *J. Dent. Res.* **2010**, *89*, 1175–1186. [CrossRef] [PubMed]
5. Besinis, A.; De Peralta, T.; Handy, R.D. Inhibition of biofilm formation and antibacterial properties of a silver nano-coating on human dentine. *Nanotoxicology* **2014**, *8*, 745–754. [CrossRef]
6. Hannig, M.; Hannig, C. Nanomaterials in preventive dentistry. *Nat. Nanotechnol.* **2010**, *5*, 565–569. [CrossRef]
7. Allaker, R.P.; Memarzadeh, K. Nanoparticles and the control of oral infections. *Int. J. Antimicrob. Agents* **2014**, *43*, 95–104. [CrossRef]
8. Beyth, N.; Houri-Haddad, Y.; Domb, A.; Khan, W.; Hazan, R. Alternative antimicrobial approach: Nano-antimicrobial materials. *Evid.-Based Complement. Altern. Med.* **2015**, *2015*, 246012. [CrossRef]
9. Cochrane, N.J.; Cai, F.; Huq, N.L.; Burrow, M.F.; Reynolds, E.C. New approaches to enhanced remineralization of tooth enamel. *J. Dent. Res.* **2010**, *89*, 1187–1197. [CrossRef]
10. Nongonierma, A.B.; Fitzgerald, R.J. Biofunctional properties of caseinphosphopeptides in the oral cavity. *Caries Res.* **2012**, *46*, 234–267. [CrossRef]

11. Grychtol, S.; Basche, S.; Hannig, M.; Hannig, C. Effect of cpp/acp on initial bioadhesion to enamel and dentin in situ. *Sci. World J.* **2014**, *2014*, 512682. [CrossRef]
12. Najibfard, K.; Ramalingam, K.; Chedjieu, I.; Amaechi, B.T. Remineralization of early caries by a nano-hydroxyapatite dentifrice. *J. Clin. Dent.* **2011**, *22*, 139–143. [PubMed]
13. Lelli, M.; Putignano, A.; Marchetti, M.; Foltran, I.; Mangani, F.; Procaccini, M.; Roveri, N.; Orsini, G. Remineralization and repair of enamel surface by biomimetic Zn-carbonate hydroxyapatite containing toothpaste: A comparative in vivo study. *Front. Physiol.* **2014**, *5*, 333–340. [CrossRef] [PubMed]
14. Lu, K.L.; Meng, X.C.; Zhang, J.X.; Li, X.Y.; Zhou, M.L. Inhibitory effect of synthetic nano-hydroxyapatite on dental caries. *Key Eng. Mater.* **2007**, *336*, 1538–1541. [CrossRef]
15. Tschoppe, P.; Zandim, D.L.; Martus, P.; Kielbassa, A.M. Enamel and dentine remineralization by nano-hydroxyapatite toothpastes. *J. Dent.* **2011**, *39*, 430–437. [CrossRef]
16. Zhang, M.; He, L.B.; Exterkate, R.A.M.; Cheng, L.; Li, J.Y.; ten Cate, J.M.; Crielaard, W.; Deng, D.M. Biofilm layers affect the treatment outcomes of NaF and nano-hydroxyapatite. *J. Dent. Res.* **2015**, *94*, 602–607. [CrossRef]
17. Nedeljkovic, I.; De Munck, J.; Slomka, V.; Van Meerbeek, B.; Teughels, W.; Van Landuyt, K.L. Lack of buffering by composites promotes shift to more cariogenic bacteria. *J. Dent. Res.* **2016**, *95*, 875–881. [CrossRef]
18. Guggenheim, B.; Giertsen, E.; Schupbach, P.; Shapiro, S. Validation of an in vitro biofilm model of supragingival plaque. *J. Dent. Res.* **2001**, *80*, 363–370. [CrossRef]
19. Brambilla, E.; Ionescu, A.C.; Cazzaniga, G.; Ottobelli, M.; Samaranayake, L.P. Levorotatory carbohydrates and xylitol subdue *Streptococcus mutans* and *Candida albicans* adhesion and biofilm formation. *J. Basic Microbiol.* **2016**, *56*, 480–492. [CrossRef]
20. Ionescu, A.; Brambilla, E.; Wastl, D.S.; Giessibl, F.J.; Cazzaniga, G.; Schneider-Feyrer, S.; Hahnel, S. Influence of matrix and filler fraction on biofilm formation on the surface of experimental resin-based composites. *J. Mater. Sci. Mater. Med.* **2015**, *26*, 58. [CrossRef]
21. Cazzaniga, G.; Ottobelli, M.; Ionescu, A.C.; Paolone, G.; Gherlone, E.; Ferracane, J.L.; Brambilla, E. In vitro biofilm formation on resin-based composites after different finishing and polishing procedures. *J. Dent.* **2017**, *67*, 43–52. [CrossRef] [PubMed]
22. Ionescu, A.C.; Brambilla, E.; Hahnel, S. Does recharging dental restorative materials with fluoride influence biofilm formation? *Dent. Mater.* **2019**, *35*, 1450–1463. [CrossRef] [PubMed]
23. Huang, S.B.; Gao, S.S.; Yu, H.Y. Effect of nano-hydroxyapatite concentration on remineralization of initial enamel lesion in vitro. *Biomed. Mater.* **2009**, *4*, 034104. [CrossRef] [PubMed]
24. Li, L.; Pan, H.; Tao, J.; Xu, X.; Mao, C.; Gu, X.; Tang, R. Repair of enamel by using hydroxyapatite nanoparticles as the building blocks. *J. Mater. Chem.* **2008**, *18*, 4079–4084. [CrossRef]
25. Roveri, N.; Battistella, E.; Bianchi, C.L.; Foltran, I.; Foresti, E.; Iafisco, M.; Lelli, M.; Naldoni, A.; Palazzo, B.; Rimondini, L. Surface enamel remineralization: Biomimetic apatite nanocrystals and fluoride ions different effects. *J. Nanomater.* **2009**, *2009*, 746383. [CrossRef]
26. Aykut-Yetkiner, A.; Attin, T.; Wiegand, A. Prevention of dentine erosion by brushing with anti-erosive toothpastes. *J. Dent.* **2014**, *42*, 856–861. [CrossRef]
27. De Melo Alencar, C.; de Paula, B.L.F.; Ortiz, M.I.G.; Magno, M.B.; Silva, C.M.; Maia, L.C. Clinical efficacy of nano-hydroxyapatite in dentin hypersensitivity: A systematic review and meta-analysis. *J. Dent.* **2019**, *82*, 11–21. [CrossRef]
28. Orsini, G.; Procaccini, M.; Manzoli, L.; Giuliodori, F.; Lorenzini, A.; Putignano, A. A double-blind randomized-controlled trial comparing the desensitizing efficacy of a new dentifrice containing carbonate/hydroxyapatite nanocrystals and a sodium fluoride/potassium nitrate dentifrice. *J. Clin. Periodontol.* **2010**, *37*, 510–517. [CrossRef]
29. Brambilla, E.; Ionescu, A.; Cazzaniga, G.; Edefonti, V.; Gagliani, M. The influence of antibacterial toothpastes on in vitro *Streptococcus mutans* biofilm formation: A continuous culture study. *Am. J. Dent.* **2014**, *27*, 160–166.
30. Hannig, C.; Basche, S.; Burghardt, T.; Al-Ahmad, A.; Hannig, M. Influence of a mouthwash containing hydroxyapatite microclusters on bacterial adherence in situ. *Clin. Oral Investig.* **2013**, *17*, 805–814. [CrossRef]
31. Kong, M.; Chen, X.G.; Xing, K.; Park, H.J. Antimicrobial properties of chitosan and mode of action: A state of the art review. *Int. J. Food Microbiol.* **2010**, *144*, 51–63. [CrossRef] [PubMed]
32. Li, X.; Wang, J.; Joiner, A.; Chang, J. The remineralisation of enamel: A review of the literature. *J. Dent.* **2014**, *42*, S12–S20. [CrossRef]

33. Dabsie, F.; Gregoire, G.; Sixou, M.; Sharrock, P. Does strontium play a role in the cariostatic activity of glass ionomer?: Strontium diffusion and antibacterial activity. *J. Dent.* **2009**, *37*, 554–559. [CrossRef] [PubMed]
34. Guida, A.; Towler, M.R.; Wall, J.G.; Hill, R.G.; Eramo, S. Preliminary work on the antibacterial effect of strontium in glass ionomer cements. *J. Mater. Sci. Lett.* **2003**, *22*, 1401–1403. [CrossRef]
35. Bollen, C.M.; Lambrechts, P.; Quirynen, M. Comparison of surface roughness of oral hard materials to the threshold surface roughness for bacterial plaque retention: A review of the literature. *Dent. Mater.* **1997**, *13*, 258–269. [CrossRef]
36. Marsh, P.D. In sickness and in health—What does the oral microbiome mean to us? An ecological perspective. *Adv. Dent. Res.* **2018**, *29*, 60–65. [CrossRef]

16

Novel Orthodontic Cement Comprising Unique Imidazolium-Based Polymerizable Antibacterial Monomers

Hui Lu * and Xiaoming Jin *

Dentsply Sirona, R&D—Consumables Product Group, 38 W Clarke Ave, Milford, DE 19963, USA
* Correspondence: Hui.Lu@dentsplysirona.com (H.L.); Xiaoming.Jin@dentsplysirona.com (X.J.)

Abstract: White spot lesions (WSLs) can develop quickly and compromise the successful outcome of the orthodontic treatment. Orthodontic bonding cement with the capability to prevent or mitigate WSLs could be beneficial, especially for patients with high risk of caries. This study explored novel mono- and di-imidazolium-based polymerizable antibacterial monomers and evaluated orthodontic cement compositions comprising such novel monomers. Their antibacterial potentials, mechanical properties, and shear bond strength (SBS) to bovine enamel were investigated. Statistical tests were applied to SBS and mechanical tests (one-way ANOVA and Tukey's test). For antibacterial resins C (ABR-C) and E (ABR-E), their minimum inhibitory concentration (MIC) and minimum bactericidal concentration (MBC) against cariogenic *Streptococcus mutans* bacterial strain UA159 were found to be 4 μg/mL and 8 μg /mL, respectively. The loss of dry mass from completely demineralized dentin beams in buffer solutions pre-dipped into ABR-C and ABR-E resins is much less than that in control buffer (artificial saliva) only. For unfilled resins comprising up to 12 wt % ABR-C, no significant decreases in flexural strength or modulus were observed. For experimental cements incorporating 1–4 wt % ABR-C, there was no drastic compromise to the SBS to enamel except for 3 wt % ABR-C. Furthermore, their SBS was all comparable to the commercially available orthodontic cements. The ISO-22196 antimicrobial test against *S. aureus* showed significant levels of antibacterial effects—up to over 5 logs of microorganism reduction exhibited by ABR-C-containing experimental cements. The imidazolium-based polymerizable monomers could be utilized to functionalize orthodontic bonding cement with steady antibacterial activity and develop a potential strategy to counteract WSLs.

Keywords: white spot lesions; antibacterial; biofilms; dental; orthodontic

---

1. Introduction

Beyond just straightening teeth and achieving better esthetics, proper orthodontic intervention can result in greatly improved oral and psychological health [1,2]. A major undesirable outcome during orthodontic treatment is the development of white spot lesions (WSLs) around orthodontic brackets, especially near the gingival margin [3–6]. The boosted accumulation of biofilms around the brackets further lowers pH around these sites. Despite advancements in patient education, WSLs can still develop rapidly and could compromise the successful outcome of the treatment, even resulting in premature termination of treatment in severe cases [7–9]. It has been reported that between roughly 26% and 70% of patients using fixed orthodontic appliances exhibited various levels of WSLs during the orthodontic treatment [4,6,7]. In another study, the prevalence of WSLs was reported to be 38% in the 6-month group, whereas it was 46% in the 12-month group [9].

Due to the more retentive, complicated surfaces around brackets and higher occurrences for plaque or biofilm adherence, it has become quite challenging to maintain good oral hygiene, especially for less compliant patient groups [8,10–12]. It has been reported that fixed orthodontic appliances can affect the self-cleansing capabilities of the intraoral system, owing to the interactions of saliva and teeth surfaces. Even for patients with clear aligners, wearing aligners 20~22 h daily could limit the natural cleansing and neutralizing effects of saliva [13]. The fixed orthodontic appliances can even alter the oral microflora and increase the levels of acidogenic plaque bacteria, i.e., *Streptococcus mutans* (*S. mutans*), and *lactobacilli* in saliva and dental biofilm during active wearing of such appliances throughout lengthy orthodontic treatment procedures, with an average duration around two to three years [14–19] .

The interface between tooth and orthodontic bonding adhesive or cement, many of them based on (meth)acrylate chemistry, could also become the victim of bacterial attack and subsequent degradation [20,21]. Finer et al.'s findings revealed increased degradation of resin-based composite and bonding agent by *S. mutans* UA159 vs. control. Esterase activities at levels that could degrade adhesives and resin composite have also been linked to *S. mutans* [20]. While bonding the irregularly shaped orthodontic appliances onto the tooth surface, the residual excess of orthodontic cements can also stimulate the extra accumulation of dental biofilm around brackets. The biofilm degradation of this important tooth–cement–bracket interface may contribute to the premature debonding of the brackets, especially given the compounding interactions with the microorganisms that could lead to biocorrosion on the surfaces of metal-based brackets and appliances [22].

Given the extensive prevalence of WSLs occurring during orthodontic treatments, various strategies have been utilized to prevent or mediate demineralization and occurrence of WSL formation. The use of fluoride via various forms, i.e., mouth rinse, gel, topical varnish, toothpaste, etc., has been the predominant remedy applied and studied [7,14,23,24]. Fluoride ions have been well documented to enhance remineralization of enamel and mitigate mineral loss during acid dissolution, by replacing the hydroxyl groups in hydroxyapatite and forming more acid-resistant fluorapatite [25]. The findings consolidated by Bergstrand and Twetman concluded that the use of topical fluoride varnish along with fluoride toothpaste has been the best evidence-based approach to prevent WSLs. The mean prevented portion based on six clinical trials was 42.5% with a range from 4% to 73% [23]. These studies provided convincing support for routine professional applications of fluoride varnish around the bracket base during orthodontic treatment [24–28].

The application of quaternary ammonium compound (QAC) has been actively investigated to introduce antibacterial activity into the orthodontic bonding system. A unique type of antimicrobial polymer is demonstrated by incorporating quaternary ammonium polyethyleneimine (QPEI) nanoparticles. QPEI nanoparticle-containing composites have been reported to exhibit antibacterial activity against salivary bacteria and in vivo antibiofilm activity [29]. Experimental orthodontic bonding cements with 1% incorporated insoluble QPEI and polycationic polyethyleneimine nanoparticles were reported to exhibit stable, long-lasting antibacterial properties against *S. mutans* [30,31]. A variety of QAC-containing functional monomers have been systematically studied, including the widely studied methacryloyloxydodecylpyridinium bromide (MDPB) [32,33] ; dimethylaminohexadecyl methacrylate (DMAHDM), a mono-methacrylate QAC with an alkyl chain length of 16 [34,35]; dimethylaminododedecyl methacrylate (DMADDM), a mono-methacrylate QAC with an alkyl chain length of 12 [36–38]; and 2-methacryloxylethyl hexadecyl methyl ammonium bromide (MAE-HB), a crosslinkable, di-methacrylate QAC with an alkyl chain length of 16 [39,40]. Significant antibacterial activities and biofilm reductions have been demonstrated.

Recently, a series of polymerizable imidazolium-based antibacterial resins (ABRs) were successfully designed in our laboratory [41,42]. To the best of our knowledge, no such novel crosslinkable imidazolium-based monomers have been investigated for their application towards an orthodontic bonding system with the potential to prevent and mitigate WSLs. The aims of this study were to investigate imidazolium-based ABR's antibacterial activities and impacts on the adhesive and mechanical properties of experimental orthodontic bonding cement formulations.

2. Results

By coupling with different mono-ols, diols, polyols (such as triols), monoamines, diamines, and/or polyamines, a range of methacrylate resins with (poly)imidazole moieties were prepared. During the processes of synthesizing imidazolium-based polymerizable resins from imidazole-containing monomers, a facile process based on imidazole and (meth)acrylated resins was developed. As demonstrated in Schemes 1 and 2, a variety of imidazole-containing polymerizable monomers were able to be prepared accordingly.

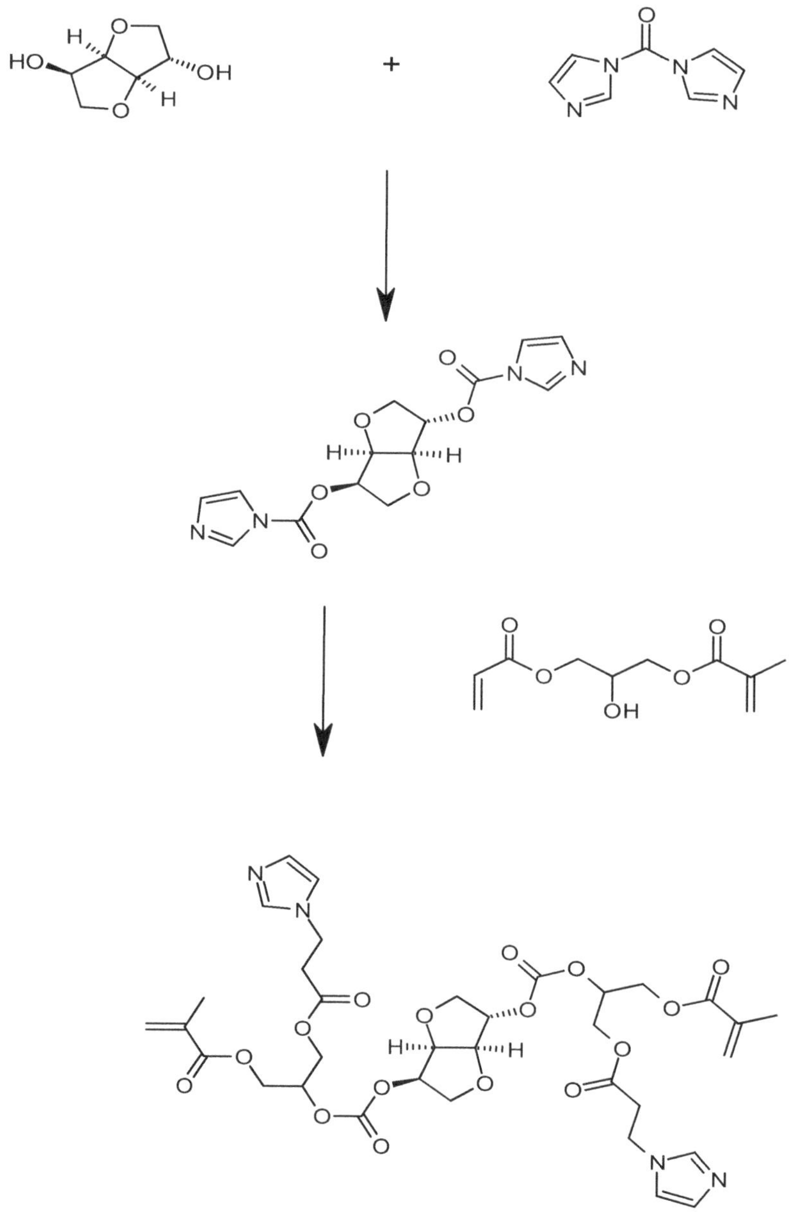

Scheme 1. Isosorbide-based bisimidazole–dimethacrylate resins.

The polymerizable imidazole-based resins were further converted into polymerizable imidazolium-based monomers by reacting them with a variety of halogenated alkyls. A variety of polymerizable imidazolium-based antibacterial resins (ABRs) were successfully synthesized as exhibited in Schemes 3 and 4. The primary evaluations of these novel ABRs' antibacterial activity include the determination of minimum inhibitory concentration (MIC) and minimum bactericidal concentration (MBC) against cariogenic *S. mutans* bacterial strain UA159.

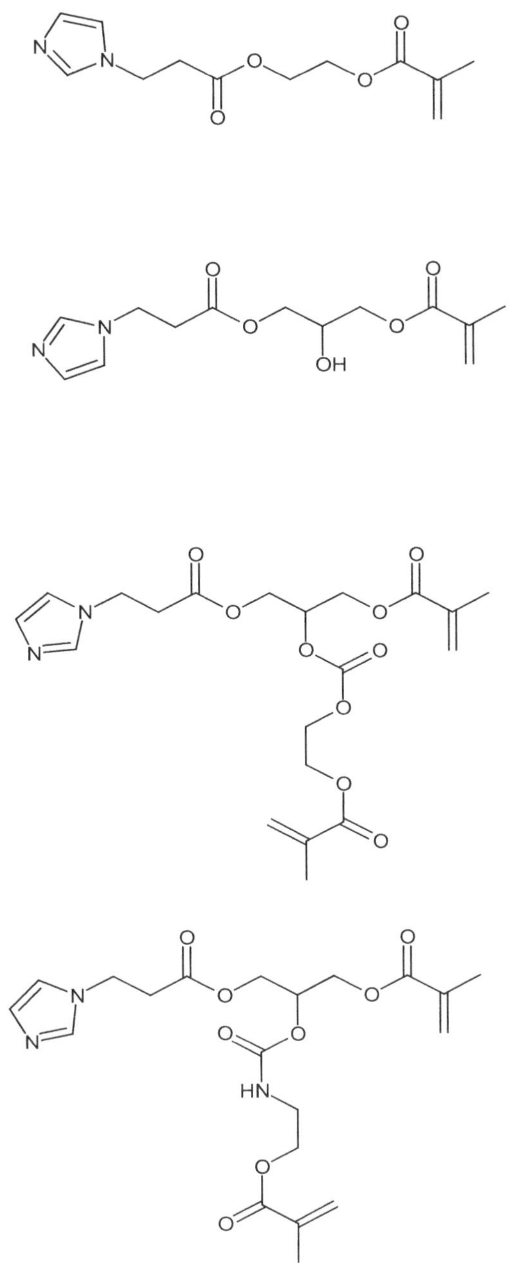

Scheme 2. Various polymerizable mono-imidazole monomers synthesized.

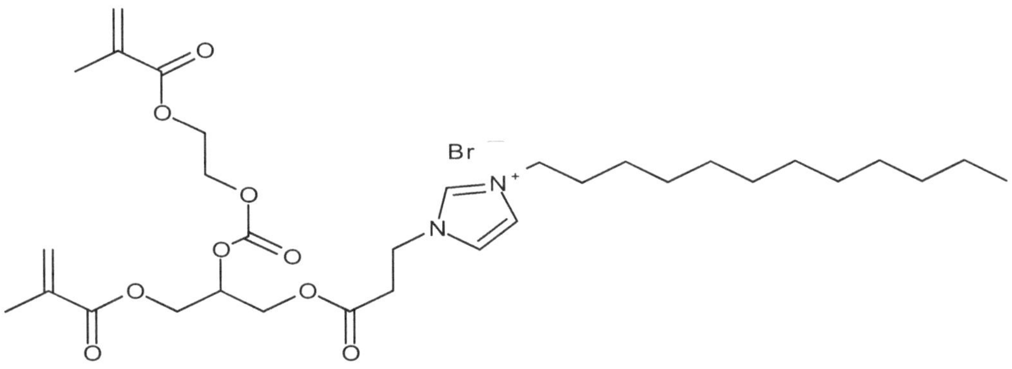

Scheme 3. Polymerizable alkylimidazoliumbromide–dimethacrylate monomer, antibacterial resin C (ABR-C).

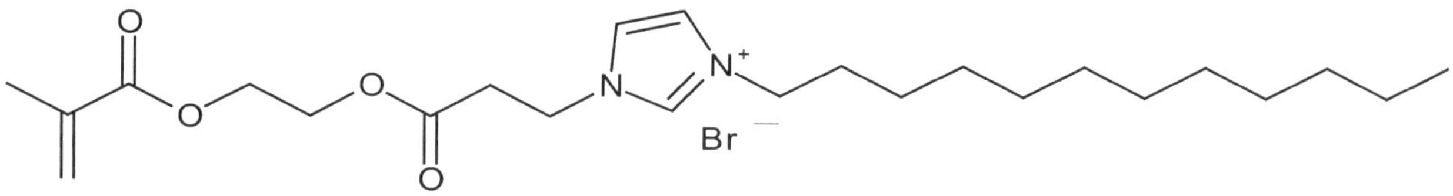

Scheme 4. Polymerizable alkylimidazoliumbromide–methacrylate monomer ABR-E.

Table 1 presents the results of MIC and MBC for representative ABR resins and SDR Resin (a proprietary dimethacrylate monomer, without imidazole moiety, synthesized by Dentsply Sirona) in comparison to frequently used controls, namely chlorhexidine (CHX) as wide-spectrum antimicrobial agent and triethylene glycol dimethacrylate (TEGDMA). TEGDMA was chosen as control monomer because it is widely used in the composition of resins for dental-related applications, including but not limited to restorative, adhesive, and orthodontic compositions. In addition, it was not known to have antibacterial potencies against common cariogenic oral bacteria strains. Furthermore, by using a modified JIS Z 2801 test method, a preliminary antibacterial test against *S. mutans* strain UA159 was used to evaluate the antibacterial effectiveness for such formulated compositions. After 24 h contact, a bacterial reduction of 99.88% was exhibited by test sample containing ABR-E (Scheme 4), as compared to control. This indicated that imidazolium-based polymerizable resin could be highly effective in suppressing the growth of bacteria such as *S. mutans*.

Table 1. Minimum inhibitory concentration (MIC) and minimum bactericidal concentration (MBC) of novel antibacterial resins ABR-E and ABR-C against *Streptococcus mutans* strain UA159, as compared to SDR Resin, triethylene glycol dimethacrylate (TEGDMA), and chlorhexidine.

Test Compound	Stock Solution	Tested Concentrations	Bacterial Inoculum Size (CFU/mL)	MIC	MBC
ABR-E	2.5%	0–0.1%	9×10^7	4 µg/mL (0.0004%)	8 µg/mL (0.0008%)
ABR-C	1%	0–0.1%	9×10^7	4 µg/mL (0.0004%)	8 µg/mL (0.0008%)
SDR Resin	0.25%	0–0.1%	9×10^7	No bacterial growth inhibition	
TEGDMA	100%	0–0.1%	9×10^7	No bacterial growth inhibition	
Chlorhexidine	2.5 mg/mL	0–125 mg/mL	9×10^7	2 mg/mL	4 mg/mL

The loss of dry mass from completely demineralized dentin beams (2 mm × 1 mm × 6 mm) in buffer solutions pre-dipped into ABR-C and ABR-E resins, versus in control buffer (artificial saliva) without pre-dip, was studied. The amount of soluble collagen in these demineralized dentin beams was measured after 7 days of incubation at 37 °C. As Figure 1 indicates, dentin beams without pre-dip lost about 15.5% of their dry mass due to degradations of endogenous matrix metalloproteinases (MMPs) and cathepsins. When the dentin beams were pre-dipped in 1–4% of imidazolium-based ABR resins (ABR-C, ABR-E) for 30 s and then dropped in incubation medium, the dentin beams only lost about 3.5–5% of their dry mass. Furthermore, the hydroxyproline (HYP), an amino acid unique to collagen, content in the medium was also measured. The collagen peptide fragments that were solubilized by the endogenous proteases of the dentin matrix were hydrolyzed to amino acids in 6N HCl and then analyzed for hydroxyproline. In the control group, the proteases released about 10.5 µg HYP/mg dry dentin after 7 days; beams pre-dipped in 1% or 4% of ABR-C released less than half as much hydroxyproline and the beam treated with ABR-E yielded a similar result.

As the designed imidazolium-based resin still comprises a methacrylate functional group, no compatibility or copolymerization issues were found when mixed with typical dimethacrylate-type dental resins, such as 1,6-bis[methacryloyloxyethoxycarbonylamino]-2,4,4-trimethylhexane (UDMA), ethoxylated bisphenol A dimethacrylate (EBPADMA), and TEGDMA. Even with 16 wt % loading of ABR-C into the control orthodontic resin, no mixability issue was observed and the resulting resin mixture was found uniform. The 3-point bending flexural strength and modulus of unfilled orthodontic resins containing 4~16 wt% ABR-C, along with control, were measured following ISO-4049 method and the results are presented in Table 2.

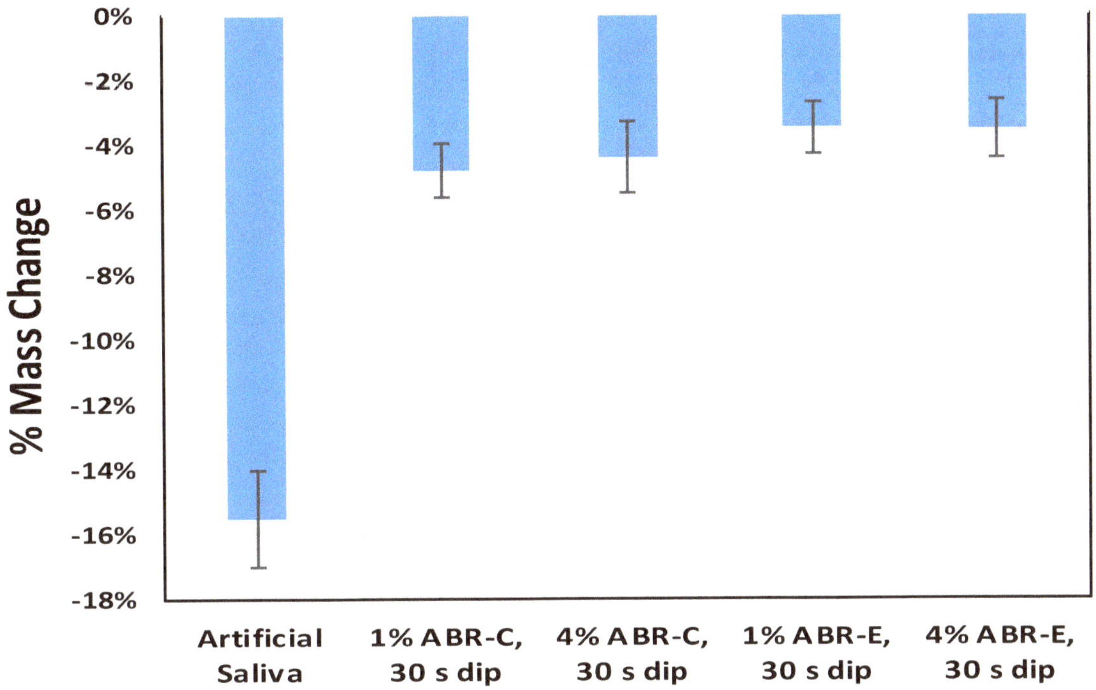

Figure 1. Effect of pre-dipping in antibacterial resins ABR-C and ABR-E on loss of dry mass of demineralized dentin beams after incubation for 7 days at 37 °C.

Table 2. Flexural strength and flexural modulus of exp. orthodontic resins (unfilled) that contain various concentrations of imidazolium-based polymerizable antibacterial monomer ABR-C.

Resin Sample	Control	4%_ABR-C	8%_ABR-C	12%_ABR-C	16%_ABR-C
Antibacterial Monomer in Resin	0	4 wt%	8 wt%	12 wt%	16 wt%
Flexural Strength, MPa (s.d.)	97 (8) ^{A}	88 (5) ^{A,B}	91 (4) ^{A}	95 (3) ^{A}	81 (4) ^{B}
Flexural Modulus, MPa (s.d.)	2443 (87) ^{a}	2388 (183) ^{a}	2394 (139) ^{a}	2293 (82) ^{a,b}	2125 (125) ^{b}

Within the same row, means that do not share the same superscript(s) are significantly different ($\alpha = 0.05$).

The 75 wt % filled experimental orthodontic cements incorporating various concentrations of antibacterial monomer ABR-C were also studied. The current investigation examined flexural and compressive strengths, flexural modulus, ambient light sensitivity, and notched-edge shear bond strength (NE-SBS) to bovine enamel. Results along with statistical analysis are presented in Table 3. For reference, the shear bond strength to bovine enamel, using the same NE-SBS method, and ambient light sensitivity of five commercially available orthodontic bonding cements were also evaluated, as presented in Figures 2 and 3, respectively.

Antibacterial testing was also conducted at an independent and good laboratory practice (GLP) complied testing institution. As shown in Table 4, for orthodontic cement paste formulations that incorporated imidazolium-based dimethacrylate antibacterial monomer (ABR-C), the ISO-22196 antimicrobial testing results against ATCC 6538 showed significant levels of antibacterial effects—up to over 5 logs of microorganism reduction—when compared with control. Such highly effective bactericidal effects for the imidazolium-based polymerizable resins were promising due to a relatively low-level loading and significantly reduced probability of leaching out owing to the dimethacrylate functional groups.

Table 3. Adhesive and physical properties of orthodontic cements (filled with 75% inorganic filler) that contain various concentrations of imidazolium-based polymerizable antibacterial monomer ABR-C.

Orthodontic Cement	Control	1%_ABR-C	2%_ABR-C	3%_ABR-C	4%_ABR-C
Antibacterial Monomer in Cement	0	1 wt%	2 wt%	3 wt%	4 wt%
Resin Conc.	25.0%	25.0%	25.0%	25.0%	25.0%
Ambient Light Sensitivity	2:35"	2:00"	2:05"	2:00"	2:15"
Compressive Strength, MPa (s.d.)	373 (25) [A]	361 (12) [A,B]	346 (10) [B]	352 (5) [A,B]	307 (15) [C]
Flexural Strength, MPa (s.d.)	150 (14) [A]	139 (6) [A]	114 (10) [B]	114 (10) [B]	88 (7) [C]
Flexural Modulus, MPa (s.d.)	11165 (531) [a]	10848 (383) [a,b]	10319 (549) [a,b]	10607 (629) [a,b]	10066 (445) [b]
NE-SBS to Etched Enamel, MPa (s.d.)	32.8 (2.7) [A,B]	36.7 (4.5) [A]	28.8 (4.3) [B,C]	25.4 (3.5) [C]	31.0 (5.8) [A,B,C]
SBS to Enamel Range, MPa	29.5 ~ 37.2	31.9 ~ 43.4	21.9 ~ 32.7	21.5 ~ 29.5	23.1 ~ 38.0
SBS to Enamel C.V.	8.1%	12.1%	14.8%	14.0%	18.7%

Within the same row, means that do not share the same superscript(s) are significantly different ($\alpha = 0.05$).

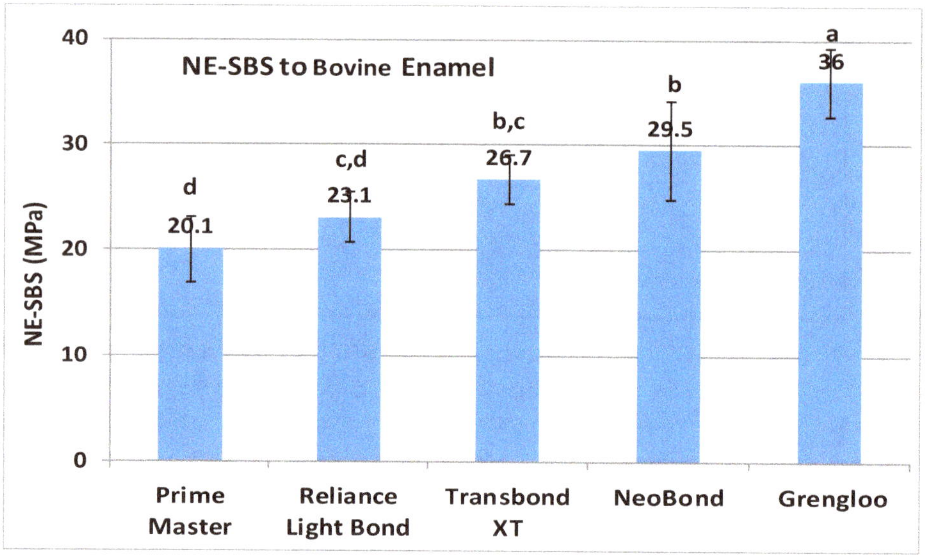

Figure 2. Notched-edge shear bond strength to bovine enamel of commercial orthodontic cements. Values that do not share the same superscript(s) are significantly different ($\alpha = 0.05$).

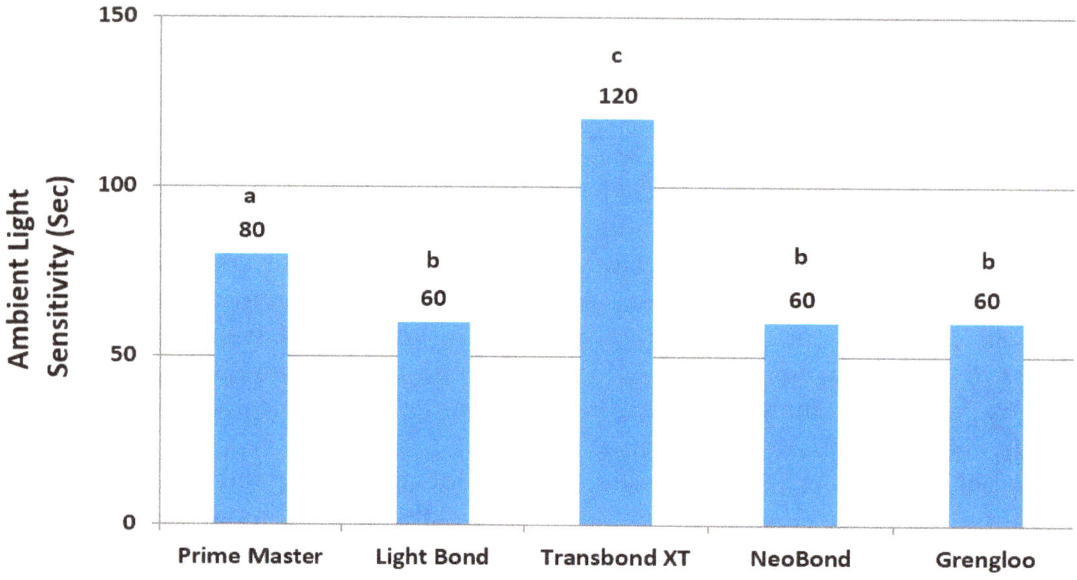

Figure 3. Ambient light sensitivity of commercial orthodontic cements. Values that do not share the same superscript are significantly different ($\alpha = 0.05$).

Table 4. ISO-22196 antimicrobial test of orthodontic cements (filled with 75 wt % inorganic filler) that contain various concentrations of imidazolium-based polymerizable antibacterial monomer using *S. aureus* 6538. The limit of detection for this assay is 5 CFU/carrier.

Test Micro-Organism	Contact Time	Carrier Type	Anti-Bacterial Monomer in Cement	CFU/Carrier	Percent Reduction Compared to Control at Contact Time	Log_{10} Reduction Compared to Control at Contact Time
S. aureus 6538	Time Zero	Control	0	1.00×10^6	N/A	
	24 h	ATL Control	0	8.50×10^5		
		2%_ABR-C	2 wt%	1.00×10	99.9988%	4.93
		4%_ABR-C	4 wt%	1.50×10	99.998%	4.75
		1%_ABR-C	1 wt%	4.72×10^3	99.44%	2.26
		3%_ABR-C	3 wt%	<5.00	> 99.9994%	> 5.23

3. Discussion

As demonstrated by MIC and MBC test results reported in Table 1, ABR-C and ABR-E displayed distinct antibacterial activities against cariogenic *S. mutans* cells. Not surprisingly, the MIC values of ABR-C and ABR-E were higher than that of benchmark wide-spectrum bactericidal chlorhexidine, which is also highly leachable and does not offer sustained antibacterial activity once leached out. Also as expected, the 8 μg/mL MBC of ABR-C and ABR-E is higher than CHX's MBC of 4 μg/mL, whereas no bactericidal activities were observed at all for SDR Resin and TEGDMA. It has been shown that, for an organic QAS compound, 10~14 carbon atoms for the N-alkyl group are associated with higher antimicrobial activity [43,44]. Another study also showed that imidazolium's N-alkyl's chain length can play a critical role in antitumor activity and cytotoxicity; C-12 was found exhibiting high antitumor activity against ~60 tumor cell lines as well as low cytotoxicity in most cases. Longer chain length could improve antitumor potency but also increase imidazolium's cytotoxicity [45]. As demonstrated in their chemical structures in Schemes 3 and 4, respectively, both ABR-C and ABR-E have a 12-carbon atom chain length on their N-alkyl group, which helps in explaining their identical MIC and MBC values.

The dentin mass loss results (Figure 1) indicate that the ABR resins, even at low concentrations, are effective against matrix metalloproteinases (MMPs) for minimizing the collagen degradation. MMPs belong to a larger group of proteases known as the metzincin superfamily. These collagenases are capable of degrading triple-helical fibrillary collagens, such as those in dentin, into distinctive fragments. More specifically, certain MMPs are considered to contribute to the gradual degradation of collagen fibrils in hybrid layers established during dentin bonding. A wide range of MMPs, including MMP-2, MMP-8, MMP-9, and MMP-20, have been detected in the human dentin matrix [46]. It is well reported that CHX has broad anti-MMP activity in addition to antimicrobial capability. However, the long-term *in vivo* anti-MMP activity of CHX may not be as effective, which has been attributed to possible leaching out of the CHX [47,48]. It has also been reported that cationic quaternary ammonium methacrylates may exhibit dentin MMP inhibition comparable with that of CHX but that higher concentrations were required [49].

The synthetic strategy in this investigation focused on covalently linking antibacterial compounds that contain functional groups with strong antibacterial activities to a variety of backbones and polymerizable groups compatible with conventional dental resin systems. The antibacterial capability of the active compound could be either enhanced or reduced by polymerization. This depends on how the compound eradicates bacteria, either by disrupting bacterial membrane or via depleting the bacterial food supply. In order for an antibacterial resin to be a viable option for industrial-scale production and application, there are several essential requirements that need to be fulfilled: (1) synthesis of ABR should be straightforward and not cost-prohibitive; ideally, well-established synthetic routes are preferred; (2) ABR should have good storage stability (sufficient shelf life); (3) end products that contain ABR should be able to maintain their antibacterial activities through recurrent bacterial challenges; (4) ideally, the antibacterial effect can be achieved with relatively small dosing and minimum bacterial resistance in the target pathogenic microorganisms; (5) no drastic compromises to the other vital properties should be introduced by ABR. As shown in Table 2, even at up to 12 wt % loading level, there are no significant decreases in flexural strength or flexural modulus with the incorporation of the imidazole-based polymerizable antibacterial monomer ABR-C, as compared to control. The flexural strength of the resin mixture with 16 wt % antibacterial monomer showed lower flexural strength, but flexural modulus still retained 84% value as compared to control.

During this investigation, it was found that a group of polymethacrylate resins containing at least one imidazole moiety could be readily prepared via appropriate hybrid methacrylate–acrylate resins or polyacrylate resins with proper control of the conversion of the imidazole addition. This is an effective approach to incorporating an imidazole moiety into a polymerizable resin as novel acid-free functional resins. Moreover, such imidazole-containing polymerizable resins may be further chemically modified by reacting with a variety of halogenated alkyls to form polymerizable resins with ionic moiety of imidazolium, which results in a unique class of polymerizable ionic liquid resins.

Sufficient mechanical properties of the orthodontic bonding cement are important as the bending force and torque during teeth straightening and aligning could be quite significant. There is a slight reduction of flexural strength with a higher loading amount of ABR-C; however, flexural modulus can be maintained with up to 3 wt % of ABR-C loading (Table 3). A similar trend was also observed for compressive strength. Ambient light sensitivity (ALS) is another important property for light curable orthodontic cement or adhesive, as adequate ALS is needed for the bracket to be carefully placed and aligned at the correct position and angle, before it is light cured. As also exhibited in Table 3, the ALS values of ABR-C-containing orthodontic cements are all at 2 min or higher, which compared well with commercially available orthodontic cements, as shown in Figure 3.

Orthodontic cement with the capability to prevent the development of WSLs without compromising enamel bond strength would be desirable. Orthodontic treatments last an average of two to three years, during which time orthodontic cement must be capable of bonding to the enamel with high bond strength in order to resist masticatory loads. As demonstrated in Table 3, for experimental orthodontic cements incorporating 1–4 wt % ABR-C, there is no drastic compromise to the SBS to enamel except for 3 wt % ABR-C. More importantly, their SBS values are all comparable to those of the commercially available orthodontic cements products (Figure 2), with mean SBS ranging from 20.1 MPa to 36.0 MPa. However, this bond strength to enamel should not be too high either, to prevent damages to the enamel while removing the bracket.

The strong effectiveness in eradicating bacteria for the imidazolium-based polymerizable resins was further demonstrated by the formulated experimental orthodontic cements. As exhibited in Table 4, even at a low-level loading (1 wt %) of such imidazolium-based polymerizable monomer, a reduction of over 2 logs of microorganisms can be achieved by ABR-C. When the loading level of ABR-C was increased from 2 wt % to 4 wt %, reductions of around 5 logs or higher were observed. Moreover, with optimized compositions, not only can a highly effective antibacterial capability be achieved, but balanced mechanical properties can also be maintained (Table 3). The potent antibacterial property of this novel polymerizable imidazolium resin offers another crucial benefit—no severe cytotoxicity was introduced [50]. Conventional QAS-based polymerizable resins, on the other hand, could be less effective and a high dose loading (up to 30 wt %) is needed, which frequently leads to significant drops in mechanical properties and elevated cytotoxicity [51,52].

Effective antimicrobial agents are expected to regulate the oral biofilm at levels compatible with good oral health while not sacrificing the beneficial properties of the resident oral microflora. Compounds comprising imidazolium moieties have exhibited various antibacterial, antioxidant, and antifungal properties; imidazolium salts' overall mechanism of antibacterial function is similar to that of QAS—mainly by disturbing the planktonic cell membrane [52]. Nonetheless, comprehensive studies by Koo et al. have shown that ABR-MC (ABR-modified composite) impaired biofilm initiation by disrupting bacterial accumulation, cell colonization, and subsequent biofilm development, if left unintervened [50]. The anti-biofilm properties of ABR-MC were assessed using an EPS-matrix producing *S. mutans* in an experimental biofilm model. Using high-resolution confocal fluorescence imaging and biophysical methods, they observed severely reduced biomass, remarkable disruption of bacterial accumulation, and defective 3D matrix structure on the surface of ABR-MC. Mechanism-wise, it was speculated that the distinct difference in the basicity between N-substitute imidazole (pK_{aH} of 7.20 for 1-methylimidazole) and aliphatic tertiary amine (pK_{aH} of 10.7 for triethylamine) might be the major contributor to the increased polarity and higher potential in its charged conjugated moiety (imidazolium). However, the exact mechanism contributing to the much more pronounced bactericidal effects as compared to conventional QAS compounds will require further investigation. Other areas of relevant investigation include the further study of the hydrolytical stability of these antibacterial monomers.

4. Materials and Methods

4.1. Materials

Antibacterial resins (ABR-C and ABR-E) were prepared in house; the detailed preparation route can be found in a previous paper [50]. SDR Resin and adhesion-promoting resin (APR, Dentsply proprietary resin) were supplied by Dentsply Sirona's internal production (Milford, DE, USA). Other conventional dental resins and ingredients used in formulations were purchased from commercial sources, including 1,6-bis [methacryloyloxyethoxycarbonylamino]-2,4,4-trimethylhexane (UDMA), ethoxylated bisphenol A dimethacrylate (EBPADMA), trimethylolpropane trimethacrylate (TMPTMA), camphorquinone (CQ), dimethylaminobenzonitrile (DMABN), diphenyl (2,4,6-trimethylbenzoyl) phosphine oxide (TPO), and butylated hydroxytoluene (BHT). Inorganic fillers were milled and silanated in house, including barium fluoroalumino borosilicate glass (BFBG), bariumalumino borosilicate glass (BABG), and AEROSIL fumed silica OX-50 (silanated OX-50). All fillers were surface treated by γ-methacryloxypropyl-trimethoxysilane.

Commercially available orthodontic cements studied include the following: Prime Master (Sun Medical Co., Shiga, Japan), Light Bond (Reliance Orthodontic Products, Alsip, IL, USA), Transbond XT (3M Unitek, Monrovia, CA, USA), NeoBond (Dentsply Sirona, Milford, DE, USA), and Grengloo (Ormco, Glendora, CA, USA).

Preparation of experimental orthodontic resin and cement. Experimental dental resin mixture with various concentrations of polymerizable antibacterial resin (0 (control), 4, 8, 12, 16 wt %) was mixed with other resins, namely UDMA (28~34 wt %), EBPADMA (20~26 wt %), APR (28~32 wt %), TMPTMA (6~8 wt %), CQ (~0.1 wt %), DMABN (~0.2 wt %), and BHT (~0.07 wt %), to a uniform resin blend at 55 °C using an overhead mechanical stirrer (Fisher Scientific, Pittsburgh, PA, USA). Experimental orthodontic cements were compounded with 75 wt % of inorganic filler mixture using a Ross double planetary mixer at 55 °C to a uniform paste (Ross Mixer, Charles Ross & Son Company, Hauppauge, NY, USA). The inorganic filler used in this study consists of three types of fillers in the filler blend: ~33 wt % BABG, ~65 wt % BFBG-2, and ~2 wt % silanated OX-50.

4.2. Evaluation Methods

MIC and MBC Testing. Three monomers were tested against controls, i.e., ABR-E, ABR-C, and SDR Resin (a proprietary dimethacrylate monomer, without imidazole moiety, synthesized by Dentsply Sirona). The monomers were diluted in UltraPure distilled water (Gibco, Gaithersburg, MD, USA) before use. Different concentrations of the three tested monomers, along with two controls, i.e., wide-spectrum antimicrobial agent chlorhexidine (CHX) and conventional monomer TEGDMA, were incubated statically with the cariogenic organism *S. mutans* strain UA159 using mid-exponential cells for 48 h at 37 °C in the presence of 5% CO_2. A fixed initial inoculum size of 9×10^7 CFU/mL of bacterial cells was inoculated per well and 2-fold dilutions of the experimental monomers, CHX, and TEGDMA were added. The following concentrations were tested: 0 to 125 μg/mL for CHX; 0 to 0.1% for the experimental monomers ABR-E, ABR-C, SDR Resin, and the control monomer TEGDMA. The MIC was determined as the lowest test concentration needed to ensure that culture did not grow over 10% of the relative cell, as determined by visual inspection of the growth inhibition of each well compared to that of the control well (without test compounds). For the MBC test, cells were serially diluted and spot-plated on agar plates; MBC values were determined by using the actual reduction of the bacterial viable cell counts. The MBC was determined as the lowest concentration that allows less than 0.1% of the original inoculum to survive.

Dentin Mass Loss. Completely demineralized dentin beams (2 mm × 1 mm × 6 mm) were prepared. Dentin beams were obtained from extracted molars after removing the enamel and superficial dentin. The beams were then submerged in 10% phosphoric acid for 18 h at 25 °C to completely demineralize the dentin. They were incubated in a control buffer (artificial saliva) to see how much of the insoluble collagen in demineralized dentin could be solubilized in 7 days of incubation at 37 °C. The loss of dry mass from completely demineralized dentin beams (2 mm × 1 mm × 6 mm) in buffer solutions pre-dipped into ABR-C and ABR-E resins for 30 s, versus in control buffer (artificial saliva) without pre-dip, was studied. The amount of soluble collagen in these demineralized dentin beams was measured after 7 days of incubation at 37 °C.

Flexural Strength. Specimens were prepared based on ISO 4049:2019. Samples were carefully injected into 25 mm × 2 mm × 2 mm stainless steel molds, then covered by Mylar film and cured with a Spectrum 800® (Dentsply Sirona, Milford, DE, USA) halogen lamp uniformly across the entire length of the specimen, using an irradiance of 850 mW/cm^2 for 5 × 20 s. After curing, specimens were immersed in DI water for 24 h at 37 °C prior to the 3-pt bending flexural test. Flexural test was performed on an Instron Universal Tester (Model 4400R, Norwood, MA, USA countr using a crosshead speed of 0.75 mm/min. Six specimens per sample set were prepared and tested.

Compressive Strength. Samples were carefully injected into Ø4 mm × 7 mm stainless steel molds, sandwiched between two Mylar films. Light curing of the specimen was carried out with a Spectrum 800® (Dentsply Sirona) halogen lamp at an irradiance of 850 mW/cm^2 for 20 s on both ends. After curing, specimens were immersed in DI water for 24 h at 37 °C, before being polished to Ø4 mm × 6 mm specimen size with 600 grit sand paper. The compression test was performed on an Instron Universal Tester (Model 4400R) using a crosshead speed of 5 mm/min. Six specimens per sample set were prepared and tested.

Ambient Light Sensitivity (ALS). ALS was tested on a Suntest unit (model CPS 56007014, Heraeus Noblelight, Buford, GA, USA) with a UV filter that was calibrated to provide illuminance of 8000 ± 1000 lux tested by a Lux Meter HD400 (Extech, Nashua, NH, USA). A spheroidal mass of approximately 0.03 gm of the material was weighed to be tested on a glass microscope slide, and the slide was positioned with a matte black cover on top of the cell with a UV filter in place. The Suntest light was turned on, and one should wait at least 10 s until the light output has stabilized. The matte black cover was removed and the timer was started simultaneously. After exposure, the slide with the sample was removed and the second microscope slide was immediately pressed against the material with a slight shearing action to produce a thin layer. The material was visually inspected to see whether it was physically homogeneous. If the material has begun to set, clefts and voids appear in the specimen when the thin layer is being produced. The time was recorded when the sample started to set and appeared physically non-homogeneous. In all, 3 runs were conducted for each sample.

Notched-Edge Shear Bond Strength. Caries-free and freshly extracted bovine incisors were carefully sectioned longitudinally through the distal, occlusal, and mesial surfaces using a precision low speed saw (TechCut 4™, Allied High Tech Products, Rancho Dominguez, CA, USA). The sectioned bovine incisors, with buccal surface exposed, were then mounted in a cylindrical block using cold-cure acrylics. The exposed surface was then coarse ground on a model trimmer until a flat enamel surface was exposed, followed by wet ground on a grinding wheel under running water using 120-grit and 320-grit SiC sanding papers until the surface was even and smooth when visually inspected. Enamel was acid etched using 34% phosphoric etching gel for 15 s, then thoroughly rinsed for 20 s. The notched-edge bonding jig contained a cylindrical plastic mold, resulting in samples with a defined bonding area (diameter of 2.38 mm). The antibacterial orthodontic cement restorative composite was then carefully placed into the center of the mold and good contact with the substrate was ensured. After light curing with a Spectrum 800® (Dentsply Sirona) halogen lamp at 850 mW/cm^2 for 20 s, the specimen was then carefully removed from the mold. Specimens were stored in DI water for 24 h at 37 °C prior to SBS testing. The SBS test was performed on an Instron Universal Tester (Model 4400R) using a crosshead speed of 1 mm/min. Seven specimens per sample set were prepared and tested.

JIS Z 2801. This test was conducted at Antimicrobial Test Laboratories (ATL, Round Rock, TX, USA), an independent and GLP complied testing institution. JIS Z 2801 was adopted as ISO standard (ISO-22196). This test is designed to quantitatively test the ability of hard surfaces to inhibit the growth of microorganisms over a 24-h period of contact. The test microorganism selected for this test was *Streptococcus mutans* (*S mutans*, ATCC® 25175). The following protocol was used by ATL: (1) test microorganism *S mutans*, ATCC® 25175 was prepared by growth in tryptic soy broth for 24 h; (2) the suspension of the test microorganism was standardized by dilution in a Dey-Engley neutralizing broth (D/E Broth) at 0.9 mL blanks; (3) control and test surfaces were inoculated with microorganisms, and then the microbial inoculum was covered with a thin sterile film; (4) microbial concentrations were determined at "time zero" by elution followed by dilution and plating to tryptic soy agar (Difco); (5) a control was run to verify that the neutralization/elution method effectively neutralized the antimicrobial agent in the antimicrobial surface being tested; (6) the inoculated covered control and antimicrobial test surfaces were allowed to incubate undisturbed in a humid environment for 24 h at 36 ± 1 °C; and (7) after incubation, microbial concentrations were determined and the reduction of microorganisms relative to the control surface was calculated as follows:

$$\text{R (Average Log Reduction)} = \text{Log}\,(B/C), \tag{1}$$

where

B = Average number of viable cells on the control pieces after 24 h.
C = Average number of viable cells on the test pieces after 24 h.

ISO-22196 Antimicrobial Test. This test was conducted at Antimicrobial Test Laboratories (ATL, Round Rock, TX, USA), an independent and GLP complied testing institution. ISO method 22196 is a quantitative test designed to assess the performance of materials' antimicrobial capabilities on hard non-porous surfaces. The method can be conducted using contact times ranging from 10 minutes up to 24 h. For the ISO 22196 test, non-antimicrobial control surfaces are used as the baseline for calculations of microbial reduction. The test microorganism selected for this test was *Staphylococcus aureus* 6538 (*S. aureus* 6538). This bacterium is a Gram-positive, spherical-shaped, facultative anaerobe. *Staphylococcus* species are known to demonstrate resistance to antibiotics such as methicillin and is commonly used in standard test methods as a model for Gram-positive bacteria. *S. aureus* pathogenicity can range from commensal skin colonization to more severe diseases such as pneumonia and toxic shock syndrome (TSS). The following protocol was used by ATL: (1) *S. aureus* 6538 prepared by growth in tryptic soy broth for 18 h and the suspension of the test microorganism was standardized by dilution in broth at 1:500 by volume; (2) control and test surfaces were inoculated with microorganisms, and then the microbial inoculum was covered with a sterile thin film; (3) microbial concentrations were determined at "time zero" by elution, followed by dilution and plating to tryptic soy agar; (4) a control was run to verify that the neutralization/elution method effectively neutralized the antimicrobial agent in the antimicrobial surface being tested; (5) the inoculated covered control and test surfaces were allowed to incubate undisturbed in a humid environment at 36 ± 1 °C for 24 h; and (6) after incubation, microbial concentrations were determined and the reduction of microorganisms relative to the control surface was calculated as follows:

$$Percent\ Reduction = \left(\frac{B-A}{B}\right)\times 100$$

$$Log_{10}\ Reduction = Log\left(\frac{B}{A}\right)$$

where

B = Number of viable test microorganisms on the control carriers after the contact time.
A = Number of viable test microorganisms on the test carriers after the contact time.

Statistical Analysis. Statistical analysis was conducted with Minitab 17 Statistical Software (Minitab®, State College, PA, USA). Normality of data was checked using the Anderson–Darling test. Mechanical properties and shear bond strength data were analyzed with one-way analysis of variance (ANOVA) and Tukey's test. Significance levels of 0.05 were used for ANOVA and Tukey's tests.

5. Conclusions

This study explored the potential of incorporating unique imidazolium-based polymerizable antibacterial monomers into orthodontic bonding cements. For unfilled resins comprising up to 12 wt % ABR-C, no significant decreases in flexural strength or modulus were observed. For experimental cements incorporating 1–4 wt % ABR-C, there is no drastic compromise to the SBS to enamel except for 3 wt % ABR-C; moreover, their SBS values are all comparable to those of the commercially available orthodontic cements. The ISO-22196 antimicrobial test against *S. aureus* showed significant levels of antibacterial effects—up to over 5 logs of microorganism reduction exhibited by ABR-C-containing experimental cements. Although MIC and MBC were identified, and a range of antibacterial activities of imidazolium-based orthodontic cements were demonstrated, clinical and long-term studies are still important to validate the efficacy of this unique series of imidazolium resins towards preventing and mitigating WSLs for patients.

Author Contributions: H.L. and X.J. contributed equally to conceptualization; methodology; validation; formal analysis; investigation; resources; data curation; writing—original draft preparation; writing—review and editing; visualization; supervision; and project administration. All authors have read and agreed to the published version of the manuscript.

Acknowledgments: We would like to thank Anuradha Prakki and her team at University of Toronto for assistance with the MIC and MAC tests. We would also like to thank David Pashley and his team at Augusta University for the dentin mass loss and HYP content study. We also greatly appreciate the laboratory assistance provided by Donna Reid and Brandon Zhang.

References

1. Nascimento, V.; Conti, A.; Cardoso, M.; Valarelli, D.; Almeida-Pedrin, R. Impact of orthodontic treatment on self-esteem and quality of life of adult patients requiring oral rehabilitation. *Angle Orthod.* **2016**, *86*, 839–845. [CrossRef] [PubMed]
2. Grewal, H.; Sapawat, P.; Modi, P.; Aggarwal, S. Psychological impact of orthodontic treatment on quality of life—A longitudinal study. *Int. Orthod.* **2019**, *17*, 269–276. [CrossRef]
3. Wishney, M. Potential risks of orthodontic therapy: A critical review and conceptual framework. *Aust. Dent. J.* **2017**, *62*, 86–96. [CrossRef] [PubMed]
4. Heymann, G.C.; Grauer, D. A contemporary review of white spot lesions in orthodontics. *J. Esthet. Restor. Dent.* **2013**, *25*, 85–95. [CrossRef] [PubMed]
5. Chapman, J.A.; Roberts, W.E.; Eckert, G.J.; Kula, K.S.; González-Cabezas, C. Risk factors for incidence and severity of white spot lesions during treatment with fixed orthodontic appliances. *Am. J. Orthod. Dentofac. Orthop.* **2010**, *138*, 188–194. [CrossRef]
6. Buschang, P.H.; Chastain, D.; Keylor, C.L.; Crosby, D.; Julien, K. Incidence of white spot lesions among patients treated with clear aligners and traditional braces. *Angle Orthod.* **2019**, *89*, 359–364. [CrossRef]
7. Tasios, T.; Papageorgiou, S.N.; Papadopoulos, M.A.; Tsapas, A.; Haidich, A.B. Prevention of orthodontic enamel demineralization: A systematic review with meta-analyses. *Orthod. Craniofac. Res.* **2019**, *22*, 225–235. [CrossRef]
8. Leeper, D.K.; Noureldin, A.; Julien, K.; Campbell, P.M.; Buschang, P.H. Risk assessments in orthodontic patients developing white spot lesions. *J. Investig. Clin. Dent.* **2019**, *10*, e12470. [CrossRef]

9. Tufekci, E.; Dixon, J.S.; Gunsolley, J.C.; Lindauer, S.J. Prevalence of white spot lesions during orthodontic treatment with fixed appliances. *Angle Orthod.* **2011**, *81*, 206–210. [CrossRef]
10. Khalaf, K. Factors affecting the formation, severity and location of white spot lesions during orthodontic treatment with fixed appliances. *J. Oral Maxillofac. Res.* **2014**, *5*. [CrossRef]
11. Joen, D.; An, J.; Lim, B.; Ahn, S. Orthodontic bonding procedures significantly influence biofilm composition. *Prog. Orthod.* **2020**, *21*, 1–9. [CrossRef] [PubMed]
12. Baeshen, H.A.; Rangmar, S.; Kjellberg, H.; Birkhed, D. Dental Caries and Risk Factors in Swedish Adolescents about to Start Orthodontic Treatment with Fixed Appliances. *J. Contemp. Dent. Pract.* **2019**, *20*, 538–562. [CrossRef]
13. Srivastava, K.; Tikku, T.; Khanna, R.; Sachan, K. Risk factors and management of white spot lesions in orthodontics. *J. Orthod. Sci.* **2013**, *2*, 43–49. [CrossRef]
14. Sonesson, M.; Svensäter, G.; Wickström, C. Glucosidase activity in dental biofilms in adolescent patients with fixed orthodontic appliances—A putative marker for white spot lesions—A clinical exploratory trial. *Arch. Oral Biol.* **2019**, *102*, 122–127. [CrossRef] [PubMed]
15. Sinclair, P.M.; Berry, C.W.; Bennett, C.L.; Israelson, H. Changes in gingival and gingival flora with bonding and banding. *Angle Orthod.* **1987**, *57*, 271–278. [PubMed]
16. Ristic, M.; Svabic, M.V.; Sasic, M.; Zelic, O. Clinical and microbiological effects of fixed orthodontic appliances on periodontal tissues in adolescents. *Orthod. Craniofac. Res.* **2007**, *10*, 187–195. [CrossRef]
17. Paolantonio, M.; Festa, F.; Di Placido, G.; D'Attilio, M.; Catamo, G.; Piccolomini, R. Site-specific subgingival colonization by Actinobacillus actinomycetencomitans in orthodontic patients. *Am. J. Orthod. Dentofac. Orthop.* **1999**, *115*, 423–428. [CrossRef]
18. Lucchese, A.; Bondemark, L.; Marcolina, M.; Manuelli, M. Changes in oral microbiota due to orthodontic appliances: A systematic review. *J. Oral Microbiol.* **2018**, *10*, 1476645. [CrossRef]
19. Freitas, A.; Marquezan, M.; Nojima, M.; Alviano, D.; Maia, L. The influence of orthodontic fixed appliances on the oral microbiota: A systematic review. *Dent. Press J. Orthod.* **2014**, *19*, 46–55. [CrossRef]
20. Bourbia, M.; Ma, D.; Cvitkovitch, D.; Santerre, J.P.; Finer, Y. Cariogenic Bacteria Degrade Dental Resin Composites and Adhesives. *J. Dent. Res.* **2013**, *92*, 989–994. [CrossRef] [PubMed]
21. Stewart, C.A.; Finer, Y. Biostable, antidegradative and antimicrobial restorative systems based on host-biomaterials and microbial interactions. *Dent. Mater.* **2019**, *35*, 36–52. [CrossRef] [PubMed]
22. Mystkowska, J.; Niemirowicz-Laskowska, K.; Łysik, D.; Tokajuk, G.; Dąbrowski, J.R.; Bucki, R. The Role of Oral Cavity Biofilm on Metallic Biomaterial Surface Destruction–Corrosion and Friction Aspects. *Int. J. Mol. Sci.* **2018**, *19*, 743. [CrossRef]
23. Bergstrand, F.; Twetman, S. A review on prevention and treatment of post-orthodontic white spot Lesions—Evidence-based methods and emerging technologies. *Open Dent. J.* **2011**, *5*, 158–162. [CrossRef] [PubMed]
24. Sandra, C.D.; Maria, D.; Ingrid, M.D.; Vanessa, H.D.; Katia, V.R.; Leandro, C. Preventing and Arresting the Appearance of White Spot Lesions around the Bracket by applying Fluoride Varnish: A Systematic Review. *Dentistry* **2018**, *8*, 1–7. [CrossRef]
25. Aghoutan, H.; Alami, S.; Quars, F.E.; Diouny, S.; Bourzgui, F. White Spots Lesions in Orthodontic Treatment and Fluoride—Clinical Evidence. In *Emerging Trends in Oral Health Sciences and Dentistry*, 1st ed.; Virdi, M., Ed.; IntechOpen Limited: London, UK, 2015. [CrossRef]
26. Sonesson, M.; Brechter, A.; Abdulraheem, S.; Lindman, R.; Twetman, S.S. Fluoride varnish for the prevention of white spot lesions during orthodontic treatment with fixed appliances: A randomized controlled trial. *Eur. J. Orthod.* **2019**, 1–5. [CrossRef] [PubMed]
27. Höchli, D.; Hersberger-Zurfluh, M.; Papageorgiou, S.N.; Eliades, T. Interventions for orthodontically induced white spot lesions: A systematic review and meta-analysis. *Eur. J. Orthod.* **2017**, *39*, 122–133. [CrossRef] [PubMed]
28. Paula, A.B.; Fernandes, A.R.; Coelho, A.; Marto, C.M.; Marques-Ferreira, M.; Caramelo, F.; Vale, F.; Carrilho, E. Therapies for White Spot Lesions-A Systematic Review. *J. Evid. Based Dent. Pract.* **2017**, *17*, 23–38. [CrossRef]
29. Beyth, N.; Yudovin-Farber, I.; Perez-Davidi, M.; Domb, A.J.; Weiss, E.I. Polyethyleneimine nanoparticles incorporated into resin composite cause cell death and trigger biofilm stress in vivo. *Proc. Natl. Acad. Sci. USA* **2010**, *107*, 22038–22043. [CrossRef]

30. Zaltsman, N.; Shvero, N.D.; Polak, D.; Weiss, E.I.; Beyth, N. Antibacterial orthodontic adhesive incorporating polyethyleneimine nanoparticles. *Oral Health Prev. Dent.* **2017**, *15*, 245–250. [CrossRef]
31. Varon-Shahar, E.; Sharon, E.; Zabrovsky, A.; Houri-Haddad, Y.; Beyth, N. Orthodontic cements and adhesives: A possible solution to streptococcus mutans outgrowth adjacent to orthodontic appliances. *Oral Health Prev. Dent.* **2019**, *17*, 49–56. [CrossRef]
32. Imazato, S.; Ehara, A.; Torii, M.; Ebisu, S. Antibacterial activity of dentine primer containing MDPB after curing. *J. Dent.* **1998**, *26*, 267–271. [CrossRef]
33. Oz, A.Z.; Oz, A.A.; Yazicioglu, S.; Sancaktar, O. Effectiveness of an antibacterial primer used with adhesive-coated brackets on enamel demineralization around brackets: An in vivo study. *Prog. Orthod.* **2019**, *20*, 15. [CrossRef] [PubMed]
34. Feng, X.; Zhang, N.; Xu, H.H.K.; Weir, M.D.; Melo, M.A.S.; Bai, Y.; Zhang, K. Novel orthodontic cement containing dimethylaminohexadecyl methacrylate with strong antibacterial capability. *Dent. Mater. J.* **2017**, *36*, 669–676. [CrossRef] [PubMed]
35. Wang, X.; Zhang, N.; Wang, B.; Park, S.R.; Weir, M.D.; Xu, H.H.K.; Bai, Y. Novel self-etching and antibacterial orthodontic adhesive containing dimethylaminohexadecyl methacrylate to inhibit enamel demineralization. *Dent. Mater. J.* **2018**, *37*, 555–561. [CrossRef]
36. Cheng, L.; Weir, M.D.; Zhang, K.; Arola, D.D.; Zhou, X.; Xu, H.H. Dental primer and adhesive containing a new antibacterial quaternary ammonium monomer dimethylaminododecyl methacrylate. *J. Dent.* **2013**, *41*, 345–355. [CrossRef] [PubMed]
37. Melo, M.A.S.; Wu, J.; Weir, M.D.; Xu, H.H.K. Novel antibacterial orthodontic cement containing quaternary ammonium monomer dimethylaminododecyl methacrylate. *J. Dent.* **2014**, *42*, 1193–1201. [CrossRef]
38. Wang, S.; Zhang, K.; Zhou, X.; Xu, N.; Xu, H.H.K.; Weir, M.D.; Ge, Y.; Wang, S.; Li, M.; Li, Y.; et al. Antibacterial effect of dental adhesive containing dimethylaminododecyl methacrylate on the development of Streptococcus mutans biofilm. *Int. J. Mol. Sci.* **2014**, *15*, 12791–12806. [CrossRef]
39. Huang, L.; Xiao, Y.H.; Xing, X.D.; Li, F.; Ma, S.; Qi, L.L.; Chen, J.H. Antibacterial activity and cytotoxicity of two novel cross-linking antibacterial monomers on oral pathogens. *Arch. Oral Bio* **2011**, *56*, 367–373. [CrossRef]
40. Yu, F.; Dong, Y.; Yu, H.-H.; Lin, P.-T.; Zhang, L.; Sun, X.; Liu, Y.; Xia, Y.-N.; Huang, L.; Chen, J.-H. Antibacterial Activity and Bonding Ability of an Orthodontic Adhesive Containing the Antibacterial Monomer 2-Methacryloxylethyl Hexadecyl Methyl Ammonium Bromide. *Sci. Rep.* **2017**, *7*, 41787. [CrossRef]
41. Jin, X. Method and Antibacterial/Antimicrobial Compositions in Dental Compositions. U.S. Patent 8747831, 2014.
42. Jin, X. Imidazole and Imidazolium Resins and Methods for Preparing Curable Imidazolium Antimicrobial Resins. U.S. Patent RE47512, 2016.
43. De Almeida, C.M.; Da Rosa, W.L.O.; Meereis, C.T.W.; Ribeiro, J.S.; Da Silva, A.F.; Lund, R.G.; De Almeida, S.M. Efficacy of antimicrobial agents incorporated in orthodontic bonding systems: A systematic review and meta-analysis. *J. Orthod.* **2018**, *45*, 79–93. [CrossRef]
44. Garcia, M.T.; Ribosa, I.; Perez, L.; Manresa, A.; Comelles, F. Aggregation Behavior and Antimicrobial Activity of Ester-Functionalized Imidazolium-and Pyridinium-Based Ionic Liquids in Aqueous Solution. *Langmuir* **2013**, *29*, 2536–2545. [CrossRef]
45. Malhotra, S.V.; Kumar, V. A profile of the in vitro anti-tumor activity of imidazolium-based ionic liquids. *Bioorganic Med. Chem. Lett.* **2010**, *20*, 581–585. [CrossRef]
46. Mazzoni, A.; Tjäderhane, L.; Checchi, V.; Di Lenarda, R.; Salo, T.; Tay, F.; Pashley, D.; Breschi, L. Role of dentin MMPs in caries progression and bond stability. *J. Dent. Res.* **2015**, *94*, 241–251. [CrossRef]
47. Sadek, F.T.; Braga, R.R.; Muench, A.; Liu, Y.; Pashley, D.H.; Tay, F.R. Ethanol wet-bonding challenges current anti-degradation strategy. *J. Dent. Res.* **2010**, *89*, 1499–1504. [CrossRef] [PubMed]
48. Gostemeyer, G.; Schwendicke, F. Inhibition of hybrid layer degradation by cavity pretreatment: *Meta-* and trial sequential analysis. *J. Dent.* **2016**, *49*, 14–21. [CrossRef]
49. Ge, Y.; Wang, S.; Zhou, X.; Wang, H.; Xu, H.H.K.; Cheng, L. The use of quaternary ammonium to combat dental caries. *Materials* **2015**, *8*, 3532–3549. [CrossRef] [PubMed]
50. Hwang, G.; Koltisko, B.; Jin, X.; Koo, H. Nonleachable imidazolium-incorporated composite for disruption of bacterial clustering, exopolysaccharide-matrix assembly, and enhanced biofilm removal. *ACS Appl. Mater. Interfaces* **2017**, *9*, 38270–38280. [CrossRef] [PubMed]

Permissions

All chapters in this book were first published by MDPI; hereby published with permission under the Creative Commons Attribution License or equivalent. Every chapter published in this book has been scrutinized by our experts. Their significance has been extensively debated. The topics covered herein carry significant findings which will fuel the growth of the discipline. They may even be implemented as practical applications or may be referred to as a beginning point for another development.

The contributors of this book come from diverse backgrounds, making this book a truly international effort. This book will bring forth new frontiers with its revolutionizing research information and detailed analysis of the nascent developments around the world.

We would like to thank all the contributing authors for lending their expertise to make the book truly unique. They have played a crucial role in the development of this book. Without their invaluable contributions this book wouldn't have been possible. They have made vital efforts to compile up to date information on the varied aspects of this subject to make this book a valuable addition to the collection of many professionals and students.

This book was conceptualized with the vision of imparting up-to-date information and advanced data in this field. To ensure the same, a matchless editorial board was set up. Every individual on the board went through rigorous rounds of assessment to prove their worth. After which they invested a large part of their time researching and compiling the most relevant data for our readers.

The editorial board has been involved in producing this book since its inception. They have spent rigorous hours researching and exploring the diverse topics which have resulted in the successful publishing of this book. They have passed on their knowledge of decades through this book. To expedite this challenging task, the publisher supported the team at every step. A small team of assistant editors was also appointed to further simplify the editing procedure and attain best results for the readers.

Apart from the editorial board, the designing team has also invested a significant amount of their time in understanding the subject and creating the most relevant covers. They scrutinized every image to scout for the most suitable representation of the subject and create an appropriate cover for the book.

The publishing team has been an ardent support to the editorial, designing and production team. Their endless efforts to recruit the best for this project, has resulted in the accomplishment of this book. They are a veteran in the field of academics and their pool of knowledge is as vast as their experience in printing. Their expertise and guidance has proved useful at every step. Their uncompromising quality standards have made this book an exceptional effort. Their encouragement from time to time has been an inspiration for everyone.

The publisher and the editorial board hope that this book will prove to be a valuable piece of knowledge for researchers, students, practitioners and scholars across the globe.

List of Contributors

Fabiola Vaca-Cornejo, Sergio H. Dueñas Jiménez and Judith M. Dueñas Jiménez
Department of Physiology, University Center of Health Sciences, University of Guadalajara, Guadalajara, Jalisco 44100, Mexico

Héctor Macías Reyes
Department of Clinical Surgery, Fray Antonio Alcalde Hospital, University of Guadalajara, Guadalajara, Jalisco 44100, Mexico

Ricardo A. Llamas Velázquez
Sophia Laboratories, Guadalajara 45010, Jalisco, México

Chen Chen
State Key Laboratory of Oral Diseases, West China Hospital of Stomatology, Sichuan University, Chengdu 610041, China
Department of Prosthodontics, Endodontics and Operative Dentistry, University of Maryland School of Dentistry, Baltimore, MD 21201, USA

Junling Wu
Department of Prosthodontics, Endodontics and Operative Dentistry, University of Maryland School of Dentistry, Baltimore, MD 21201, USA
Shandong Provincial Key Laboratory of Oral Biomedicine, Jinan 250012, China

Michael D. Weir
Department of Prosthodontics, Endodontics and Operative Dentistry, University of Maryland School of Dentistry, Baltimore, MD 21201, USA

Lin Wang
Department of Prosthodontics, Endodontics and Operative Dentistry, University of Maryland School of Dentistry, Baltimore, MD 21201, USA
VIP Integrated Department, Stomatological Hospital of Jilin University, Changchun 130011, China

Xuedong Zhou
State Key Laboratory of Oral Diseases, West China Hospital of Stomatology, Sichuan University, Chengdu 610041, China

Hockin H. K. Xu
Department of Advanced Oral Sciences and Therapeutics, School of Dentistry, University of Maryland, Baltimore, MD 21201, USA
Center for Stem Cell Biology & Regenerative Medicine, University of Maryland School of Medicine, Baltimore, MD 21201, USA
Marlene and Stewart Greenebaum Cancer Center, University of Maryland School of Medicine, Baltimore, MD 21201, USA
Department of Prosthodontics, Endodontics and Operative Dentistry, University of Maryland School of Dentistry, Baltimore, MD 21201, USA
Department of Mechanical Engineering, University of Maryland, Baltimore County, MD 21250, USA

Mary Anne S. Melo
Department of Advanced Oral Sciences and Therapeutics, School of Dentistry, University of Maryland, Baltimore, MD 21201, USA
Division of Operative Dentistry, Department of General Dentistry, University of Maryland School of Dentistry, Baltimore, MD 21201, USA
Department of Prosthodontics, Endodontics and Operative Dentistry, University of Maryland School of Dentistry, Baltimore, MD 21201, USA

Gina Quiram and Danieli C. Rodrigues
Department of Bioengineering, University of Texas at Dallas, 800 W Campbell, Richardson, TX 75080, USA

Francisco Montagner
Department of Conservative Dentistry, Dental School, Federal University of Rio Grande do Sul, Rua Ramiro Barcelos 2492, 90460-001 Porto Alegre, Brazil

Kelli L. Palmer
Department of Biological Sciences University of Texas at Dallas, 800 W Campbell, Richardson, TX 75080, USA

Mihaela C. Stefan
Department of Bioengineering, University of Texas at Dallas, 800 W Campbell, Richardson, TX 75080, USA
Department of Chemistry, University of Texas at Dallas, 800 W Campbell, Richardson, TX 75080, USA

Katherine E. Washington
Department of Chemistry, University of Texas at Dallas, 800 W Campbell, Richardson, TX 75080, USA

Omar Rodriguez, Adel Alhalawani, Saad Arshad and Mark R. Towler
Department of Mechanical & Industrial Engineering, Ryerson University, Toronto, ON M5B 2K3, Canada
Li Ka Shing Knowledge Institute, St. Michael's Hospital, Toronto, ON M5B 1W8, Canada

Evgeniy Papynov, Oleg Shichalin, Igor Buravlev and Anton Belov
Institute of Chemistry, Far Eastern Branch of Russian Academy of Sciences, 159, Prosp. 100-letiya Vladivostoka, Vladivostok 690022, Russia
Far Eastern Federal University, 8, Sukhanova St., Vladivostok 690091, Russia

Arseniy Portnyagin, Vitaliy Mayorov, Evgeniy Merkulov and Taisiya Kaidalova
Institute of Chemistry, Far Eastern Branch of Russian Academy of Sciences, 159, Prosp. 100-letiya Vladivostoka, Vladivostok 690022, Russia

Yulia Skurikhina, Vyacheslav Turkutyukov and Vladimir Apanasevich
Pacific State Medical University, 2, Ostryakov Aven., Vladivostok 690990, Russia

Alexander Fedorets
Far Eastern Federal University, 8, Sukhanova St., Vladivostok 690091, Russia

Thomas E. Paterson, Caroline J. Harrison, Paul V. Hatton and Ilida Ortega
School of Clinical Dentistry, University of Sheffield, Shefield 0114, UK

Rui Shi
Beijing Laboratory of Biomedical Materials, Institute of Traumatology and Orthopaedics, Beijing Jishuitan Hospital, Beijing 100083, China

Jingjing Tian
Beijing Key Laboratory of Micro-nano Energy and Sensor, Beijing institute of Nanoenergy and Nanosystems, Chinese Academy of Sciences, Beijing 100083, China
Central Laboratory, Peking Union Medical College Hospital, Peking Union Medical College and Chinese Academy of Medical Sciences, Beijing 100730, China

Mailys De Sousa Mendes
Certara, Simcyp division, Sheffield 0114, UK

Zhou Li
Beijing Key Laboratory of Micro-nano Energy and Sensor, Beijing institute of Nanoenergy and Nanosystems, Chinese Academy of Sciences, Beijing 100083, China

Nikos N. Lygidakis and Paul F. Ashley
Unit of Paediatric Dentistry, Department of Craniofacial Growth and Development, UCL Eastman Dental Institute, London WC1X 8LD, UK

Elaine Allan
Division of Microbial Diseases, UCL Eastman Dental Institute, London WC1X 8LD, UK
Department of Microbial Diseases, UCL Eastman Dental Institute, London NW3 2QG, UK

Wendy Xia and Anne M. Young
Department of Biomaterials and Tissue Engineering, UCL Eastman Dental Institute, London WC1X 8LD, UK
Department of Biomaterials and Tissue Engineering, UCL Eastman Dental Institute, London NW3 2QG, UK

Paola Andrea Mena Silva
Dental Materials Laboratory, School of Dentistry, Federal University of Rio Grande do Sul, 90035-003 Porto Alegre-RS, Brazil
Universidad Central del Ecuador, 170129 Quito, Ecuador
Postgraduate Department, Universidad Regional Autónoma de Los Andes, 170129 Quito, Ecuador

Isadora Martini Garcia, Vicente Castelo Branco Leitune, Susana Maria Werner Samuel and Fabrício Mezzomo Collares
Dental Materials Laboratory, School of Dentistry, Federal University of Rio Grande do Sul, Rua Ramiro Barcelos 2492, Rio Branco, Porto Alegre, RS 90035-003, Brazil

Julia Nunes and Fernanda Visioli
Oral Pathology Department, School of Dentistry, Federal University of Rio Grande do Sul, 90035-003 Porto Alegre-RS, Brazil

Mary Anne Melo
Operative Dentistry Division, General Dentistry Department, University of Maryland School of Dentistry, Baltimore, MD 21201, USA
Ph.D. Program in Biomedical Sciences, University of Maryland School of Dentistry, Baltimore, MD 21201, USA

Rayan B. Yaghmoor
Department of Biomaterials and Tissue Engineering/ Department of Microbial Diseases, UCL Eastman Dental Institute, London, NW3 2QG, UK
Department of Restorative Dentistry, Umm Al-Qura University, College of Dental Medicine, Makkah 24381, Saudi Arabia

Paul Ashley
Unit of Paediatric Dentistry, UCL Eastman Dental Institute, London WC1E 6DE, UK

Antonio Shigueaki Takimi
Laboratory for Electrochemical Processes and Corrosion, Engineering School, Federal University of Rio Grande do Sul, Bento Gonçalves, 9500, Prédio 43427, Sala 216, Porto Alegre, RS 91501-970, Brazil

Carlos Pérez Bergmann
Laboratory of Ceramic Materials, Federal University of Rio Grande do Sul, Avenida Osvaldo Aranha 99, Porto Alegre, RS 90035-003, Brazil

Hamid Mortazavian, Jānis Lejnieks and Kenichi Kuroda
Department of Biologic and Materials Sciences & Prosthodontics, School of Dentistry, University of Michigan, Ann Arbor, MI 48109, USA

Guillaume A. Picquet, Lynette A. Zaidel and Carl P. Myers
Oral Care Early Research, Colgate-Palmolive Company, Piscataway, NJ 08855, USA

Anthony A. Giuseppetti, Stanislav A. Frukhtbeyn and Drago Skrtic
ADA Foundation, Research Division, Frederick, MD 21704, USA

Rochelle D. Hiers, Fernando L. Esteban Florez and Sharukh S. Khajotia
College of Dentistry, University of Oklahoma Health Sciences Center, Oklahoma City, OK 73117, USA

Heba Mitwalli
Program in Dental Biomedical Sciences, University of Maryland School of Dentistry, Baltimore, MD 21201, USA
Department of Restorative Dental Science, College of Dentistry, King Saud University, Riyadh 11451, Saudi Arabia

Abdulrahman A. Balhaddad
Program in Dental Biomedical Sciences, University of Maryland School of Dentistry, Baltimore, MD 21201, USA
Department of Restorative Dental Sciences, College of Dentistry, Imam Abdulrahman bin Faisal University, Dammam 31441, Saudi Arabia

Rashed AlSahafi
Program in Dental Biomedical Sciences, University of Maryland School of Dentistry, Baltimore, MD 21201, USA
Department of Restorative Dental Sciences, College of Dentistry, Umm Al-Qura University, Makkah 24211, Saudi Arabia

Thomas W. Oates and Michael D. Weir
Department of Advanced Oral Sciences and Therapeutics, School of Dentistry, University of Maryland, Baltimore, MD 21201, USA

Leopoldo Torres Jr and Diane R. Bienek
ADA Science & Research Institute, LLC, Innovative & Technology Research, Frederick, MD 21704, USA

Andrei C. Ionescu, Gloria Cazzaniga, Marco Ottobelli and Eugenio Brambilla
Oral Microbiology and Biomaterials Laboratory, Department of Biomedical, Surgical and Dental Sciences, University of Milan, via Pascal 36, 20133 Milan, Italy

Franklin Garcia-Godoy
Bioscience Research Center and Clinical Research, College of Dentistry, University of Tennessee Health Science Center, 875 Union Avenue, Memphis, TN 38163, USA

Hui Lu and Xiaoming Jin
Dentsply Sirona, R&D—Consumables Product Group, 38WClarke Ave, Milford, DE 19963, USA

Index

www.ingramcontent.com/pod-product-compliance
Lightning Source LLC
LaVergne TN
LVHW060517210926
848485LV00005B/1098